Absolutely Phenomenal Medical Treatments

By Anthony di Fabio and Dr. Curt Maxwell

Publisher certifies that this is an independent news report made as accurately as possible, and that all treatments should be through a licensed physician, and that we cannot be responsible for mal-application or mis-application or inappropriate treatment of any kind

Published in the U.S.A. by The Arthritis Trust of America, 7111 Sweetgum Road, Fairview, TN 37062-9384.

INTRODUCTION

You'll be amazed at the treatments described!

At least one of them is more than one hundred years old. Some will appear entirely new, yet have at least a generation or more of good science behind them. It's possible that most of them are practiced by your nearest alternative/complementary practitioner.

Words of caution before you proceed. When you take the methodology of these treatments to your family physician, be prepared to be either pooh poohed or to receive a lecture on "science based medicine."

If it were me and my doctor used either the "pooh pooh" tactic or started lecturing on "science based medicine," I'd quickly pick up my hat and check book and walk away.

Why?

Because in the case of the "pooh pooh" doctor, s/he's stuck in a rut of authoritarianism and apparently doesn't have time to look for actual causes of your ailment but, instead, is well trained in pushing drugs according to thoughtless recipes designed by patent medicine huxters.

In the case of the "science based medicine" doctor, s/he doesn't realize that a few college courses in chemistry, physics and mathematics do not a scientist make. S/he is incapable of — as a practitioner of medicine who follows the recipes of patented medicine drug pushers — evaluating the so-called scientific studies (double-blind) that are repeatedly funded by those with a huge dollar stake in their outcomes.[6]

You can find many excellent books on how those so-called scientific studies are compromised.[1] We shan't go into the almost total corruption that surfaces between our governmental regulatory agency, the FDA, and the patented medicine drug pushers. The point will be adequately made when one of us summarizes personal experience with the "science based medicine" bullhocky, as to be described.

Anthony di Fabio apparently developed a disease named as "polycythemia." Too many red corpuscles were being produced. This thickened the blood leading to easy tiredness, inability to effectively utilize oxygen and several other problems.

Di Fabio had never before heard of this disease but quickly learned that the only standard of treatment was from a phlebotomist. Usually the phlebotomist will train assistants to draw a small amount of blood thus reducing the number of red blood platelets and, presumably, easing the patient's load for another three weeks. Repeated blood withdrawals then keeps the patient living just a little longer. (This is great for insuring the doctor's patient load but a little hard on your insurance agent who must pay and pay and pay for nothing more than a little symptom relief. Much longer relief was obtained by donating blood to the Red Cross because they at no cost drew more than a small vial of blood at each visit, but I suppose the doctors have a reason — or at least a justification — when they describe the Red Cross approach as not a good idea.)

Di Fabio was told that in time the cells within his bones that created red blood cells would most likely eventually wear out at which time he would suffer from an incurable leukemia.

OK! Fine! Di Fabio knew how he would die, just not when.

Di Fabio routinely also made an appointment with a practitioner of computerized electro-dermal screening, a diagnostic and often effective treatment that will be described in our last chapter.

No! He didn't get cured by this device but during the diagnostic phase the practitioner asked "Have you had any surgical procedures on your body?"

The answer was "yes." The practitioner scurried into another room and came back with a programmable laser. She read its recommended frequency setting from a small booklet, set the laser at the indicated frequency and passed it for a few minutes across the old scar tissue. Three weeks later she did the same thing.

Lo!

The polycythemia was gone! — Or at least lessened!

She'd reasoned from her studies and experience that some of the twelve up and down meridians through which chi —

life force according to early Chinese studies — passes had been blocked by di Fabio's two earlier surgeries.

By the way, this curative health practitioner was a non-degreed wife of a chiropractor who is so successful with her computerized electrodermal analysis that her appointments are always well booked far in advance. She was pretty much self-taught and she never once handed out impressive sounding words like "science based medicine." She may not have discovered the source of di Fabio's problem but in a few seconds she'd accomplished at least as much relief as had the "science-based" professional did from drawing a small amount of blood!

Getting back to "science based medicine," we must tell you of the phlebotomist's attempt to get Anthony di Fabio to take some kind of beta blocker. Beta blockers, called beta antagonists, are a class of drugs used for various indications but particularly for the management of cardiac arrhythmias, cardio protection after myocardial infarction (heart attack), and hypertension. It seems that allopathic practitioners are in love with beta blockers so many prescriptions are written for one kind of heart problem or another.

Di Fabio refused to take the drugs. The doctor with some impatience called di Fabio's son who was also a medical doctor. He'd reasoned that di Fabio's son would put pressure on his father and "by gosh, the patient would become a *good* patient."

Unknown to the phlebotomist di Fabio's son was a practitioner of both alternative and general medicine. The son quietly listened, thanked the phlebotomist and went on his way, never saying a word to his father.

To add to the pressure the phlebotomist then gave a nice lecture on "science based medicine." Di Fabio asked, "Can you prove those benefits?"

"Yes," the doctor answered. "I'll send you some scientific studies."

After three weeks, sure enough, a big, brown envelope arrived in the mail with reports of a dozen or so double-blind studies. Di Fabio went through each one very carefully. Each study was a report of one company's double-blind study showing that one beta blocker was just a touch better than another company's beta blocker -statistically insignificant comparisons. There was no study whatsoever showing that a beta blocker was superior to the use of absolutely essential heart nutrients — magnesium, Lcarnitine, d-ribose and coenzyme Q10. In addition to a whole host of bad side effects, these patented drugs often deprive specific organs of nutrients making symptoms worse so that new patented drugs have to be given to counteract the new symptoms. This second drug will also have side effects and so more patented drugs are prescribed to relieve the new side effects, and so it will go ad nauseum until some old folks are gulping down dozens of damaging drugs daily all the while commenting on what a nice doctor they have — if they can rise above a drug induced stupor!. Or, maybe that opinion is their stupor!! Consider just one consequence among several of taking beta blockers. It rapidly uses up the heart's necessary coenzyme Q10 thus bringing about additional heart problems in the long run!

As of this writing a drug company is saturating television with a new patented "breakthrough" drug that combines coenzyme Q10 with their beta blocker. You see, all beta blocker huxters have long known that beta blockers use up coenzyme Q10 thus causing additional dangerous side effects to your heart. Once the market had been saturated with beta blockers it became economically sensible to add in the coenzyme Q10 to their beta blockers. Lo! A "breakthrough!"

The patient is never served by drug pushers, only the dollar!

Among other destructive side effects of statin drugs, Duane Graveline, M.D. reports nerve damage, mood disorders, personality changes, muscle problems, polyneuropathy, degenerative muscle tissue, sexual dysfunction, immune suppression, pancreas or liver dysfunction, and cataracts.[5] Joseph Mercola, D.O. (http://www.mercola.com) states that beta blockers also cause plaque buildup in the teeth.

Paraphrasing Jonathan Wright, M.D. of Renton, Washington, this highly educated and trained phlebotomist does not suspect that recently patented drugs are foreign to the cellular tissue that evolved in our human body for millions of years sans exposure to synthetic drugs; but we did evolve throughout millions of years of exposure daily to surrounding natural substances.

Our bodies have no idea what to do with totally synthetic chemical structures such as beta blockers. The human body only knows how to respond to a limited range of natural substances. No matter how you view modern medicine, the body cannot adapt to new patented drugs in just a few years. Perhaps in another million or so years during which time the human body is repeatedly saturated with unnatural, damaging patented drugs a kind of bodily adaptation will take place in our 24th descendent, but patented medicine manufacturers develop new drugs so fast that it's doubtful there will ever be a catch-up. Evolution normally proceeds much more slowly. The constant exposure of absolutely foreign newly invented chemicals is more likely to be a killer disease of its own.

There are two paradigms in the practice of medicine. (A "paradigm" is a thought pattern in a scientific discipline or in an epistemological context. It's a philosophical or theoretical framework for practice of a discipline such as medicine.)

"Allopathic" medical practitioners are the common garden variety of medical doctor. With a few exceptions they are versed (we should say brainwashed) in the treating of symptoms. A good example of the treating of a symptom is their response to the complaint of a headache. A headache might be caused by one or more causations: allergy, improper nutrition, tumor of the brain, unbalanced hormones, and so on.[2] On first complaining of a headache to your "science based" physician they will more often than not prescribe an NSAID, that's a non-steroidal anti-inflammatory drug — or perhaps they'll prescribe an aspirin.

Note that none of these drugs, patented or unpatented, does anything more than reduce the pain — the symptom. No drug scrambles throughout the body and comes up breathing hard to exclaim, "Ah ha! I've found you've a nutritional allergy! Stop eating white bread!"

The doctor gets paid for your office visit. S/he's sure to

have you back again because s/he knows she's just treated a symptom and the true cause of your disease will drive you back to her/his office.

Medicare is equally happy because the doctor's clerk has inked in the proper symptom code for treating your symptom. The government is happy because you've filled in all the proper documents. And, if you're as blind as most patients who've not been taught truth in medicine, you're very happy that you've got a magic pill that you can swallow whenever the headache returns — while the actual cause of your headache continues to create additional problems compounded by the problems created by side effects of the patented drug just conned on you.

If your doctor has a positive, outgoing doctor-to patient personality you'll continue believing "s/he's a wonderful doctor!"

Headaches are rather common. Let's look at a more serious problem. You have a tumor called by some fancy medical name ending with the word "cancer."

Have you ever wondered why after more than half a century of "research" and literally billions of dollars expended there's so little improvement in the life-span of cancer victims?[3]

Look it up for yourself, but one of the biggest problems is the cozy relationship between patented drug pushers and our FDA that's supposed to guard us from the fox. Treatments that act as a disincentive to the creation of more patented drugs by the pharmaceutical companies are normally squashed by the FDA — or the person touting such beneficial treatments is flattened!

One of our former referral physicians, Bruce Halstead, M.D., was always welcome as a cancer expert behind the former iron curtain of Soviet Russia such was his expertise in cancer. He'd written academic books on the use of herbals in medicine. Dr. Halstead was an advisor to the famed Jacques

Yves Cousteau. Before his death in 1997, according to Wikipedia, Yves Cousteau was known in the

USA as "Jacques Cousteau." Cousteau was a French naval officer, explorer, ecologist, filmmaker, innovator, scientist, photographer, author and researcher who studied the sea and all forms of life in water. He co-developed the aqua-lung and pioneered marine conservation.

Bruce Halstead was an advisor to this famous man!

Before he died in 2002, Dr. Halstead practiced medicine in California. He was approached by a lady who did not want the California politically dictated “standard of treatment.” Bruce asked her to sign a statement stating that she was not being treated for cancer but, rather, was taking Pau d’Arco tea to help strengthen her immune system.

The patient’s statement was ignored by ignorant governmental authorities and Dr. Halstead lost his license. He was jailed for six years for not using destructive surgery, chemotherapy or radiation![4] We’ve been told that this disgraceful and improper use of governmental authority has ceased in California as there are now a number of alternative/ complementary cancer treatment centers there.

Except for occasions when a tumor is interfering with the proper functioning of a bodily organ, surgery is certainly not an answer. But then certainly neither is chemotherapy or radiation for any reason. In California, for example, the patented drug pushers together with their brain-washed doctors had influenced the government politicians to pass a law that makes it a criminal offense to use anything other than “standard of treatments.” So, what are “standard of treatments?” Easy — surgery, chemotherapy and radiation!

Any doctor or other health professional who finds a method of actually curing cancer without using the “standard of care” is usually prosecuted to the point where they not just lose their license but also end up in jail, their life and their family’s lives ruined forever.

Cancer cells of one sort or another began forming early in life. Some say even inside the womb. Certainly as children then adults we form cancer cells all of our lives. So why don’t all of us also die quickly from cancer?

Because our immune system, if normal or not disturbed, has learned a survival trait of recognizing cancer cells and cutting them out.

It's easy to reason, therefore, that the tumor — the big, ugly, bad tumor — is not the disease called "cancer," but rather is a symptom of the disease, which is obviously systemic.

So why, therefore, are billions of dollars spent by our government and private industry on treating the symptom — cutting out the symptom, radiating the symptom, or killing the symptom with every cell-damaging chemical?

The answer is clear: patented drug-pushing companies charge huge amounts for providing dangerous, damaging and deadly patented drugs for treating the symptoms; doctors, hospitals and related services make tons of money on applying these damaging drugs to treat the symptoms. A cancer cure would be a danger to a large, lying industry!

This book is not about cancer. Treatment of cancer is cited as an example of a whole insane, paranoic system that cheats and lies to folks in need primarily so a class of sickening professionals can (1) maintain "higher" autocratic prestige; and, so that another class (2) will be assured of lots and lots of profits for stock holders and pharmaceutical managers.

There's a simple test. Ask your doctor if s/he would take the same recommended cancer treatment. If your doctor is honest you'll be somewhat shocked at her/his negative answer.

So, that's what our dominating allopathic medicine is about — the lucrative business of normally and merely treating symptoms.

Alternative/complementary medical practitioners are supposed to search for causes. At least that's our definition of alternative/complementary medical practitioners. Not everyone who practices alternative medicine is well-versed in this search. The majority are at least able to think outside the allopathic medical paradigm. And, just as not all preachers are godly creatures, not all doctors of any kind are equally knowledgeable or of good intent.

There are, of course, many excellent, well-meaning practitioners of allopathy. According to Joseph Mercola D.O.[67] in an article titled "Why It's Economically Unfeasible for Most Doctors to Spend More Than 2 Minutes with you . . . ," a recent poll showed that over a third of doctors are unhappy about aspects of the current state of health care which impedes their ability to provide a quality health care. Mercola says, "Think about it — they are in a model that does not work, as they never treat the cause. They are unknowing pawns of the drug companies and make relatively little money. Sure, they might rake in a few hundred thousand at best, but then they have to pay expenses like malpractice insurance and their income dives — unless they are among those who conspire to steal from insurance or government with overpriced procedure. . . . Then they have to deal all day long with complaining patients, who are all failing to get better from use of the doctors' ignorant recommendations.

"[Doctors give] almost 4 prescriptions per child (age 0-18), and more than 31 prescriptions per senior, aged 65 and over! . . . That's practically the only advice left for doctors to give, between the pressure put on their office visits — brief and inexpensive — and the pressure put on them by the drug companies."

Allopathically trained doctors are excellent for emergencies or necessary surgeries, but don't ever be satisfied with a health practitioner who is not willing to rise above the box lid!

We wish we had the space and time to describe all of the wonderful treatments we've heard about. We've written about just a small portion of those treatments that seem to have a great beneficial effect on most people and most of these treatments are suppressed or are often misunderstood.

But — even so, while some of our recommended treatments can be found with most any alternative/ complementary health professional, not all of the treatments described herein are easily available. Some folks have managed to obtain them even in the face of strong FDA disapproval. We're not recommending that you defy our government's laws of ignorance and greed, but we surely believe that you should be running the government's FDA not the FDA running you! The FDA should not be ruled by the conflict-of-interest patented drug pushers as they are presently. At least toward that goal you can join with others who seek to bring about the end of corruption in our "guardian" agencies.

Do your own research and thinking, please!

The Proper Way to Use Vitamin C

The two scientists who stand out above all others in the twentieth century are Albert Einstein and Linus Pauling. Both men received the Nobel Prize, Pauling twice. Both men brought about revolutions in thought and the practice of science that changed the world forever. Everyone, it seems, has heard the name "Einstein" especially in connection with his influencing President Franklin Delano Roosevelt to set up the Manhattan project during WWII to create the first atomic bomb. If you haven't seen or heard that E = mc2 then you've lived on Mars several years before NASA plans to be there. You should talk to them. That development brought about the atomic and hydrogen bombs which, little by little has leaked to unstable countries. Although Albert Einstein's lifetime of mathematical physics contributed to a wide range of scientific disciplines, he received the Nobel Prize for equations developed earlier than his equation describing conversion of mass to energy and vice versa.

While almost everyone has heard or read of Einstein, few have heard mention of Linus Pauling, Ph.D. — except associated with derogatory comments from patent medicine pushers and their duped or ignorant shills, allopathic practitioners — about Pauling's claim that Vitamin C can prevent or perhaps even cure the common cold.

There is no modern textbook in high school or college in any country on earth that doesn't teach chemistry and physics according to some of Pauling's theories and research work!

Linus Carl Pauling was born in 1901. He was an American chemist, peace activist, author and educator. He was among the first scientist to work in the fields of quantum chemistry and molecular biology. He was one of only four people to win two Nobel Prizes in different fields (chemistry and peace) and the only person to be awarded two unshared prizes.

Pauling's last two years in school were focused on the electronic structure of atoms and their bonding to form molecules; he related how physical and chemical properties of substances were determined by structure. His graduate work involved the use of X-ray diffraction to determine the structure of crystals. From this springboard he made discoveries that are also now found in textbooks on minerals. He became one of the first scientists in the field of quantum chemistry and pioneered in the application of quantum theory to the structure of molecules. He had published more than fifty scientific papers, was awarded the Langmuir Prize for the most significant work in pure science in his age class.

Many other discoveries, theories and research could be listed for Pauling. If you're interested, do a look up through Google. You won't be disappointed.

Linus Carl Pauling, PhD was a first rank scientist, indeed! Where he got caught in the medical webof-deception began on his lecture of "Molecular Medicine" in the late 1950s. He worked on the role of enzymes in brain function believing that mental illness was partly caused by enzyme dysfunction. When he read *Niacin Therapy in Psychiatry* by Abram Hoffer, he theorized that vitamins might have important biochemical effects unrelated to their prevention of associated deficiency diseases. This began the controversial but popular megavitamin craze. In 1968 Pauling published "Orthomolecular Psychiatry." These ideas also formed the basis to modern orthomolecular medicine, that is, use of the "right" molecule — "ortho" means "right."

Following up (or taking advantage of) his many years of successful research, Pauling published the lay book *Vitamin C and the Common Cold* in 1970. This brought about collaboration with Ewan Cameron, a British cancer surgeon. Additional lay publications followed such as *How to Live Longer and Feel Better* in 1987.

By this time all of those who had their financial dog running in the medical race were jumping up and down on the figurative chest of this brilliant scientist, and doing so with all four of their canine feet!

The so-called prestigious Mayo Clinic ran clinical trials that seemed to show that this brilliant scientist was totally wrong.[1] We don't need to describe all of the ways in which they attempted to shaft Pauling's research work. A brief analogy will suffice.

Supposing you were told that the proper use of medicinal vitamin C was to use a dosage of X number of grams three times a day and you wanted to disprove their claims. Pauling wrote that you must use intravenous vitamin C, so immediately you change the study to oral pills with all their disadvantage of absorbability patient by patient. Also you read Pauling saying that you must continue the treatment for Y number of days, so again you, in your own arrogance, change it to something considerably less than Y number of days.

Yea gad!

You don't have to be a rocket scientist to begin to see the flaws in studies from people without integrity and each with a long string of academic degrees after their last names.

A man sells you a car, saying that if you'll fill the tank up with gas you should be able to travel 300 miles. You, however, fill it up with one gallon and then run out of gas. While riding back home in the wrecker truck you rant and fume. "He told me I'd get 300 miles." You shout this again and again until the truck driver raps you on the mouth with his wrecking bar — or until he finally believes you and begin shouting out the same falsehood.

So much for the Mayo Clinic, in-bed-with legalized drug pushers and like-twisted "professionals" of evil intent.

During Linus Pauling's later days many other alternative/complementary doctors began to make sense of the dispute. We're about to tell you of the findings of one of these doctors, Robert F. Cathcart III, M.D.

It is of great significance that humans, other primates, guinea pigs and a very small number of bird species are unable to synthesize Vitamin C. An easy conclusion to reach is that all of these mammals passed through an evolutionary period where each lost the ability to synthesize Vitamin C. Irwin Stone described the genetic defect — whereby higher primates lost the ability to synthesize ascorbate — as caused by a mutated defective gene for the liver enzyme L-gulonolactone oxidase. All higher mammals except primates, guinea pigs and the few bird species mentioned developed a biochemical feedback mechanism which causes an increase in ascorbate synthesis under the influence of external or internal stresses.

Robert F. Cathcart, M.D.[11], of California, in his paper "Vitamin C, Titrating to Bowel Tolerance, Anascorbemia, and Acute Induced Scurvy", presents his brilliantly developed clinical findings demonstrating rather clearly how the body tolerates increasing amounts of Vitamin C when it is under the stress of various diseases. He shows from his clinical findings on 9,000 patients that the body's ability to absorb Vitamin C is directly proportional to the severity of stress and/or disease. Diseases improve or are cured by his "bowel tolerance" measuring technique for determining the exact amount of Vitamin C required by the body at the moment, and he will label a "100 gram cold," for example, when the cold requires 100 grams of vitamin C to be rid of its symptoms, a "50 gram cold" when it takes but 50 grams, and so on.

Mammals that do not have the ability to synthesize Vitamin C are at a distinct disadvantage, and obviously can be affected by external organisms and stress more easily than those that can synthesize their Vitamin C. Those that do so synthesize Vitamin C with a precision that would shame most scientific laboratories. They manufacture and meter out throughout their bodily systems exact quantities of Vitamin C dependent upon their present degree of stress and their degree of need for a given set of infections. The more infection and/or stress the more Vitamin C is manufactured. The less infection and/or stress the less Vitamin C is manufactured. Haven't you ever wondered how it is that certain pets, like dogs and cats, can eat bacteria-ridden garbage and, providing they are not poisoned, they have no difficulty in staying healthy?

Whether establishment physicians accept the fact or not, tens of thousands — no hundreds of thousands — have already verified good results through usage of Vitamin C. Many alternative/complementary physicians know and use these techniques to fight off patient infection, reduce stress and to assist the patient's immune system.

Vitamin C can be used intravenously by itself in sufficiently large dosages to reverse a number of otherwise intransigent disorders that have a causation based on free-radical pathology[12]. Cathcart says: "Well nourished humans contain not much more than 5 grams of Vitamin C in their bodies. The majority of people have much less and therefore are at risk for many problems related to failure of metabolic processes that depend on ascorbate. Stone calls this condition 'chronic subclinical scurvy'[9].

"Some of the increased need for ascorbate," Cathcart relates, "occurs in areas of the body not primarily involved in the disease and can be accounted for by such functions as the adrenals producing more adrenalin and corticoids; the immune system producing more antibodies, interferon, and other substances to fight infection; the macrophages utilizing more ascorbate with their increased activity; and production and protection of a substance called c-AMP and c-GMP with subsequent increased activity of other endocrine glands, and so on." Cathcart continues with "... there must be a tremendous draw on ascorbate locally by increased metabolic rates in the primarily infected tissues. The infecting organisms themselves liberate toxins which are neutralized by ascorbate, but in the process destroy ascorbate. The levels of ascorbate in the nose, throat, Eustachian tubes and bronchial tubes locally infected by a 100 gram cold must be very low, indeed. With this acute induced scurvy localized in these areas it is a small wonder that healing can be delayed and complications such as chronic sinusitis, otitis media and bronchitis, etc. develop."

For a cold in the nose, there is a lack of vitamin C in that portion of the anatomy. Linus Pauling recommends 3.1 grams of sodium ascorbate in 100 ml of water. Use 20 drops into each nostril with an eye dropper. This gives local concentration of 1000 times more than oral dosages would provide[9].

Cathcart adds that from his personal experience and from that of patients, it is apparent that the adrenals are capable of utilizing large amounts of ascorbate with benefit if made available. According to Cathcart, the following medical problems should be expected with increased incidence as ascorbate is depleted: "disorders of the immune system such as secondary infections, Rheumatoid Arthritis and other collagen disease, allergic reactions to drugs, foods and other substances, chronic infections such as herpes, or sequelae of acute infections such as Guillain-Barre' and Reye's syndromes, rheumatic fever, or scarlet fever; disorders of the blood coagulation mechanisms such as hemorrhage, heart attacks, strokes, hemorrhoids, and other vascular thrombosis; failure to cope properly with stresses due to suppression of the adrenal functions such as phlebitis, other inflammatory disorders, asthma and other allergies; problems of disordered collagen formation such as impaired ability to heal, excessive scarring, bed sores, varicose veins, hernias, stretch marks, wrinkles, perhaps even wear of cartilage or degeneration of spinal discs; impaired function of the nervous system such as malaise, decreased pain tolerance, tendency to muscle spasms, even psychiatric disorders and senility; and cancer from the suppressed immune system and carcinogens not detoxified; etc."

Cathcart does not say that ascorbate depletion is the only cause for the diseases above, but that a lack of the Vitamin can predispose to these diseases and that each one of the systems involved in the above diseases are known to be dependent upon ascorbate to function properly. Further, that patient improvement has been noted when Vitamin C has been provided in proper amounts by himself and others, including A. Kalokerinos and F.R. Klenner[10].

All readers should rush out to the local health food store and purchase Vitamin C tablets. Right? Wrong! The problem with tablets is this: Tablets contain ascorbic acid or Sodium or Calcium ascorbate crystals held together by binders — supposedly neutral substances that help to hold the crystals together in the form of a tablet. If you were to take a sufficient amount of ascorbic acid in this form to alleviate most conditions, you would discover yourself with diarrhea from some of the binders, and this would happen long before you determined the correct "bowel tolerance level" dosage of Vitamin C for your present condition.

Vitamin C is also often quite expensive when purchased in tablet form in large quantities from retail health products outlets. You need to find a source of ascorbate that is reasonably low cost, without binders, and purchase it in large quantity so that you feel free to add the Vitamin C to your diet as a supplement each day. How much you should take is to be determined by your physical condition, amount of stress, whether or not seriously ill, and so on. The means of determining the proper amount will be described via Cathcart's "Bowel Titration" technique.

Another fact you should know is that ascorbic acid, sodium ascorbate and calcium ascorbate are physiologically equivalent with ascorbic acid being, weight for weight, slightly more concentrated. One good source for all three of the above is from Bronson Pharmaceuticals. You can order soluble, fine crystals of Vitamin C in 1 kilo quantities for ascorbic acid and sodium ascorbate, and in one pound quantity for calcium ascorbate. You will find it to your advantage to have all three, as the ascorbic acid can be added to fruit drinks and other fluids where the sodium and calcium ascorbate would not taste quite right, and vice versa. The two ascorbates are virtually tasteless (with a very light salty flavor, if anything), and the ascorbic acid is tart, as an acid should be. All three can be mixed in water. Note, however, that only the ascorbic acid itself should be used to determine proper amount to take for the moment via the Cathcart Bowel Tolerance Method.

To avoid overbalancing mineral ratios, by taking too much sodium as compared to calcium, one can mix the two ascorbates, sodium and calcium — and one can also supplement with magnesium and whatever minerals that your physician recommends, the magnesium in dosages of equal weight to the calcium intake.

Cathcart's Bowel Tolerance Method

Cathcart's "Bowel Tolerance" technique is simple to apply. A normal person can probably get by very well on between 4 and 15 grams of vitamin C per 24 hour period. This includes, of course, the amount you consume via green peppers, lettuce, fruits and so on. According to Dr. Cathcart, when one comes down with a sickness, or has been under unusual stress, one increases the amount of Vitamin C consumed each 24 hours to the point where diarrhea just begins — then one backs off to the dosage used the day prior to the day of the diarrhea. That "dosage just lower than required to produce diarrhea," is the exact amount your body needs for that illness for the time being. ***Only ascorbic acid can be used for determining by bowel tolerance the correct amount of Vitamin C that is required!***

It may be necessary to increase your dosages by amounts of 5, 10, 15, . . . grams per 24 hour period until you find the correct dosage. These are monitoring matters best left up to you and your personal experiences. We usually take 2 grams in the morning and evening or between 3 and 5 grams per day, as a regular maintenance routine. It's easy and convenient — using a 1/4 measuring teaspoon lying beside one of the Vitamin C containers — to quickly slip 1 gram into our water or cold drink, whether it is fruit or soda pop. (One quarter teaspoon approximates 1 gram of powdered or crystalline Vitamin C.) You can add the same quantity, or more, to a glass of orange juice, or any other fruit juices, but we would recommend using ascorbic acid, as it is the natural taste of fruits. You should know that the amount of Vitamin C that you consume in a commercially prepared fruit drink is insignificant and not really enough to talk about, and certainly not sufficient to produce a disease cure! As presented at the Second Annual Rheumatoid Disease Foundation Medical Seminar, Cathcart's findings were shown, as follows:

USUAL BOWEL TOLERANCE DOSES

Condition	**Grams Per 24 Hours**	**Number of Doses Per 24 Hours**
Normal	4-15	4
Mild Cold	30-60	6-10
Severe Cold	60-100	8-15
Influenza	100-150	8-20
ECHO, Coxsackievirus	100-150	8-20
Mononucleosis	150-200+	15-25
Viral Pneumonia	100-200+	15-25
Hay Fever, Asthma And Food Allergy	0.5-50	4-8

Burn, Injury, Surgery	25-150	6-20
Anxiety, Exercise and Other Mild Stress	15-25	4-6
Cancer	15-100	4-15
Ankylosing Spondylitis	15-100	4-15
Reiter's Syndrome	15-60	4-10
Acute Anterior Uveitis	30-100	4-15
Rheumatoid Arthritis	15-100	4-15
Bacterial Infections	30-200+	10-25
Infectious Hepatitis	30-100	6-15
Candida Infections	15-200+	6-15

According to Cathcart, disease symptoms will persist until the amount of Vitamin C reaches about 80-90% of bowel tolerance dosages. Perhaps it is only near this tolerance that the ascorbate is pushed into the primary sites of the disease. Further, suppression of symptoms in some instances may not be total, but usually it is very significant and often the amelioration is complete and rapid.

If you try this procedure and find that your bowels emit a great deal of gas to the point of discomfort as you increase daily dosages, then you are one who has "gas-forming" microflora throughout your intestines, such as, but not only as, *Candida albicans*. The gas is usually non-odorous carbon dioxide, and usually a by-product of yeast organisms. This indicates a separate problem that should be handled if you are to have good absorption of digested foods, and if you are to successfully use the Cathcart technique.[8]

Repeating again, according to Cathcart, ***the Bowel Tolerance test should be made only with ascorbic acid***, but once the tolerance dosage is learned for your particular problem, and then you can use the other ascorbates. Technically one should determine the relative proportion of ascorbic acid in calcium and sodium ascorbate; that is, when using calcium or sodium ascorbic instead of ascorbic acid, one should determine the molecular weight of ascorbate. For general maintenance dosages, approximations of either ascorbic acid or the sodium or calcium ascorbates are O.K. As we've mentioned earlier, every person responds to substances differently. Vitamin C is no exception. According to Cathcart, at least 80% of his patients tolerated ascorbic acid well. Perhaps among those who did not are those who also had the gas generation problem from organisms that did not belong to the human symbiote family. (See "Candidiasis: Scourge of Arthritics," http:www.arthritistrust.org)

Evidently Vitamin C when taken properly can provide an important supplement to restoring the body's natural health.

While degenerative arthritis will sometimes be improved, it is the various inflammatory Rheumatoid Diseases where most improvement shows, using Vitamin C therapy. There are probably several reasons why. There is, first, the general free-radical scavenging effect of Vitamin C that can temporarily, at least, clean-out damaging inflammatory products and toxins. Then there is the fact that Vitamin C when placed in all organs and tissues in appropriate amounts for a given person will permit the bodily functions to behave properly. Third, there is the fact of eliminating altogether, or at least reducing attacks on, tissues by foreign invaders, thus helping ourselves in the restoration of health or to maintain health. There is also a related factor where Vitamin C can block allergic reactions with augmented adrenal functions, and allergic reactions may be prevalent in a large number of Rheumatoid Arthritis patients as well as in Candidiasis patients. Remember, Candidiasis almost certainly accompanies many who have one or more of the 100 Rheumatoid Diseases. Finally, and maybe most importantly, Vitamin C in proper dosages has the ability to relieve stress that produces continuous and damaging cortisol via the adrenal glands.

Maintenance dosages are difficult for a physician to state properly, as the individual needs of the patient varies greatly and, also, the needs vary considerably in terms of degree of stress and sickness of the moment. Each Rheumatoid Arthritis victim must learn and make quantity determinations for him/herself.

In addition to a multiplicity of uses that the human body has for Vitamin C, its concentration "directly determines the stability of the tissues. It does so primarily via the protein collagen, which has a similar function in the human body as the iron reinforcement has in a skyscraper. As a consequence of acute Vitamin C deficiency the connective tissue dissolves and the body literally breaks apart, as we know from the sailors' disease scurvy[11]." This is of immediate concern to every kind of sickness. "While acute and complete Vitamin C depletion are essentially unknown today, chronic dietary Vitamin C deficiency is widespread. The consequences of insufficient Vitamin C intake over decades on the tissues of the body, in particular on the wall of the blood vessels, are disastrous. The sequence of events is

"a. decrease of stability and elasticity of the blood vessel walls by Vitamin C deficiency

"b. loss of the cellular barrier between bloodstream and vessel wall,

"c. increased infiltration and massive deposition of dangerous blood constituents in the vessel wall,

"d. development of atherosclerosis, in particular at those sites where high pressure and turbulences prevail (e.g. at those arteries close to the heart),

"e. narrowing of the vessel diameter and decrease of the blood circulation,

"f. eventually heart attack and stroke occur. . . . Heart disease is an early stage of scurvy, a chronic Vitamin C deficiency of the body tissues[5]."

Our intake of Vitamin C has been either excreted or utilized within 24 hours of ingestion, according to Jeffrey Bland, Ph.D., President of Health-Comm, Inc. It is important, therefore, that we eat foods containing this essential vitamin daily, or supplement with a good source.

One of us (Curt Maxwell) has successfully used IV vitamin C for various conditions as outlined in the "Clinical Guide summarized and annotated by Lendon H. Smith, M.D. (forward by Linus Pauling, Ph.D.) and as described in Dr. Klenner's book *Curing the Incurable: Vitamin C, Infectious Diseases, and Toxins*. Dr. Maxwell has also successfully treated some forms of cancer using IV Vitamin C and Laetrile as part of the treatment protocol.

One last point, from personal experience: One of us (Anthony di Fabio) once poo-poohed use of large quantities of Vitamin C as he was taught by very well meaning "establishment" physicians that one got sufficient vitamins and minerals in his daily foods. He didn't question at the time how others could know this when they did not follow him about daily to see how badly he ate or how lacking in nutrition was the food available for purchase. Di Fabio took Vitamin C in tablet form only a few milligrams per day, and saw absolutely no effect on colds. Not until reading Cathcart, Pauling, Stone and others did he realize how truly ignorant and almost superstitious we are in protecting "establishment" medical Authoritarianism.

Di Fabio had suffered from colds and flu as a child, throughout his teens, and throughout the next forty years, until he began following Pauling's advice with sufficient quantities of Vitamin C. Di Fabio is almost never sick from those diseases, at most, perhaps once a year or less. And even then, it lasts but several days and he's well again. Vitamin C in large dosages may not cure your particular ailment, but it will sure make life easier— and protect your body while doing so!

Bill Burke writes:

"I have had osteoarthritis (known that is) for 23 years, manifesting itself in the following sequence: neck, hands, left hip, left knee. I lived on aspirin and Indocin until early 1978, when a piece in the *Saturday Review* by Norman Cousins prompted me to give high-dose Vitamin C a secret trial. (I was a complete skeptic, and didn't want to look like a fool if the stuff didn't work). Reading between the lines, I picked 10 grams per day as a large dose; being a total neophyte and naive, I had to feel my way in the dark. On the 4th day the improvement was so marked that I experimentally dropped Indocin and did not miss it at all. In time I experimentally dropped aspirin for a week; it was a miserable week, and I went back on aspirin thankfully. Sometime later I read (*Chemtech*, Feb. 1978) an interview with Robert F. Cathcart, III, M.D., an orthopedic-surgeon-turned-general-practitioner, who had discovered the boweltolerance phenomenon: i.e., that instead of being a nuisance side effect encountered by some people taking larger-than-vitamin-like doses of ascorbic acid, diarrhea is a God-given indicator that any person has taken more than he can absorb, and therefore more than he needs at any given time. Having learned how to establish my needed intake I quickly found that on about 30 grams per day I was without pain and essentially without discomfort. That was in May of 1978. From that time (to June 1984) I have never taken an aspirin or other painkiller and have needed none. (Which is not to say that I have never had discomfort since but rather that when I have it either more C will help or nothing will help.)

"Wanting to know what was the rationale, if any, behind this dramatic relief (and freeing from synthetic drugs), and also why my doctor didn't know about it (I having previously been a leading exponent of the If-it's-any-good-my-doctor-will-tell-me-about-it school of thought), I began to read and correspond intensively. In the ensuing six years I have learned that there are at least two ways in which C encompasses the relief of arthritic (or any inflammatory) pain: (1) By competitively inhibiting the enzyme phosphodiesterase, it protects the cyclonucleotide cyclic AMP and thus makes more of the latter available to mediate the production of cortisone — which, being home-made does not have the undesirable side effects of the synthetic steroids; and (2) by maximizing the conversion of dietary linoleic acid into steroids; and (3) by maximizing the conversion of dietary linoleic acid into PGE-2, which among other things governs the inflammatory process. (Aspirin and the prescription anti-inflammatory drugs are prostaglandin blockers, but they do so rather indiscriminately so that in suppressing the semi-Bad Guy E-2 they also tend to suppress the super Good Guy E-1. Since E-1, among other things, governs the production of T-lymphocytes, this accounts for the fact that these drugs depress the immune system.) (E-2 is by no means all bad, so it should not be suppressed totally. It is involved in protecting the stomach against ulceration, which explains why the prostaglandin blockers so often cause ulcers. One Rheumatoid Disease patient was — before I got to her — on Motrin, and had to have emergency surgery for a perforated ulcer. She later got the [recommended Arthritis Trust of America] treatment from Dr. Plagenhoef, and is now free of Rheumatoid Disease.) [See "Essential Fatty Acids are Essential," http://www.arthritistrust.org.]

"It is probably significant that my left knee was the last joint to become arthritic, and was the one that had bothered me least.

"It appears to me that Dr. Paul Pybus' treatment [See *Intraneural Injections for Rheumatoid Arthritis and Osteoarthritis & The Control of Pain in Arthritis of the Knee,* Kindle at Amazon.com or Nook at Barnes & Noble] is designed to interrupt a source of stress on the knee long enough to allow nutrients (essentially protein and ascorbic acid) access to the cartilage so that repair may proceed. It would then seem that [your] "other health-improvement programs" should above all include a bowel-tolerance intake of Vitamin C not only for the repair aspects, but also for the relief of residual inflammation. (A recent paper states that L-arginine considerably speeds up the deposition of collagen in healing wounds in rats and might well do the same in humans, so perhaps adding L-arginine to the regimen might be prudent.)

"It was thanks to Dr. Cathcart that I learned about [Roger] Wyburn-Mason. Cathcart's paper asserts that while Rheumatoid Arthritis significantly increases bowel tolerance, Osteoarthritis doesn't. I wrote, about a year ago to argue that point on the basis of my own high intake. He replied that he stood by his observation, and that if my allergies were not enough to account for my large need then perhaps there was an unsuspected rheumatoid component in my arthritis; and he referred me to Wyburn-Mason's *Medical Hypotheses* paper of 1979. [See *Causation of Rheumatoid Disease and Many Human Cancers*, Roger Wyburn-Mason, M.D., Ph.D. Kindle at Amazon.com or Nook at Barnes & Noble.] So in time I went to Dr. Plagenhoef and said I wanted to be tested for Rheumatoid Disease. All tests were negative. I said I wanted the [treatment] anyway. He resisted. I prevailed. In the 4th and 5th weeks I had an unmistakable Herxheimer reaction. After the 6th week my arthritis was significantly improved — about 50%. More to the point, my bowel tolerance for C plummeted by 40%, showing that a chronic source of stress had been removed from my body. (See *Arthritis: Osteoarthritis and Rheumatoid Disease Including Rheumatoid Arthritis* Amazon.com at Kindle or Nook at Barnes & Noble.)

"While I was on the metronidazole treatment [early Arthritis Trust of America treatment], incidentally, I used no prednisone. I simply increased my intake of Vitamin C as necessary to control the discomfort, which meant going as high as 4 grams an hour on the Herxheimer days. Exogenous steroids are not necessary — not when Vitamin C so well facilitates the endogenous stuff."

Hydrogen Peroxide Therapy

Since our friendly neighborhood allopathic physicians know virtually nothing about the health benefits of vitamin C it's nearly a certainty that they know nothing about its function in the mammalian body. It may also come as a surprise to the reader to learn that Vitamin C, among other uses, assists portions of the immune system to produce hydrogen peroxide (H2O2) and, that the hydrogen peroxide forms oxidative enzymes which kill invasive microorganisms.

Some countries sell the hydrogen peroxide in weaker solutions, Americans usually purchase 3% over-the-counter hydrogen peroxide in dark, plastic bottles — light weakens the mixture. As a topical treatment for open wounds — scrapes and cuts, etc. — it's a wonderful disinfectant. The revelation to most, though, is that also it can be used for intravenous injections in its pure form.

Hydrogen peroxide has been in use for more than a century for medical purposes, the abstracts of articles and research reports published from 1966 through 1988 reaches 2" high when printed on 8-1/2"X11" paper. From 1818 to 1966 the abstracts reach higher. First isolated in 1818 by Louis Jacques Thénard, it soon became a standard for sterilization of equipment. In aerospace research, H2O2 has been used to sterilize satellites and space probes. It's an oxidizer also often used as a bleach to whiten clothing and hair. About fifty percent of the world's production of hydrogen peroxide in 1994 was used for pulpand paper-bleaching. H2O2 had numerous industrial applications. As an oxidizer it does a magnificent job of creating oxidative enzymes inside the human blood stream that helps keep down our enormous population of invasive microorganisms.

A complete list of uses — both biological and industrial — for H2O2 would fill a large book, indeed! A number of clinics in the United States and Mexico use hydrogen peroxide therapy, as well as other treatment modalities on a routine basis usually given by intravenous injection (IV).

Hydrogen peroxide is an essential metabolite, meaning that it is necessary to life's process according to William Campbell Douglass, M.D. of Georgia.[16]

As we age our immunological system weakens which permits organisms of opportunity to spread thereby breeding colonies of organisms whose presence is anathema to good health. Killing these organisms should permit at least temporary respite from microbial warfare and give your system time to heal.

According to William Campbell Douglass, M.D.[15], not only is H2O2 involved in phagocytosis (killing and absorption of foreign germs), but also "it acts like insulin in that it aids the transport of sugar through the body." It is also at least as important, or perhaps more so, than thyroid for heat generation because it creates "intracellular thermogenesis, a warming of your cells which is absolutely essential to life's processes."

Various physicians also use hydrogen peroxide therapy for various ailments. Physicians have independently discovered such treatments to be effective against some types of cancer, leukemia, arthritis, coronary heart disease, arterial circulation disorders, colitis, gum diseases, and assorted children's diseases. The American Cancer Society states that "there is no scientific evidence that hydrogen peroxide is a safe, effective or useful cancer treatment," and advises cancer patients to "remain in the care of qualified doctors who use proven methods of treatment and approved clinical trials of promising new treatments." Since allopathic approaches have failed to significantly increase survival time for cancer victims for more than sixty years at the cost of billions of dollars one can only wonder at the temerity of such recommendations. But then changes to allopathic medical approaches using only surgery, chemotherapy or radiation occurs as fast as changes in the use of phlebotomy (bleeding) and constant, persistent applications of deadly mercury for every ailment. Robin Hood, you may recall, died of excessive bleeding from standard of care phlebotomy while Lewis Carroll's Mad Hatter was mad because of his use of mercury in blocking hats!

The First International Conference of Bio-oxidative Medicine[23] was held February 17-19, 1989 in Dallas/Ft. Worth, TX. Physicians presented papers on the efficacy and safety of hydrogen peroxide infusions.

According to Dr. William Campbell Douglass, II[16], also the Baylor University Medical Center may "have gone a long way toward proving that H2O2 dripped into the leg and carotid vessels of patients known to have severe arteriosclerosis will clear those arteries of disease. When these patients died, autopsies were done to compare arteries that had been treated with H2O2 with those not treated. They reported: 'The elution [separation] of lipids from the arterial wall by dilute hydrogen peroxide has been accomplished. . . .' In simple English that means the plaque buildup was removed by injecting H2O2 into the blood vessels. . . . That was over 20 years ago[2]" [now nearly 30 years ago.] Dr. Douglass added that, "The investigators also reported that the improvement is not temporary."

While H2O2 has been used to good advantage for hardening of the arteries, temporal arteritis, shingles, chronic obstructive pulmonary disease, the yeast syndrome, various viral infections, including AIDS, certain forms of cancer, dental gum diseases, colds (35% H2O2 in cold humidifier), growing better food, purifying water without chlorine complications, increasing thyroid activity, arthritis, depression, emphysema, lupus erythematosis, multiple sclerosis, . . ., a list of claims made would exceed our space limitations[24].

There are also many important forgotten facts in the past medical literature. For example, William Campbell Douglass, M.D. reports on "Dr. Edward C. Rosenow, author of 450 published medical papers — an associate at the Mayo Clinic for over 60 years — proved [more than] 90 years ago (1914) that bacteria could be found consistently in the lymph nodes that drain joints (*J.A.M.A.*, April 11, 1914). He was probably the first scientist to postulate that H2O2 would help arthritis . . . " because of *Streptococcus viridans*."

Charles H. Farr, M.D., Ph.D. (deceased), said, "Perhaps we have become myopic about biological oxidation! The majority of investigational studies seem to concentrate on the damaging effects of biological oxidation and the production of free radicals. Hydrogen peroxide is usually treated as a[n] intermediate or by-product of metabolism and considered of minor significance in metabolic pathways except as it relates to biochemical disruption, tissue or cellular damage.

"We feel the physiological effects of bio-oxidation and, in particular hydrogen peroxide should be investigated with a new prospect.

"From the 2,500 or more references on hydrogen peroxide we have collected and reviewed we have come to appreciate this physiological product as a[n] extremely important molecule in metabolism. Hydrogen peroxide is produced by all cells of the body for many different physiological reasons. The granulocytes produce H2O2 as a first line of defense against bacteria, yeast, virus, parasites, macrophages, and most fungi. It is involved in any metabolic pathway which utilizes oxidases, peroxidases, cyclo-oxygenase, lipoxygenase, myeloperoxidase, catalase and probably many other enzymes. Hydrogen peroxide is involved in protein, carbohydrate and fat metabolism, immunity, vitamin and mineral metabolism or any other system you might wish to explore.

"Our studies demonstrate a positive metabolic effect to intravenous infusion of H2O2 . Its ability to oxidize almost any physiological or pathological substance, in addition to producing increased tissue and cellular oxygen tensions, has proven it to have therapeutic value.

"We feel the evidence presented should stimulate a new appreciation in the study of the potential therapeutic application of bio-oxidative mechanisms."

Considering the all-encompassing role played by hydrogen peroxide in our bodies, one can now understand why Vitamin C is so very important, as it furnishes molecules for us to construct hydrogen peroxide!

Two Means of Administration

There are two ways to administer hydrogen peroxide for medical purposes. Both means require a pure grade of hydrogen peroxide which is something different than one can purchase at the drug store for topical treatment of sores and wounds. The 3% drugstore hydrogen peroxide also contains tin and phosphate compounds that are dangerous to consume either by means of IV (intravenous) or orally.

We must caution at the outset that Dr. Farr and some other physicians do not approve of use of H2O2 for oral treatment, as so many treatment modalities describe[11].

Dr.Farr told us — and some other physicians agree — that hydrogen peroxide used orally produces free-radicals in the stomach and these free-radicals are not safe. Combinations of fatty acids which are likely to be in the stomach in the presence of iron and ascorbate may reduce hydrogen peroxide to hydroxyl and superoxide free radicals. These may have a deleterious effect upon the gastric and duodenal mucosa, with an increase of glandular stomach erosion, duodenal hyperplasia (abnormal increase in number of cells), adenoma and carcinoma, although in rats there seems to be inconsistencies in the studies related to carcinogenesis using 0.8% concentration for ten weeks versus 1% concentration for 32 weeks, the former indicating carcinogenesis, the latter not so.

Since some clinics are using both intravenous and oral techniques with patients successfully, or to some good advantage, apparently not all possible research is in on the subject of oral versus IV administration.

We have twice tried the oral method and have failed to continue onward because of a terrible, revolting nausea. Some folks react similarly, others don't, and some persevere despite all. As stated earlier, Dr. Farr's research demonstrates that hydrogen peroxide stimulates oxidative enzymes which increases the metabolic rate. Intravenous use rapidly relieves allergenic reactions, influenzal symptoms, chronic systemic candidiasis, acute viral reactions as a result of the oxidation of antigenic substances and regulation of immune system functions.

To prepare the IV (intravenous) solutions, Dr. Farr begins with 30% H2O2 of USP food or cosmetic grade. Thirty percent H2O2 is a powerful oxidizer and should be handled with extreme caution.

The 30% solution is diluted with equal amounts of sterile distilled water to make a 15% stock solution. The stock solution is passed through a Millipore 0.22mm medium flow filter for sterilization and removal of particulate matter. The stock solution is stored in 100 ml sterile containers and kept refrigerated for future use.

His infusion solutions are then prepared using sterile 5% dextrose in water. The addition of 1/4 ml sterile of the 15% H2O2 stock solution to each 100 ml of carrier solution produces a 0.0375% concentration that is finally used for the intravenous infusions.

Dr. Farr further warns that "caution must be exercised that nothing is added to the H2O2 solution because of its tremendous oxidizing power. Even ascorbic acid (Vitamin C) is rapidly oxidized to the mono-dehydroascorbate radical, an unstable compound which degrades into numerous other chemical fragments.... Vitamins, minerals, peptides, enzymes, amino acids, heparin, EDTA, or other injectable materials should never be mixed with the H2O2 solution," according to Dr. Farr, but later use by other physicians found that certain substances could be introduced simultaneously.

By far the widest use for hydrogen peroxide, whether wisely or not, seems to be that of oral usage where a 35% "food grade" is diluted to a 3% concentration by use of 1 ounce of 35% H2O2 to 11 ounces of distilled water. The 3% concentration is then used by quantities of drops in distilled water, increasing the dosages and number of oral treatments daily throughout a number of weeks.

Many have made the claim that a "die-off" effect is observed similar in nature to the Herxheimer Effect. (Whenever a microorganism more complex than a simple bacteria is killed in massive quantities, fever and chills may occur, called "The Herxheimer." (See "The Herxheimer Effect," http://www.arthritistrust.org.)

Other Uses for H2O2

Use 3% solution, except where 35% is highlighted.

Vegetable soak: Add 1/4 cup to a full sink of cold water. Soak light-skinned (like lettuce) 20 minutes, thicker skinned (like cucumbers) 30 minutes. Drain, dry and refrigerate. Prolongs freshness. If time is a problem, spray vegetables (and fruits) with a solution of 3%. Let stand for a few minutes, rinse and dry.

Leftover tossed salad: Spray with a solution of 1/2 cup water and 1 Tbls. 3%. Drain, cover and refrigerate.

To freshen kitchen: Keep a spray bottle in the kitchen. Use it to wipe off counter tops and appliances. It will disinfect and give the kitchen a fresh smell. Works great in the refrigerator and kid's school lunch boxes.

Marinade: Place meat, fish, or poultry in a casserole (avoid using aluminum pans). Cover with hydrogen peroxide. Place loosely covered in refrigerator for 1/2 hour. Rinse and cook.

In the dishwasher: Add 2 ozs to your regular washing formula.

Sprouting seeds: Add 1 oz. to a pint of water and soak the seeds overnight. Add the same amount of hydrogen peroxide each time you rinse the seeds.

House and garden plants: Put 1 oz. in 1 quart of water. Water or mist plants with this solution.

Humidifiers and steamers: Mix 1 pint to 1 gallon of water.

Laundry: Add 8 ozs. to your wash in place of bleaches.

Shower: Keep a spray bottle of hydrogen peroxide in the shower. Spray your body after washing to replace the acid mantle of your skin that soap removes.

Facial: Use on a cotton ball as a facial freshener after washing. (Remember: do not use 35% grade!)

Rejuvenating detoxifying bath: Add 6 ozs. to 1/2 tub of water. May increase hydrogen peroxide up to 2 cups per bath. Soak at least 1/2 hour.

Alternate bath: Add 1/2 cup 35% H2O2, 1/2 cup sea salt, and 1/2 cup baking soda or Epsom salts to bath water and soak.

Foot soak: Add 1-1/2 ozs. 35% H2O2 to 1 gallon water and soak.

Athlete's foot: Soak feet nightly until condition is improved.

Mouthwash: Add a dash of liquid chlorophyll for flavoring if desired.

Toothpaste: Use baking soda and add enough to make a paste. Or just dip your brush in it and brush.

Douche or enema: Add 6 Tbls. to a quart of distilled water. 6 Tbls. is the maximum amount to use.

Pets: For small animals (dogs & cats) use 1 oz. to 1 qt. of water.

Agriculture: Use 8 ozs. 35% H2O2 per 1000 gallons of water. If you do not have an injector, start out by using 1 tsp. 35% H2O2 in the drinking cup at the stanchion.

Drinking water of ailing cows: Use 1 pt., to 5 gallons of water. To drench sick calves, put 1/3 pt. bottle and fill remainder with water. Do this twice a day. For an adult cow, use the same procedure, but use a quart.

Foliage feed crops: put 5 to 16 ozs. of 35% H2O2 into 20 gallons of water. This is sufficient for 1 acre. Spray on plants early in the morning when the dew is still on them and the birds are singing.

Hydrogen peroxide has been a recognized medicinal source since at least the 1800's, has gone into disrepute, and now seems to lie in a sort of limbo so far as allopathic medical practitioners are concerned.

However, research has progressed forward on its use throughout the world, and American doctors of a more open-minded view are persisting in learning its good effects.

Again we caution the reader that there is controversy between the use of oral hydrogen peroxide and use of IV (intravenous) treatment. You must study the issues and come to your own judgment. But please make an educated decision, and whichever you decide, find a physician who knows what s/he is doing.

Stimulation of Oxidative Enzymes

Charles H. Farr, M.D., Ph.D. has used hydrogen peroxide clinically, and has reported on research that he performed that sheds a great deal of light on how H2O2 functions. Contrary to popular belief the use of H2O2 by either infusion or orally cannot supply as much oxygen as a good, deeply inhaled breath.

Instead, it is the stimulation of oxidative enzymes that does the useful trick. Dr. Farr's conclusions are appropriate and follow:

Dr. Farr[20] says, "There are a number of commercial products [that] claim to contain more oxygen on a volumes percent basis than Hydrogen Peroxide and consequently this has been interpreted as meaning they would somehow have more biological activity. There is a great deal of confusion about the difference between the terms `Oxygenation' and `Oxidation' when applied to biochemical reactions. A product which contains more oxygen per molecule may or may not have any biological activity.

"We reported Intravenous Hydrogen Peroxide has an oxidative stimulatory effect when administered to man which appears to be independent of the amount of oxygen produced.

"Hydrogen Peroxide is a very simple molecule produced by almost every cell in the body. This amazing molecule, essential for life in both plant and animal, has been generally overlooked for its role in oxidative metabolism. Every chemist knows any reaction must have an opposite reaction to balance the equation. This applies equally to reactions in the test tube and in living cells. The world seems to have been caught up in the idea all biological oxidation is harmful because free-radicals may be produced. Free-radicals can cause lipid peroxidation and membrane damage. Consequently many products, containing anti-oxidants, are being promoted to prevent peroxidation. Some researchers, including this author, feel peroxidation serves a useful purpose in the biochemical balance and may need stimulating at times instead of preventing.

"Hydrogen Peroxide as an oxidizer, under certain catalytic conditions, can degrade into water and oxygen.

"The fact that Hydrogen Peroxide may increase oxygen tension in the tissue is of secondary importance. Any student of biochemistry knows the principal reaction of an oxidizer, such as Hydrogen Peroxide, is to accept electrons in the RedOx [reduction/oxidation] reactions of the body and has nothing to do with "Oxygen" or "Oxygenation." It is true Hydrogen Peroxide increases the *rate of oxidation* in the body[22], but this is not because it produces oxygen but rather it *stimulates oxidative enzymes*.

"Hydrogen Peroxide is a naturally produced purposeful molecule in the body. It functions to aid membrane transport, acts as a hormonal messenger, regulates thermogenesis (heat production), stimulates and regulates immune functions, regulates energy production and many other important metabolic functions. These effects can occur without increasing the amount of oxygen. It is purposely used by the body to produce Hydroxyl Radicals to kill bacteria, virus, fungi, yeast and a number of parasites. This natural killing or protective system has nothing to do with increasing the amount of available oxygen. "The amount of oxygen produced by a therapeutic infusion of Hydrogen Peroxide is very small. A single breath of fresh air contains many times more oxygen than found in either a therapeutic infusion or in a few drops of 35% Food Grade Hydrogen Peroxide taken orally.

"Claims are being made that molecules containing Oxygen and Chlorine, or Chlorite ions will sterilize water, milk and almost anything to which they have been added. Chlorine is added to almost all public water supplies for the same purpose. The small amount of oxygen in these molecules have very little to do with this sterilization process. There are many more aerobic (requires oxygen) than anaerobic (does not use oxygen) bacteria and increasing the oxygen supply may actually stimulate the growth of the aerobic bacteria. `Oxygen supply' or `Oxygenation' is not a credible basis for the promotion of these products. *Oxidation* is the key word and not *Oxygenation.*

"Oxidation is the removal of an electron from a molecule which changes electrical energy of the molecule into an oxidized state. The oxidizing agent which accepts the electron through this reaction becomes reduced. This reaction takes place in many biochemical reactions in which OXYGEN is *not* involved. In oxidative reactions in which Hydrogen Peroxide is involved, oxygen is released when the Hydrogen Peroxide, acting as an oxidizer, is reduced, but it is the transfer of the electrons which is important and not the production of Oxygen.

"Manufacturers of products which claim to have the same effect as Hydrogen Peroxide may not have a good understanding of the biochemical role of Hydrogen Peroxide in the body. Some of these products claim to provide more oxygen molecules than Hydrogen Peroxide and that may be true but I know of no scientific evidence to show this enhances oxidative metabolism. Cancer and many other degenerative diseases are thought to be the results of poor cellular oxidative processes. They are not the results of a reduced supply of oxygen. Persons with anemias or severe lung disease may have an oxygen deficit but do not necessarily have a greater incidence of Cancer or chronic diseases. The problem is not the delivery of oxygen to the cells but utilization by the cells. Hydrogen Peroxide affects utilization or oxidation dramatically whereas hyper-oxygenated or chlorinated molecules have not been shown to be necessary in the body to improve oxidative metabolism[23]."

Many physicians and clinics are effectively using Hydrogen Peroxide intravenously with their patients.

There is a ton of literature favoring Hydrogen Peroxide treatment for various medica conditions[10].

We suggest that your study of H2O2 may be an important step in your search for good health. It's worth looking into!

A Closer Look at Intravenous Hydrogen PeroxideH2O2

(c)BY GORDON N. JOSEPHS, DO, HOMEOPATHIC PHYSICIAN[27]

In 1988, satisfied chelation patients began sending me lots of referrals. My patients particularly began sending me a lot of people with *emphysema, asthma, and chronic lung disease*. Well chelation therapy does have a benefit for these people, but chelation is best known for heart and circulation problems. I needed something that particularly worked well for *lung* problems.

I heard about intravenous hydrogen peroxide, and I heard that it was *terrific* for lung disease. I also heard that you had to be *very careful*, that the therapy could be *dangerous*. I heard *conflicting* stories from doctors, but *none of these doctors actually used intravenous hydrogen peroxide*. My search for the truth led me to a meeting of IBOM, the International Bio-Oxidative Medical Foundation, presided by Dr. Charles Farr, an MD in Oklahoma City.[15]

I went to Dallas to an IBOM meeting for several days. There I was taught *exactly* how to *safely* administer hydrogen peroxide intravenously. I was taught a *specific protocol*. At the meeting, IBOM doctors were speaking *from experience* about the various things for which they found peroxide useful. To my very great amazement, I learned that peroxide was good for a *great many things* beside lung problems.

General Information About Peroxide

There are lots of studies which demonstrate that peroxide does the following:

1. Peroxide *stimulated the immune system*.
2. Peroxide *killed* a dozen different *pathogenic bacteria*, and killed many *viruses*, and *yeast and fungus* too!
3. Peroxide even *improved circulation* and *unblocked arteries*, like chelation did!
4. It caused debris deep down in the lungs to be *expelled*!
5. It got rid of all kinds of *chronic pains*, but nobody was certain why.
6. It *oxygenated the body*, better than if you got into a $100,000 hyperbaric oxygen chamber!
7. Peroxide even destroyed some cancerous tumors!

And the list of things went on and on. I'd bore you to tears if I read off the list. It turns out that there are over 6000 articles in the medical literature about peroxide.

So **if peroxide does so much good, why isn't it being used more by doctors**? The answer has to do with money and stupidity.

For example, drug companies would like doctors to prescribe a $60 antibiotic, not a dollars worth of peroxide! You have to understand that the drug companies fill the medical journals with expensive, and really slick advertising. Because of these ads, doctors perceive that drugs are the state of the art. Nobody advertises hydrogen peroxide. Peroxide is not patentable. Who's going to promote peroxide when *anyone* and *any drug company* can make it?

Then, some doctors are just plain stupid. They don't even wash hands between examining patients, which was proven to reduce hospital infections by Dr. Semmelweis a hundred years ago. It took doctors 40 years to accept the electrocardiogram as useful!

Well, it's been over 60 [now 82] years since peroxide was found to be miraculous. In 1929 there was a worldwide flu epidemic. There was no drug to kill the flu virus (and there still isn't), so some people with poor immune systems died from it. 84% of those who developed *influenza pneumonia* died.

Well in 1929, doctors took patients dying from influenza pneumonia, and for the first time in history gave them intravenous hydrogen peroxide. 48% of them lived! Yes, I'm telling you that there's been an antiviral remedy for over *60* [now 82] *years* and doctors seem ignorant of it all.

Dr. Charlie Farr, who I consider my *guru*, did a great **study on flu** victims just a few years ago. He gave 44 patients with the flu a peroxide treatment, and told them to return the next day if they were not better. Seven returned (note: *all seven* that returned had a prior history of lung problems). He gave them a second peroxide treatment and told them to return if they were not better. Two returned, and they required a third dose. How's that for anti-viral action? You see, if you come early to the doctor with a virus, it can be knocked out.

Asthma, Emphysema, and Chronic Lung Disease

Well, what about *emphysema, asthma, and chronic lung disease*? It turns out that IV peroxide can do something special, something that no other substance I know of can do. It can *clean* the lungs!

Ask a pathologist what color a baby's lungs are. He'll tell you they're *pink*. At autopsy, 50 or more years later, those lungs are gray-black .... filled with *soot and grime*, from the air we breathe, that could not be eliminated by the body. It's harder to transfer oxygen from the air you breathe through soot-covered air sacks. Well here's great news. . . Intravenous peroxide *burns* the soot and debris, and *lifts it off the surface* of the air sacks. Then you cough this *gunk* up, get it out of your body and you can breathe easier after that. **Nothing else in medicine has this action.**

This miracle isn't always met with joy. All the patient knows is that they took a peroxide treatment and began coughing more than ever. They've got to understand that *this coughing is good*. The coughing can begin right as the peroxide IV is dripping, or after the IV has been completed. This reaction to peroxide may occur for three to six treatments, after which it ceases. The job is done! The air sacs of the lungs have been cleaned.

The coughing doesn't always occur. Instead of coughing, the loose debris is often brought up in the sputum (the mucus and phlegm in the throat), and then swallowed, without the patient even being aware of it.

How Many Treatments Are Needed for Lung Problems?

For *asthma, emphysema, or chronic lung disease*, peroxide treatments should be taken once per week for at least ten treatments. **It takes some time for the changes to occur in chronic disease.** You must not say to yourself, "Well, I'll just try two or three treatments, and see if it's any good for me." That's not how peroxide works. And frankly, *I don't really want you to start peroxide unless you intend to finish a reasonable series*. That's because I don't want anyone condemning peroxide unless they've given it a proper try. Peroxide is good therapy, used correctly. For asthma, emphysema, and chronic lung disease, this means taking at least ten treatments over ten weeks.

How Many Treatments Are Needed for Lung Problems?

For *asthma, emphysema, or chronic lung disease*, peroxide treatments should be taken once per week for at least ten treatments. **It takes some time for the changes to occur in chronic disease.** You must not say to yourself, "Well, I'll just try two or three treatments, and see if it's any good for me." That's not how peroxide works. And frankly, *I don't really want you to start peroxide unless you intend to finish a reasonable series*. That's because I don't want anyone condemning peroxide unless they've given it a proper try. Peroxide is good therapy, used correctly. For asthma, emphysema, and chronic lung disease, this means taking at least ten treatments over ten weeks.

Most Problems? The truth . . . it just depends upon what disease we're talking about. For example, I had a man come to me who was suffering with **temporal arteritis**. Temporal arteritis causes terrible, one-sided head pain around the eye and the temple. I had a man come to me who had been to dozens of doctors and top notch pain centers. He was loaded up on every manner of drug. A smile came over this man's face as the *first IV* was dripping. He could feel his pain going away. He took a second treatment, and it was gone! That was six months ago, and he hasn't been back! So you see, for some things it *can* be a matter of a couple treatments. I hope that you will meet personally with me or with your "peroxide" doctor, and discuss how many treatments are likely to be needed for your condition.

What Diagnoses Respond to Peroxide?

Let me tell you about some other random cases, and how peroxide worked. First, let's talk about **shingles** (also called **herpes zoster**). Just one or two treatments taken for a couple days in a row, and one more a week later generally does the trick! I had a patient with AIDS and shingles. It took about six treatments over the course of two weeks, not bad considering a battered immune system. Sometimes the pain that may linger after shingles (**post herpetic neuralgia**) responds to a peroxide series. I think it's because there's still live virus deep in the nerve root.

I believe that **Bell's Palsy** (of the face) is also from a virus similar to shingles, because my peroxide treatments have relieved the condition over a week or two.

For **colds**, or **the flu**, I've already told you that one or two treatments are generally sufficient.

I had a woman with **malignant melanoma with metastasis to her lymph nodes**. She was in awful pain. She wanted one treatment every day. When she got it, she felt no pain, was active and busy. Without a daily treatment, she was miserable and could not function.

A lot of **chronic painful conditions** respond to peroxide. I believe that all chronic pain comes *ultimately* from insufficient oxygen getting into the affected area of the body. Peroxide gets the oxygen into the tissue and the pain leaves. Nevertheless, the official line is that we *don't understand why peroxide helps chronic pain*. There's no telling the best way to give the peroxide for chronic pain. One might need it once a week or once a day. I've recently learned that slowly infusing the peroxide all day long, using an infusion pump, can get rid of constant pain much better than just a short IV (my thanks to Dr. Jesse Stoff for that finding).

For disorders of **blocked arteries**, such as **angina pectoris**, or **peripheral artery blockage in the legs**, Dr. Charlie Farr says that one peroxide each week, *plus two chelation* [EDTA] *treatments each week, works the best*. I think that's a perfectly fine schedule, and about ten weeks of treatment should be considered minimal. 15-20 weeks would be really good.

If your **immune system** is down, and you get sick a lot, take one treatment a week for ten weeks or twenty, (you'll need a variety of nutritional supplements too). Here the peroxide stimulates the production of T-helper cells and causes white cells to make interferon, and lots more.

Let's talk about **chronic fatigue syndrome**. Chronic fatigue is *not* one disease. It more than likely is a name given to hundreds of *not-yet-diagnosed* problems in a person. What I mean is that there may be someone with undiagnosed parasites, dragging their body around, exhausted. Well that's chronic fatigue. And so is undiagnosed Epstein-Bar virus infection, and so is malabsorption with mineral deficiency. My point is that there obviously is no *magic bullet remedy* for what is called chronic fatigue, because the causes of chronic fatigue are varied. The underlying cause of each individual's chronic fatigue needs to be determined and treated with the most suitable remedy or remedies. Peroxide is likely to help many chronic fatigue patients, because peroxide has so many actions.

For IBOM[15] list of diagnoses for which peroxide has been found useful, please see INDEX A at the end of this [article].

Is Peroxide the Magic Bullet?

Well *if there were a magic bullet*, it might well be IV peroxide, because peroxide has so many different actions. It can kill considerable numbers of viruses, bacteria, fungi, yeast, parasites, and even some tumor cells! It can boost the immune system by improving the number and quality of various blood cells. It can improve circulation, improve heart function, and provide oxygen to the brain. It can relieve pain. It can destroy toxic environmental chemicals inside your body and quiet allergies.

Can you think of anything more likely to help an unknown, undiagnosed, hidden illness?

Mixing Other Substances in the Peroxide IV

It was once believed that the doctor could not add any other substance into the peroxide IV bottle. It was believed that either the peroxide would be destroyed, or that the added substance might be destroyed. Recently, however, studies have determined that certain vitamins and minerals can be added into a peroxide infusion. Sadly, vitamin C cannot be added. Fortunately, *magnesium* can be added.

Magnesium is my personal favorite mineral (if there is such a thing). That's because magnesium *lowers blood pressure, relaxes artery walls and thus promotes increased circulation, reduces anginal chest pains, reduces irregular heart rhythms, relaxes muscles, alleviates muscle cramps, reduces anxiety levels, and increases energy production in every cell in your body*! Also, for reasons that we do not yet fully understand, magnesium reduces the likelihood of infusion site discomfort, arm pain. As far as I'm concerned, I'm going to add magnesium to just about every peroxide IV I can.

Other *trace minerals* can be added to a peroxide IV also. And *B-Complex Vitamins and B-12* can be added. So now it is possible to give the patient more for his money. With one treatment infusion, the doctor may be able to accomplish more, by providing the body with needed nutrients as well as peroxide.

Isn't Peroxide Harmful?

Peroxide is extremely well tolerated by the human body. This may come as a surprise to you. After all, if peroxide kills so many things, then why doesn't it kill us? The answer is the enzyme CATALASE. Catalase, found throughout the human body, causes hydrogen peroxide to change into *harmless* oxygen and water. Viruses don't have catalase, so the peroxide destroys them. Humans have catalase in their cells, and are not destroyed by peroxide.

When you get an infection, your white blood cells surround the germs and kill them. Well exactly HOW does the white blood cell kill germs? Let me tell you something that 9,999 out of 10,000 MDs don't know. Your white blood cells produce a little *hydrogen peroxide*, and they bathe the germs in the peroxide, and this kills the germs! It has always been peroxide that *naturally* cured infection in your body!

Did you know that hydrogen peroxide is made in the atmosphere, and that it comes down in our rainwater and it kills off a certain amount of living organisms in the soil? If it were not for this peroxide, the earth's surface would be putrid from bacterial overgrowth. What I'm trying to convey to you, is that peroxide is a wonderfully natural, beneficial molecule.

This is not to say that peroxide cannot be harmful. Humans can tolerate just so much of the stuff, and that's why **you should have peroxide treatments only from a well trained physician**. As far as

I'm concerned, if the doctor hasn't studied the IBOM[15] protocols, he's not prepared to do a good job with peroxide.

Possible Side Effects

There are some POTENTIAL side effects to IV peroxide. I say *potential* because, in truth, I hardly ever see undesirable side effects. But I want you to know about them. Here in Arizona, where my office is located, intravenous hydrogen peroxide is considered *experimental*. I may give you peroxide treatments, but I must follow all the rules and regulations for doing *experimental medicine*. Foremost is that you be fully informed about what I am about to do, and that includes understanding potential side effects. So here goes.

1. The most common side effect is **vein inflammation**, right where the IV is going in your arm. There can be pain, and if it occurs, there's little to do except change the location of the needle. If you have a big vein, such as in the elbow crease, that's a great place to place the IV. The bigger the vein, the less likely any discomfort. Magnesium is added to the IV and this reduces the likelihood of any pain also.

2. You can get a **red streak** up your arm, starting right where the needle is inserted. There are *two kinds* of red streaks. One kind of streak is *completely harmless* and goes away within 20 minutes of finishing the IV. The other red streak *means that the vein is getting inflamed*, and we've got to change the needle insertion.

3. A few people get a **chest sensation, with a shortness of breath feeling** after the infusion has been running for a while. It was thought that this was oxygen bubbling off in the lungs . . . but that's not so. We don't know what causes this sensation, but we know that it's okay to continue the infusion. I prefer to slow the infusion down anyway, or discontinue it, if you've had most of the treatment.

4. Another side effect is **chills**. You can feel a little chilly because peroxide can throw off temperature regulation for a short while.

5. The next side effect is called a **Herxheimer Reaction**, also called **a die-off reaction [or Lucio's phenomena]**. Actually, it's a good sign, but you don't think so when it's happening. If you've got a lot of Candida (or yeast) or a lot of infection, when the peroxide kills the yeast, your body will react to the dead, disintegrating yeast until it is eliminated from the body. You can have **chills, nausea, body aches, weakness and headaches** during this time. It can happen following one, two,

or three treatments, and then it ceases. You can't predict in whom it will happen. If you get a Herxheimer reaction, why not look on the bright side? Your Candida is on the way out! You are about to feel better.

6. Finally, because **peroxide intensifies the anticoagulant action of the drug Coumadin**, the doctor has to reduce the Coumadin dose *if you're taking it.*

That's pretty much the downside of peroxide therapy.

Question: If there was nothing wrong with you, and you took peroxide therapy for no reason at all, would it be harmful? Absolutely not! It would act like a *tune-up* to your body.

Peroxide in Australia, England, and Foreign Countries

Here in the USA we use a concentration of peroxide which has been shown to be very safe. But higher concentrations (as much as *four times* higher) have been used both in the USA and in foreign countries. The results when using higher concentrations seem to be better, and I'm often tempted to use them. The problem is that higher concentrations *can irritate and cause sclerosing of veins.* **Sclerosing means that the inflamed walls of the veins develop a scar tissue within them, which makes them tender to the touch, and hard or ropy**. The condition could go away in a few weeks or may *never* go away.

Now a patient with cancer may say, "Look, I want the strongest dose that you think may help me. My life is on the line, and I don't give a damn about some tender, hard veins." On the other hand, a person with shingles or the flu may not care to risk permanent change in a vein, just to improve the likely outcome of their *temporary* dilemma. Here in Arizona, I'm sworn to go with the safer protocol *unless you sign a written waiver*, saying that you understand the risk and you desire to take the risk.

Signing Informed Consents

Regardless what concentration of peroxide is to be used, you are going to have to sign a permit before the doctor is going to perform IV peroxide on you. That's because the bulk of doctors in the USA consider peroxide *non-customary, experimental, unnecessary, weird, strange, or unusual* therapy.

So the doctor who gives peroxide needs to protect his reputation by getting full-disclosure releases called *informed consents.* I've always been honest with my patients, and told them that my permits basically say, *"I can do anything I like to you, but you can't do anything to me!"* At my office you'll be asked to sign no less than two consents!

Will Insurance or Medicare Pay?

No! Most medical insurance companies, including Medicare, have been financially depleted by paying for large numbers of expensive surgeries and procedures. Segments of the health care industry profit from these surgeries and procedures, *and* they are politically powerful. Physicians who review claims for insurance companies often favor the extremely expensive or risky procedures while refusing payment for a more beneficial, far less expensive, and often safer therapy. While insurance companies do not specifically exclude peroxide therapy in their policies, patients often have to resort to the courts in order to collect their insurance benefits. [We teach that insurance companies usually pay for treatments that don't work, but not for those that do! Ed.]

How to Begin Peroxide Therapy

Each state is different, but in general, if you're going to start peroxide therapy, you're going to have to follow some rules established for receiving an *experimental* therapy, because that's what peroxide is *usually* considered.

That means that you will likely need a *history and a physical exam* which goes somewhat beyond just your chief complaint. *Some lab work or other tests* might be needed also. You should obtain your past medical records which support your diagnosis, so that repeating tests becomes unnecessary and the diagnosis becomes clearer.

Now, if you've got the flu, for example, well then you've got the flu and there's no time or any reason to do a pile of tests. A short examination and history is all you'll need before sitting down for your treatment. But for any chronic illness, the doctor will want to talk to you for a while, and design a plan for treating the problem, using peroxide, and anything else which might be useful.

Now that you know the facts, I hope that you will schedule an appointment with your peroxide doctor real soon . . . .

GORDON N. JOSEPHS, DO ***Index A***

DIAGNOSES TREATED BY VARIOUS CLINICIANS USING I.V. PEROXIDE WITH VARYING DEGREES OF SUCCESS (c/o L.B.O.M.)[15]

1. Asthma
2. Emphysema
3. Chronic Obstructive Lung Disease (COPD)
4. Cardiovascular Disease
5. Cerbrovascular Disease
6. Alzheimer
7. Peripheral Vascular Disease
8. Arrhythmias (Irregular heart rhythms)
9. Influenza
10. Herpes Simplex (Cold Sores)
11. Herpes Zoster (Shingles)
12. Temporal Arteritis
13. Migraine headaches
14. Cluster headaches
15. Vascular headaches
16. Coronary artery spasm with angina
17. Chronic Epstein-Bar Virus infection, infectious mononucleosis
18. Diabetes Type H
19. HIV Infections
20. Hepatitis
21. Parasitic infections, various
22. Fungal infections, various
23. Bacterial infections, particularly chronic unresponsive infections
24. Candidiasis
25. Chronic pain syndromes, various
26. Pain of metastatic cancer
27. Environmental allergies
28. Early multiple sclerosis
29. Rheumatoid arthritis

Chelation Therapy

What is Chelation Therapy?

Please don't be insulted when we tell you a certain truth, that if great and well-known spiritual leaders such as K'ung-fu-tzu, Jesus Christ, Muhammad ibn 'Abdullah, Moshe Rabbenu, Shakyamuni Siddhartha Gautama, a great Brahma, or Joseph Smith were miraculously reincarnated in our times, and if any one of these defined a cure for cancer they'd be slapped in irons and incarcerated for a long time primarily for varying from the path of politically legislated "accepted treatments."

While the use of chelation therapy is not quite on a par with a potential, safe and effective cancer treatment, the evil hue and cry from allopathic physicians and their associates against its use is sometimes as loud.

Pronounced "Key-lay'-shun," Chelation Therapy is one of the most effective treatments for a wide spectrum of diseases or aging conditions. But it is more than a treatment; it is a preventive process and most certainly a treatment of the 21st century effectively practiced by many physicians. It is a therapy where physicians who practice it on patients habitually use it on themselves and their loved ones as either a curative or preventive treatment. That's a remarkable commendation, something not said about standard cancer treatments that poison, slash and burn. Critics of Chelation Therapy have never used it on themselves nor their loved ones nor on their patients, nor have they read the voluminous literature that has been compiled by various physicians and scientists who are members of the

American College of Advancement in Medicine[28] (ACAM), an organization dedicated to certification in the practice of Chelation Therapy and to further its research.

In Chelation Therapy, the imagery is often used of the lobster claw grabbing onto a cation — a positive metal ion — in the blood stream during the process of surrounding a positive (metal) ion. The chemical equivalent of the lobster claw is a protein, an amino acid called EDTA (Ethylene Diamine Tetracetic Acid). EDTA combines with cations in the blood stream, flushing them out with the flow of urine. Do not think that this is the only form of chelation that can take place within the body. The most common form of chelation is that which takes place during strenuous exercise producing lactic acid, a natural chelater.

According to James J. Julian, M.D.[29] "Chelation is a basic process of life itself. Without the chelation mechanism life as we know it would not exist on this planet.

"Chelation is the process that enables plants to take inorganic elements and change them into organic plant structure. Chlorophyll of green plants is a chelate of the mineral magnesium; blood hemoglobin (the oxygen carrier) is a chelate of iron. Chelation is the process by which the body utilizes aspirin, penicillin, vitamins, minerals and trace elements."

Chelation is a natural process found in nature. Soap is a chelator taking off grime and dirt. When you soften water through a house water-softener you use a chelating agent to take out minerals. EDTA, when used in your 100,000 miles of internal plumbing called capillaries, veins and arteries, acts in a similar manner by taking out metal ions that will otherwise damage us.

As Julian[29] further explains, "A modified copy of one of these natural amino acids called ethylene diamine tetracetic acid (EDTA) is used in Chelation Therapy. It is modified to make it more predictable and dependable in removing specific elements with [positive] electric charges such as calcium and heavy metals; namely lead, arsenic, mercury, cadmium and aluminum from the body."

In 1893, Swiss Nobel Laureate Alfred Werner proposed a theory of metal which provided the foundation for modern chelation therapy[30, 31]. In the early 1930's Germany and the United States both experimented with chemical processes for synthesizing EDTA[31]. Chelation therapy was first used by the British in WWII as an antidote to poison gas inhalation. According to John Parks Trowbridge, M.D. and Morton Walker, "The earliest reported research using EDTA for removal of plaque-producing calcium deposits was conducted in 1946 at the University of Zurich and in 1947 and 1948 at the University of Bern[32]." In 1948 the U.S. Navy used EDTA to treat lead poisoning. Dr. Norman E. Clarke, Director of Research at Providence Hospital in Detroit, observed that after a series of treatments with EDTA, patients'[28] overall health appeared to improve. Patients who had angina reported that their chest pain was gone. Others with gangrene of the legs reported healing. Memory, sight, hearing and sense of smell all improved. People treated with chelation reported increased vigor[32].

Clarke's observations stirred up interest in physicians who reported a wide-range of benefits to patients suffering from heart disease, brain disorders, and arteriosclerosis. It was clear that EDTA was effective not only in removing toxic metals but also in helping restore blood vessels blocked by plaque.

In 1952 W. Grant, M.D., in a research paper, "described the use of EDTA chelation therapy as a solution for removing calcium from the eyes of human patients with post-keratitis corneal opacities which had resulted in cataracts[32]."

During the 1960's there was demonstrated a wide-range of benefits to patients suffering from various diseases. These demonstrations included both human and animal studies. In particular, "That EDTA is able to remove calcium from the arterial wall was conclusively shown in a study by Fred Walker, Ph.D. and outlined in his doctoral thesis[32]."

But, a serious blow to EDTA study occurred in 1969 when a patient expired. This resulted in reduced motivation to establish the positive effects of EDTA in cardio-vascular and age-associated diseases[31].

During the 1970's thru 2000's there were numerous medical/legal battles surrounding chelation therapy. Some MD's were placed on probation by their State Medical Boards. (This battle continues in certain states to this day. Many states, such as Kentucky, have arbitrarily ruled against physicians using chelation therapy. In 2000 the State of Tennessee Board of Medical Examiners scheduled hearings with the same end in mind. The hue and cry from patients was so great that the Board wisely backed down. Their hearings resulted in the largest turnout of any board hearing in the history of the State of

Tennessee.) Others have won battles which allowed them to use EDTA which was approved by the FDA for metal toxicity. Other State Medical Boards either ignored the dispute or tacitly approved the use of Chelation Therapy.

Chelation Therapy is a treatment not generally accepted by the general medical establishment. In those few states where medical boards have closed down or prosecuted physicians who practice Chelation Therapy, the State Medical Boards for the most part consist of well-meaning physicians who are concerned with our welfare (and their own pocketbooks in some cases), but who know absolutely nothing about the therapy other than what they've read that was written by others who knew nothing about it. It is safe to say that every article written against Chelation Therapy and printed in "respectable" journals has been written by a physician or researcher who has assumed the mantle of Authority, yet has absolutely no knowledge of it. Up to the time of this paper a presumed exception is a study performed by Danish surgeons (with conflict of interest) and published in the 1991 *American Journal of Surgery* and in the *Journal of Internal Medicine* 231:261-267 1992. It's clear from an analysis performed by the American Institute of Medical Preventics[34] that this study was either done in total ignorance of the appropriate methodology of scientific studies or, most probably, was fraudulently designed to cast aspersions for financial gain against this otherwise wholly successful treatment. Contrary to widespread opinion, neither science nor the field of medical practice is free of fraud, dishonesty and incompetence.

In 1973 the American Academy of Medical Preventics (now the American College of Advancement in Medicine [ACAM]) developed a safe and effective protocol for this therapy. Since that time more than a million people [2002] have been helped according to documented case histories, "most of them victims of hardening of the arteries[32]."

EDTA therapy historically began with the use of Calcium EDTA as a treatment for lead poisoning, called plumbism, after the chemical name for lead, plumbum. Remember history that the Roman

Empire was gifted with great engineers, and those engineers created a gigantic system of water plumbing made of lead. Some historians have hypothesized that lead poisoning from water contacting tubes of lead and dissolving lead compounds was a contributing factor to the downfall of the Roman Empire because the lead compounds drunken daily created lead poisoning leading to mental and physical sicknesses.

But you don't have to go as far back as the Roman Empire to observe lead poisoning. It was only rather recently that the U.S. Government banned lead from automotive gasoline engines, and also from interior paints which have poisoned so many children who have unwittingly eaten peeling lead paint.

Various doctors have been called upon from time to time to use Calcium EDTA chelation to rid a patient of lead poisoning acquired by one means or another, such as inhaling the fumes from the burning of lead batteries or breathing fumes from melting lead. In this treatment process the physician inserts a needle into the bloodstream and "pushes" a one-shot substance into the veins in the recognition that a chelating chemical will grab onto poisonous lead in the body, surround it, and allow the body to flush the poison out with the patient's urine.

That's the extent of knowledge that most physicians have about Chelation Therapy. If you ask them if they know anything about Chelation Therapy, they'll say "Yes!" thinking that you mean this singlepush process developed in 1948 for ridding the body of excessive lead. Some fewer physicians will know of the use of flushing out bone-attractive radioactive materials such as plutonium.

EDTA Chelation Therapy described herein is gentler than the one-shot lead "push" and in many ways more beneficial. EDTA can surround, combine with and flush out many unwanted substances, such as calcium, lead, arsenic, aluminum and, indeed, any positive ion that is undesired and capable of being combined with this amino acid. Calcium EDTA is usually used for lead poisoning, whereas disodium EDTA is usually used in this described Chelation Therapy. Magnesium EDTA is being used with increasing frequency. At the termination of infusion of disodium EDTA, Calcium Gluconate is often placed in the infusion bottle, converting the remainder of the EDTA to Calcium EDTA, to help prevent calcium tetany — muscle spasms. However Calcium, disodium and Magnesium EDTA are all suitable for their various purposes.

Gordon E. Potter, M.D. reports that while EDTA is excellent for bivalent ions, Desferroxamine is superior for chelating out trivalent ions such as Iron (Fe^{+++}) and Aluminum (Al^{+++}). Since

Desferroxamine passes through the blood brain barrier; it may also be superior for Alzheimer's disease; i.e. in chelating out aluminum. He has no knowledge of the safety of using EDTA and Desferroxamine at the same time, however [58].

According to Warren M. Levin, M.D." EDTA binds mercury avidly *in vitro* (in the test tube), but is ineffective *in vivo* (in the human body)[35]."

There are many poisons that we breathe in, eat, drink or are exposed to by bodily contact and skin absorption. The subject of environmental pollution is entirely too big to describe here but everyone who reads newspapers, watches television, or hears radio will surely know that our bodies are currently bathed in undesirable pollutants of every kind. EDTA Chelation Therapy cannot rid us of everything foreign, of course, but it does an excellent job of chelating out many undesirable pollutants.

What Conditions Are Benefited?

Sometime after John Parks Trowbridge, Sr. retired from the U.S. Air Force, at age 70, it was discovered that he had an aortic aneurysm, a balloon-like swelling in the wall of the main artery. As this condition indicates a weakened structure that is likely to break and lead to quick death he consulted with several physicians, including his son, John Parks Trowbridge, Jr., M.D. who, along with other physicians, recommended immediate surgery, which was accomplished. It was not until several years passed that the younger Trowbridge came to understand the benefits of Chelation Therapy, learning first from Robert

Haskell, M.D., who told him, "Of all the regimens you can use to help your patients combat degenerative disease and restore their health, chelation therapy is the most powerful. It produces the greatest number of benefits to the body — far beyond those of improved blood flow. If you want to get your prescribed nutrition to those parts of the body in which they must work, John, chelation therapy is the way to do it[32]." The primary reason for recommending Chelation Therapy to you when you have degenerative disease or have aged has to do with its ability to restore your vital function

Virtually everyone has some degree of clogging up of the 100,000 miles of plumbing. Often the process of atherosclerosis begins in children's arteries and progresses through adulthood, so that even the finest physical specimens show evidence of this beginning on autopsy. It's virtually certain that you have some of this clogging, to some degree, and that it contributes to your state of health at least indirectly.

EDTA intravenous Chelation Therapy has proved to be safe and effective in the treatment of many varied disease conditions related to abnormal or diseased vascular conditions. Because this therapy involves the vascular system, and because blood flow affects every cell in the body, it's not surprising to find a wide ranging set of lack-of-health conditions improved or outright cured after its use. According to James J. Julian, M.D.[29], EDTA Chelation Therapy reduces "toxic metal deposits, abnormal calcium deposits, blood cholesterol, blood pressure, leg cramps, pigmentation, varicosities, and size of kidney stones. [It] improves circulation, skin texture and tone, vision, hearing and liver function. [It] relieves to various degrees: digitalis toxicity, lead toxicity, symptoms of senility, pain, symptoms of irregular rhythm, hypoglycemia, phlebitis, scleroderma, skin ulcers, and Wilson's Disease," a disease of the liver thought to be related to copper.

Doctors who use disodium EDTA Chelation Therapy would agree with James Julian. Morton Walker D.P.M. quotes Rudolph Alsleben, M.D. and Wilfrid E. Shute, M.D.[36] who have asserted that beneficial effects are that it: "prevents the deposit of cholesterol in the liver, reduces blood cholesterol levels, causes high blood pressure to drop in 60 percent of the cases, reverses the toxic effects of digitalis excess, converts to normal 50 percent of cardiac arrhythmias, reduces or relaxes excessive heart contractions, increases intracellular potassium, reduces heart irritability, increases the removal of lead, removes calcium from atherosclerotic plaques, dissolves kidney stones, reduces serum iron, protects against iron poisoning and iron storage disease, reduces heart valve calcification, improves heart function, detoxifies several snake and spider venoms, reduces the dark pigmentation of varicose veins, heals calcified necrotic ulcers, reduces the disabling effects of intermittent claudication, improves vision in diabetic retinopathy, decreases macular degeneration, and dissolves small cataracts."

William J. Mauer, D.O., according to Walker[36], also provided an additional listing gathered from his own and the experience of other physicians. These include: "Eliminates heavy metal toxicity, makes arterial walls more flexible, manages excess quantities of fat in the blood, prevents osteoarthritis, causes rheumatoid arthritis symptoms to disappear, has an anti-aging effect, smoothes skin wrinkles, offers psychological relief, assures the presence of adequate zinc in the blood, lowers insulin requirements for diabetics, and dissolves large and small thrombi."

Other physicians have listed other health improvements, including reversal of impotence, when impotence is caused by blockage or decreased flow of blood.

One of us (Dr. Maxwell) uses a product utilizing the 1998 Nobel Prize in medicine in which three American PhDs got the prize for discovering the extremely fast healing ability of the nitric oxide molecule in the body which, among other discoveries, will stop and reverse heart disease, including Congestive Heart Failure. It will "clean out" the arterial plaque. This is shown by before and after readings on the "Max Pulse" instrument. The ability of Arginine and Citruline as precursors for Nitric Oxide in the body is utilized in an amazing product called "ProArgi-9." (See http://www.drcurtmaxwell.com).

Heart Disease

According to Arabinda Das, M.D.[37], in speaking of heart disease "In the U.S. 600,000 sudden deaths occur each year [Reported by Das in 1992 so this figure is probably for an earlier year. Cardiovascular diseases are the world's largest killers, claiming 17.1 million lives a year, according to Who.[Reported at http://www.who.int/cardiovascular_diseases/en/: Ed.]. Das' figures represent one death from coronary heart disease every 32 seconds. Per capita expenditure for treatment of coronary artery disease was $160 per year for every individual in the U.S. Coronary artery disease is one of the foremost diseases of this country and the number one killer. This dangerous condition develops when the blood supply to the heart muscle is impaired, usually by a narrowing process leading to stenosis — an abnormal narrowing in a blood vessel or other tubular organ or structure. Stenosis may be due to plaque formation or atherosclerosis or spasming.

"In the U.S. the diagnosis is made with vast amounts of expense, money [that is provided] by the insurance companies [and the heart conditions] still carry serious complications after treatment. . . . Complications of acute heart attacks include the heart's failure to pump enough blood (congestive heart failure), acute pulmonary edema, bronchitis, cardiac asthma, collapse (shock due to arterial blood circuit with loss of blood pressure); ineffective heart rhythm, such as the multiple supraventricular extra systole, leading to ventricular tachycardia, frequent fatal ventricular fibrillation; travelling blood clots (emboli) to brain, dilations of heart muscle, and ventricular aneurysm. These are the ways patients die at home or are brought to hospitals for intensive care."

The American Heart Association[38], in its 1992 *Heart and Stroke Facts Report*, says 980,000 Americans died of cardiovascular disease in 1988, the latest year for which figures were available. Women accounted for . . . 51%. ". . . more Americans died of cardiovascular disease in 1988 than succumbed to cancer, accidents, pneumonia, influenza, suicide and, AIDS combined."

The Center for Disease Control reports that In 2006, 631,636 people died of heart disease. Heart disease caused

26% of deaths—more than one in every four—in the United States. Heart disease is the leading cause of death for both men and women. Half of the deaths due to heart disease in 2006 were women. Coronary heart disease is the most common type of heart disease. In 2005, 445,687 people died from coronary heart disease. Every year about 785,000 Americans have a first heart attack. Another 470,000 who have already had one or more heart attacks have another attack. In 2010, heart disease will cost the United States $316.4 billion. This total includes the cost of health care services, medications, and lost productivity. (http://www.cdc.gov/heartdisease/facts.htm)

Chelation vs. By-Pass Surgery and Angioplasty

According to the American Heart Association[38], "The disease cost to the nation is staggering . . . an estimated $108.9 billion in health services and lost productivity this year [1993] alone."

According to Zigurts Strauts, M.D.[39] ". . . there are close to 300,000 bypass procedures done in the

United States annually and 5,000-7,000 angioplasties. There is, an at the most conservative estimate,

a 1.4% mortality rate in the top centers of the United States for bypass surgery and a mortality rate approaching 2% for angioplasty. In California, . . . , the mortality rate on count in 1987 was 4.7%. One out of 20 people therefore do not walk out of the operating room. We are talking about 15-20 *thousand* deaths annually due to these two procedures. The morbidity statistics are no better. In fact, it is said that up to 20% of patients going through bypass surgery have at least minimal brain dysfunction and numerous other cases involving other complications have been reported in the literature. Kidney failure is one of them . . . research has been done measuring ejection fractions [of the heart] using Chelation therapy in patients and the results have shown a significant improvement. . . . This cannot be said for bypass surgery where the improvement is only minimal at best and then only in a few patients. In fact, the patients with poor ejection fractions are not accepted as bypass candidates. One could say therefore that for those patients Chelation Therapy may be the only hope that they have."

Zigurts Strauts[28] 1987 report does not seem to be affected by the passage of time. Most recent studies have concentrated on segregating out classes of patients that have averaged out to his reported 4.7% California mortality rate.

Severity of initial disease, age of patients, type of heart condition, surgeon skill, hospital surgery load and so on have all provided grist for the statistical evaluation mill.

E.L. Hannan[40], et. al. reported that "for all patients receiving coronary artery bypass surgery in New York State in 1989, . . . demonstrate that both annual surgeon volume and annual hospital volume are significantly (inversely) related to mortality rate. Coronary bypass operations performed in hospitals with annual bypass volumes of 700 or more by surgeons with annual bypass volumes of 180 or more had a risk-adjusted mortality rate of 2.67% in comparison to a risk-adjusted mortality rate of 4.29%." In other words, the more experienced the surgeon, the less the mortality rate, an obvious conclusion. So, if the mortality rate overall is still close to 4.7%, there must be something more drastic wrong with the procedure — or the vast majority of operations are being performed by inexperienced surgeons in lowvolume hospitals.

O'Connor[41] et. al. reported in 1989 that "the overall crude in-hospital mortality rate for isolated

Cardiac Artery By-pass Grafting was 4.3%." The rate varied among centers . . . but they concluded "that the observed differences in in-hospital mortality rates among institutions and among surgeons in northern New England are not solely the result of differences in case mix . . ." J. Zelen[42], et. al. reported on a variation of mortality rate from 4% for simple, 14.7% for complex, and, 3% for all Cardiac Artery By-Pass Grafting operations at a University medical center in Greater New York.From a survey of current research literature it is clear that selection of patients to improve survival outcome can be made on the basis of age, physician, hospital and type of disease, but it is equally clear that overall survival rates show very little, if any, statistical difference from those reported in 1987.

By-Pass Surgery and Angioplasty

By-pass surgery involves the replacing of a defective artery, usually near the heart, with a less defective vein from somewhere else in the body, usually the leg. The vein is thinner than the artery and not exactly the artery's equivalent as a replacement. It can be weaker. There are about 100,000 miles of tubing — capillaries, veins and arteries — in the circulatory system. Although the region near the heart, with increased turbulence of blood flow is most likely to be blocked by plaques, blockage will also be found throughout the arteries. It is unlikely that replacing one foot of 100,000 miles of blocked circulation will have more than a temporary palliative affect, except for a limited and well-defined condition.

By-pass surgery is exceedingly expensive, supporting costly hospital rooms and staffs, expensive surgical equipment, and high professional fees.

But the main reason for avoiding by-pass surgery is that it has been found to be relatively ineffective (with the exception of certain infrequent conditions). As Morton Walker D.P.M. reports, "Henry D. McIntosh, M.D., of the Methodist Hospital in Houston, Texas, said at a symposium of the American Heart Association in Miami Beach that bypass surgery should be reserved for patients with *crippling* angina who did not respond to more conservative treatment.[36]" Dr. McIntosh's statement has since been supported by many studies, including some reported by the Institute of Health, and by some of the very same physicians who pioneered in heart by-pass.

What sense, then, to have bypass surgery? And especially what sense when all of the medical literature has already demonstrated its failure except in a very limited diagnosis of crippling angina?

The diseases that chelation can improve as a matter of routine include many of the intransigents. Instead of cutting off a gangrenous leg, the leg is healed, according to Norman E. Clarke and Warren M. Levin. Instead of expensive heart bypass surgery, the patient is healed. Instead of Carotid Artery bypass, the brain is again nourished. Senility and Alzheimer's Disease can be reversed provided brain cells have not been starved of oxygen to the point where they have died. Other diseases that stem from failing organs due to lack of nourishment, including the skin, may be halted or reversed.

Retrospective Study of Chelation Therapy

Philip Hoekstra, Sr. and John M. Baron, D.O.[43], founders of Cypher, Inc. of Ohio, along with other physicians and Ph.D.s, funded one of the first objective studies, an unpublished clinical analysis on the use of Chelation Therapy from clinical data gathered over fifteen years and involving 20,000 patients. Statistical evaluations were performed by an independent organization free from all bias. Their retrospective study unequivocally proved that Chelation Therapy solves the problem in 80% of the cases of clogging in peripheral circulation and also in the Carotid Artery preventing blood from reaching the brain, intermittent claudication, and reverses Osteoporosis (a 1% sampling), placing calcium back into bones and teeth where calcium belongs. In the Chelation Study, the 20,000 patients came from many different clinical settings, and they represent patients with a wide diversity of disease conditions.

The cost of the study was funded privately, and **not** paid by any pharmaceutical company. The main ingredient, a chemical titled in brief as EDTA (Ethylene Diamine Tetracetic Acid), is not protected by patent. No pharmaceutical company can pay large returns to stockholders from its sale. No heart surgeon can assess tens of thousands of dollars applying it to heart problems. No hospital can submit bills of tens of thousands of dollars more for use of its operating rooms and services when EDTA is given.

Elmer Cranton, M.D. states that "Magnesium is a calcium antagonist, relatively deficient in many chelation patients, and is the metallic ion least likely to be removed by EDTA. In fact, EDTA is best administered as magnesium-EDTA, providing an efficient delivery system that increases magnesium stores.[47]"

Heart Study

H. Richard Casdorph, M.D., PhD.[48] reported on "18 patients with documented arteriosclerotic heart disease" using a technetium isotope to measure the left heart ventricular ejection fraction "before and after the administration of EDTA chelation therapy . . . A statistically significant improvement in left ventricular ejection fraction occurred in this group of patients."

Retrospective Study of 2,870 Patients With Atherosclerosis and Other Degenerative States

Efrain Olszewer, M.D. and James P. Carter, M.D., Dr. P.H.[33] presented a 28-month retrospective analysis of 2,870 patients with documented atherosclerosis and other degenerative, age-associated diseases who were treated with intravenous disodium magnesium EDTA chelation therapy. Marked improvement occurred in 76.9% and good improvement occurred in 17% of treated patients with ischemic heart disease. Marked improvement occurred in 91% and good improvement occurred in 8% of treated patients with peripheral vascular disease and intermittent claudication. In patients with cerebrovascular and other degenerative cerebral diseases, 24% had marked improvement, and 30% had good improvement. Of four patients with scleroderma, three had marked improvement and one had good improvement. Seventy-five percent of all patients had marked improvement in symptoms of vascular origin. Independent of pathology, 89% of all treated patients had marked or good improvement."

The First Published
Double-Blind/Single-Blind Crossover Study

Efrain Olszewer, M.D., Fuad Calil Sabbag, M.D. and James Carter, M.D., Dr.PH conducted the first study to be published involving first a double-blind and then a single-blind study, using those who were on the placebo in the single-blind after the code was broken for the double-blind. "Ten male patients with peripheral vascular disease, . . . , were randomly assigned to receive either Na2 ethylene diamine tetra acetic acid (EDTA) plus $MgSO_4$, B complex, and vitamin C, or a placebo of $MgSO_4$, B complex, and vitamin C. . . . A total of 20 Intravenous Infusions were planned for administration to each patient. Clinical and laboratory . . . tests showed dramatic improvements after 10 infusions in some patients, and thus was broken the code indicating who was receiving EDTA and who was receiving placebo. The group that improved had been receiving EDTA; there was no change in the placebo group. The trial was then completed in a single-blind fashion. Patients originally assigned to receive placebo then received 10 EDTA Infusions, while the group originally assigned to EDTA received 20 EDTA Infusions. The group that had formerly received placebo showed improvements comparable to those seen in the first EDTA group after 10 treatments[48]."

Brain Disorders

Casdorph[42] also reports on "fifteen patients with well-documented impairment of cerebral blood flow," also using technetium isotope. He says, "A highly significant improvement ($p = .0005$) in cerebral blood flow occurred following approximately twenty intravenous infusions of disodium EDTA. All fifteen patients improved clinically, including one with little or no improvement in cerebral blood flow."

Cerebral Vascular Arterial Occlusion

E.W. McDonagh, D.O., FACGP, C.J. Rudolph, D.O., Ph.D. and E. Cheraskin, M.D., D.M.D.[49] in a study of fifty-seven patients evaluated for cerebral vascular arterial occlusion "Measurements of arterial occlusion were made with the relatively simple, noninvasive oculocerebrovasculometric analysis. Cerebrovascular arterial occlusion diminished by an average of 18% (from a mean of 28% to a mean of 10%) following therapy ($P<0.001$). Eighty-eight percent of patients treated with EDTA chelation therapy showed objective improvements in cerebrovascular blood flow."

Peripheral Vascular Stenosis

McDonagh, Rudolph and Cheraskin[49] also studied "117 lower extremities in 77 elderly patients with documented occlusive peripheral vascular stenosis, diagnosed by the Doppler systolic ankle/brachial blood pressure ratio. . . ." revealing "that intravenous ethylene diamine tetraacetic acid (EDTA) chelation therapy with supportive multivitamin/trace mineral supplementation improved arterial blood flow significantly after approximately 60 days and 26 infusions ($P<0.001$)."

Peripheral Arterial Occlusion, an Alternative to Amputation

H. Richard Casdorph, M.D., Ph.D. and Charles H. Farr, M.D., Ph.D.[49] presented four patients, "each of whom represents end-stage occlusive peripheral arterial disease with gangrene of the involved extremity. These patients had exhausted all traditional forms of therapy and they had all been referred for surgical amputation. Instead of surgery, intravenous EDTA chelation therapy was instituted with complete success in each case. These gangrenous extremities all healed and were saved from amputation. Long-term follow-up, extending for more than a year, indicates that all four patients are continuing to do well, with their previously gangrenous extremities intact and pain free. Adjunctive therapies included vitamin and mineral supplementation and, in two cases, hyperbaric oxygen therapy (HBO)."

A Case of Chelation Therapy

Warren Levin, M.D[51]. says: "I guess my favorite chelation story is about the psychoanalyst who was on the staff of a major medical center — one of the institutions that I call a mosque in this Mecca of American Medicine that is New York City. I first saw him as an emergency. He was in his fifties and looked remarkably healthy, except that he was in a wheelchair. I asked him what the emergency was and he said that he had been told he needed an amputation. It turns out he had awakened the same morning that I saw him to discover that his lower leg was cold, numb, mottled, blue, with two black-looking toes. He had immediately hied [hastened] himself over to his hospital and had a consultation with the chief of vascular surgery. The recommendation was for an immediate trip to the operating room to amputate above the knee in the hope of saving the rest of his leg. I don't know where he had heard about chelation therapy, but he asked this world-renowned surgeon about the possibility of using chelation in this situation. He was told, 'Don't bother me with that voodoo,' — that if he was going to have a good result, it required surgery. Well, he decided to get a second opinion, so he just crutched down the hall a couple of doors to one of the associate professors. He, too, suggested immediate amputation, but when asked about chelation therapy, the response was, 'Well, this is not yet infected. It looks like dry gangrene, so you have a little time. You can try it if you want, but it's a waste of time.' With that as his only hope, [the psychoanalyst] showed up in my office.

"We started emergency chelation the next day, and after about nine chelations [one taken] every other day, he was pain-free and pinking up, and after about seventeen chelations, he was walking on the leg again!

"So, he never had an amputation, and he lived the rest of his life with not only two legs but all ten toes. It's incredible that I never got a phone call from either of these two surgeons who are just blocks away from my office to say, 'Hey, what the hell did you do Levin?' and I am certain that the next patient with a similar problem that showed up in their offices was told that the only thing to do is to amputate. What a tragedy."

Preventive Reduction in Cancer Mortality

Walter Blumer, M.D. and Elmer M. Cranton, M.D.[52] report that mortality from cancer was reduced 90% during an 18-year follow-up of 59 patients treated with calcium-EDTA. Only one of 59 treated patients (1.7%) died of cancer while 30 of 172 nontreated control subjects (17.6%) died of cancer ($P = 0.002$). Death from atherosclerosis was also reduced. Treated patients had no evidence of cancer at the time of entry into this study. Observations relate only to long term prevention of death from malignant disease, if chelation therapy is begun before clinical evidence of cancer occurs."

Claudication and Joint Deformation

Before trying Chelation Therapy, one 58 year old male[53] patient prepared a detailed list of symptoms, or at least perceived symptoms, of what he felt was wrong and would like to have corrected. Since the patient didn't know what the treatment would do, he simply wrote down everything he didn't like about himself or felt was physically or emotionally wrong. He also planned to have a number of periodic laboratory tests during the course of his chelation treatments. He wanted to be able to evaluate for himself what was true or not true about this new form of treatment.

There were many items listed that did not change under Chelation Therapy. But those symptoms that did change were quite striking and are among clinical signs and symptoms that no amount of traditional drug treatment would have solved. He had to lie down at three o' clock every afternoon to rest for three to six hours. He often felt like the world could come to an end, and he'd not care. Also whenever he lay down his legs cramped terribly. This kind of pain and muscle cramping is known as "claudication," and can be a product of calcium/magnesium insufficiency and/or oxygen lack, both of which can stem from lack of proper cellular nourishment.

Pain and inflammation in one joint on one little finger would not respond to various treatments and medicines encouraged by his family doctor. Probably the reason — deduced after the fact — is that iron from vascular blood leakage acted as a catalyst that cycled through a chemical reaction resulting in the decomposition of the cartilage. And, as the cartilage decomposed into various forms of free radicals, those, in turn, created additional secondary and tertiary effects, thence leaving the iron radical free to begin the cycle again. It could not have been halted without chelating out the free iron catalyst.

After three treatments by Chelation Therapy, the little finger joint inflammation disappeared entirely for the first time in two years. Muscle claudication disappeared at about 22 treatments given over eight weeks. It didn't disappear suddenly, but gradually, over several treatments, the cramping and pain lessening each time. Extreme tiredness disappeared after 30 to 40 treatments, ten to fourteen weeks. In all this patient had 81 chelations over the next 6 years.

No other known traditional treatment, no amount of taking of known drugs to control symptoms could have brought about the improvements noted.

When the patient was 67 years of age (1992) he danced with ladies a generation younger than he was every evening, 365 days per year. His dancing was not nice, sedate, "safe" ballroom dancing, but rather the modern version of the wildly active jitterbug of the forties, only now called "Bop" (East Coast and West Coast Swing). It was fascinating to watch younger ladies cave in under this strenuous exercise, while the old-timer — who was hardly fit at one time — could dance all night.

At age 73 this old-timer married a young lady of 25, and then danced but once a week! Marriage does settle one down!! After eleven years the young lady asked for a divorce and so now, at 85, he married a 31 year old Filipina. Unfortunately, due to an automobile accident his dancing days terminated, but not his new marriage!

Glaucoma

Glaucoma is traditionally treated by means of medicines that control the inflow or defects in drainage of intra-ocular fluid. In the traditional approach only symptoms are being treated, not the causation of imbalance in intra-ocular fluids. Since "simple glaucoma is the effect in the eye of a disturbance of the water-salt economy of the body, there must be a drop in the chemistry of the blood, such as a drop in sodium salts, a rise in potassium salts, and a rise in blood cholesterol.[54]"

According to John Baron, D.O. of Ohio most Glaucoma is not a problem simply of the eye, but rather a problem that is systemic; i.e., pervades the whole body — the eye being simply one physical manifestation of the total problem.

A thermograph of the neck and head will tell whether or not the patient is getting sufficient blood to her/his facial features. If s/he is not, the patient is a candidate for Chelation Therapy, as s/he most probably suffers from progressive atherosclerosis. The glaucoma can be a result of vascular disorder arteriosclerosis of the optic artery[28], which means insufficient blood to the eyeball, etc. Only Chelation Therapy has a chance of solving that problem if it has not gone too far. Again you need a doctor who specializes in this kind of treatment and uses the correct protocol.

In addition to Chelation Therapy, one needs to look after one's general health, which means decreasing stress and improving dietary and nutritional intake. If it is not a problem of blood flow, then you have a different situation, and the use of adrenal cortex hormone will be useful in any case until you have the intra-ocular pressure under systemic control.

Toenail Fungus Infection

John Parks Trowbridge, Sr., M.D. suffered from fungus infection of the toenails after trips to the Orient while serving the United States Air Force. Twenty five years of medical attention could not rid him of this scourge. Administration of Chelation Therapy alone did so, and he said, "After my chelation therapy, the big toes have grown healthy nails that came in behind and shoved the diseased nails off[32]."

Generalized Benefits

According to Morton Walker[55], D.P.M., John Sorenson is ecstatic with the changes in himself. Sorenson says, ". . . major benefits [include]: improved hair growth, freedom from headaches, a good memory, ability to think clearly, no aches and pains except from physical injuries, clear vision, the ability to walk up to eight miles a day, weight loss to a normal 175 pounds, reversal of impotency, a healthy, tough, and flexible skin, a better skin color, bright red blood color versus muddy looking blood, no skin eruptions, wounds that heal twice as quickly as before, and no hyperacidity. I have won back 25 years of my life. At age 68, I am doing more and better work than I did at age 40 . . .

"Since taking chelation therapy my life has been a constant process of improving health, happiness, and productivity."

Eliminating Pollutants and Damaging Metallic Ions

Anything you can do to better nourish (and oxygenate) individual cells, you should do, to relieve the burdens that you already carry. Anything you can do to avoid pollutants in water, food, and air you should do. One example, of a recently hidden negative, is the use of chlorine in drinking water as a disinfectant. The "Environmental Protection Agency study showed that drinking highly chlorinated water 'subtly but noticeably shifted[28] a mouse's transport of cholesterol from high-density lipoproteins (the 'good' lipoproteins) in the blood to the 'bad' low-density lipoproteins, which foster atherosclerosis." J. Peter Bercz, who headed the study, reported that hypochlorite, a very reactive by-product of standard water chlorination, "can also destroy polyunsaturated fatty acids . . . , including those essential to

Health[56]." Multiply this single effect of a standard, assumed-to-be-safe disinfectant of water, by the thousands of impurities found in air and food. Pure food, water and air are extremely important! But more — EDTA will also help you to eliminate many of these pollutants that are acquired over a lifetime, the same that contribute in so many ways to your overall condition. In addition, by stimulating a gland called the parathyroid, your body will reverse the flow of calcium to harden bones and teeth, thereby reversing Osteoporosis.

Investigative Medical Journalist

Morton Walker D.P.M. says, "Usually, the conclusion that an objective observer draws, especially someone trained in science and medicine like myself, is that . . . More often than not anecdotal medicine is nothing more than 'buffalo dew'. . . . In the past I have believed that to be true. But what must an investigative medical journalist do when . . . exposed to story after story and to one case history after another that reports potentially imminent death, blindness, amputation, paralysis and other problems among people, and upon visiting those people to check their stories, he sees them presently free of all signs of their former health problems. This has happened to me! About 200 individuals who were victims of hardening of the arteries are much changed . . . . they are vibrant, productive, youthful looking, vigorous, full of zest for life, and they enthusiastically endorse chelation therapy as the cause of their prolonged good health. "I have . . . turned up not a single untruth[55]."

How Does Chelation Therapy Work?

There are three explanations for the way EDTA Chelation Therapy works at this writing. Possibly all theories or explanations are correct, at least in part. One theory is the free radical theory; another is the calcium binding theory, the removal of calcium that binds together the ingredients of plaques in our arteries. A third and latest theory, described by Gary Gordon, M.D., D.O., M.D. (H). is the Nitric Oxide production theory.

While EDTA Chelation Therapy will "flush out" many undesirable substances, it has been said that its chief effect is to contact, combine with and to flush out calcium that is found in and acts like glue in plaques in the arteries. This theory is probably not correct, but it has been strongly advocated.

The molecules and atoms that "seek" out or have a very strong affinity for other compounds and atoms are called "free radicals." Free radicals are always formed within the body as a natural consequence of a balance between catabolism and anabolism, the building up and breaking down of cellular tissue, respectively. Free radicals also have a vital place in killing foreign microorganisms. Whenever the balance is seriously upset, and especially for extended periods, when more free radicals are formed than can be balanced off by natural bodily processes, disease and often accompanying inflammation occurs. Chelation Therapy has a definite place in the ridding of free-radicals that cause inflammation. It performs other duties that permit functioning for health, such as ridding the body of toxic pollutants which interfere with enzymal functions. Chelation Therapy operates at a level that is basic for the health of individual cells — optimally functioning cells promote optimally functioning organs, and these, in turn, optimally functioning systems — and consequent health. Because virtually all diseases have some component of production of an excess of free-radicals, Chelation Therapy can be and often is indicated as curative or supportive for many disease states, especially chronic diseases. Oxygen atoms and other chemicals within the body are attracted to other compounds and atoms forming free radicals during combinatorial stages. Free radicals damage tissues and promote cartilage decomposition and many other cascading problems for organs, systems and tissues generally. In addition, cells cannot eliminate their waste products. Cellular breakdown occurs leading to deterioration and disease. Over time, the entire arterial system is slowly disturbed, as are organs and tissues, all of them composed of individual cells with lowered reserves and capacities.

Free Radical Theory

According to the free radical theory, perhaps 80-90% of all disease process is an excess of free radical activity[31, 39, 55,

60, 61]. Excessive free radicals create havoc by damaging cells and their DNA, changing biochemicals, damaging cell membranes and sometimes killing cells outright. Every oxygen factor also has an anti-oxidant factor in our physiological systems. We, in other words, are normally capable of neutralizing the harmful effects of atoms and molecules that have a high affinity for other elements and chemicals that would otherwise damage tissue and cells in attaching to cellular components.

Whenever one side or the other of this oxidation/anti-oxidation free-radical system becomes unbalanced damage accrues. This damage leads to diseases of the circulatory system, malignancies, inflammatory conditions and immunologic disorders[63]. According to Elmer Cranton, M.D., "The free radical concept explains contradictory epidemiologic and clinical observations and provides a scientific rationale for treatment and prevention of many of the major causes of long-term disability and death: atherosclerosis, dementia, cancer, arthritis, and other age-related diseases[47]."

EDTA chelation therapy removes metals that act as catalysts for the production of excessive free radical reactions, thus halting the disease process and/ or repairing the damage. Cranton says that "EDTA can reduce the production of free radicals by a million-fold[47]."

Karl Loren says: "My opinion, and that of others, is that chelation therapy offers the brightest promise of health help on the medical horizon today!" (see http://www.karlloren.com)

"Probably the foremost authority and expert on chelation therapy today is Dr. Elmer Cranton, author of *Bypassing Bypass*, and other Books. Cranton writes: 'The field of free radical biochemistry is as revolutionary and profound in its implications for medicine as the germ theory was for the science of microbiology. It has created a new paradigm for viewing the disease process. Emerging knowledge in this field gives us a compelling scientific rationale for treatment and prevention of major causes of long-term disability and death with EDTA chelation therapy.(98-107).[28]'

"It is increasingly being accepted that free radicals are the SOLE cause of heart disease and cancer. These two diseases are responsible for over 70% of all death in Western Society. Most doctors do not yet acknowledge this truth.

"There is no direct equivalent between intravenous chelation and oral chelation. I consider Dr. Cranton the foremost expert on intravenous chelation therapy. Yet he claims that oral chelation is quackery! I disagree with him. So, I mostly quote his explanations of IV chelation, and try to compare it with oral chelation — here.

"You can get an approximate relationship between the two. "First let's look at the word *chelate*. "The word means to *bind* or to *grab*. Chelation is the process of some substance (such as EDTA, Cysteine or N Acetyl Cysteine) grabbing a heavy metal. "Metals are grabbed in a sequential sequence, per Dr. Cranton: "The affinity of EDTA to bind various metals at physiologic pH, in order of decreasing stability, is listed below. In the presence of a more tightly bound metal, EDTA releases metals lower in the series and binds to the metal for which it has a greater affinity. Calcium is near the bottom of the list. Chromium2+ Iron 3+ Mercury 2+ Copper 2+ Lead 2+ Zinc 2+ Cadmium 2+ Cobalt 2+ Aluminum 3+ Iron 2+ Manganese 2+ Calcium 2+ Magnesium 2+.

"Thus the chelating substance start off bound to calcium, so it cannot pick up any new calcium. This, incidentally, is the proving evidence that chelation does NOT remove calcium blockage from the arteries — as many IV chelation doctors still claim!.

"But it is the nature of a chelating substance to 'let go' of the lighter mineral in order to grab the heavier metal, or more accurately, the metals in the sequence shown in the above list provided by Dr. Cranton.

"Thus the chelating substance starts off bound to calcium, but it would let go of the calcium if it 'bumps into' iron, or even aluminum. It would then let go of the aluminum if it bumps into lead. Then, bound to lead if it bumps into iron, it would NOT let go of the lead to bind to the iron.

"When you are dealing with the artificial amino acid, EDTA, about half of it stays in the blood stream for an hour or so — so it is binding to, and letting go of, heavy metals during that hour, then it is ejected from the body through the kidneys and urine. The body considers it a 'foreign substance' from the very start and wants to get rid of it. That is why it stays active in the body for such a short time.

"Cysteine and N Acetyl Cysteine (NAC), however, are natural amino acids. They can stay active in the blood stream for many hours (until they are used for chelating, used for protein structure building, or converted to sugar). When EDTA is taken orally it works to bind to metals in the stomach and intestine. It can also attract metals from inside the body, through the intestinal wall, to be bound to the EDTA in the intestine. This EDTA would remain active as long as it is in the stomach and intestine. Since the contents of the stomach would usually stay inside the body for about 24 hours or so, EDTA is active longer when taken orally than when taken intravenously.

"Thus, oral chelation 'works' in the body for more hours than does IV chelation using EDTA only. "Those particles of Cysteine and NAC that bind to metals? They would then be considered a 'foreign

Particle[28] by the body and processed through the kidney for elimination in the urine. The same would be true of the small amount of EDTA that is absorbed into the body when taken orally. "Intravenous chelation generally relies only on the artificial Amino Acid, EDTA, and generally about 2,000 mg of the EDTA is put into a water solution and dripped into one of your veins over a two or three hour period. Sometimes 3,000 mg of EDTA is used. Generally 100% of this EDTA would be in the blood stream, since it is put directly there.

"Oral chelation depends on nutrients being useful when taken through the mouth. Generally the 'chelating substances' are EDTA, Cysteine and N Acetyl Cysteine. Cysteine and NAC are easily absorbed through the mouth into the body and blood stream, Since EDTA is an 'artificial amino acid' it is not readily absorbed into the body when taken through the mouth. The Cysteine and NAC would do their chelating in the normal fashion of any chelating substance, when taken through the mouth. Since only about 5% of EDTA taken orally gets into the blood, the 95% moves through the stomach and intestines — where the 'chelating action' is different than when the chelating substances is in the blood stream.

"The one or two hours are called the 'half life' of the EDTA. In about 2 hours, half of the EDTA has been processed out of the blood stream, through the kidneys, and into the bladder, in the urine, awaiting elimination. The other half of the EDTA would be working longer, but you can see that if half of the EDTA is 'used up' every two hours, there would be very, very little left after say 8 hours.

"Now, if you just put EDTA in water, there would normally not be any metals in the water and it might hang on to calcium or it might let go of calcium — depending on what WAS in the water.

"But, in your body we don't want the EDTA to grab calcium, so the calcium and EDTA are deliberately included in the same dose — and in most cases the EDTA will let go of the calcium it came in with, and grab something heavier.

"So you now have this interesting action — oral EDTA is removing metals from the food you have just eaten, but it is also removing metals from inside the body — attracting them from inside the body to move through the wall of the intestine, into the feces in the intestine, to bind with the EDTA that is still there.

"The other ingredients in the formula, mostly cysteine and NAC, bind to metals from inside the body — and do it in the same sequential fashion.

"The only minerals that could be removed during chelation would be those that are heavier than calcium — most of them are harmful. Zinc is heavier, and not harmful, but my formula provides lots of zinc anyway.

"The EDTA which is moving through the stomach? Well, it is NOT going to be eliminated through the kidneys, but through the feces. Thus, THIS EDTA will actually have a longer time of effectiveness. The EDTA will remain effective in the intestine as long as it is still in the intestine — that would usually be about 24 hours. During that time it is constantly grabbing metals, letting go of the lighter ones and switching to the heavier metals.

'"In this sense EDTA taken orally is much more effective than EDTA taken intravenously.

"When you chelate with Cysteine, or NAC, or intravenous EDTA, you would look in the urine to test for how much metal is being dumped from the body. A urine test before using the chelating materials, and another urine test (for metals) within a couple days after starting the chelating — would tell you how much of an increase in metal there is. It would not be unusual for the increase in metal in the urine to be as much as FIFTY TIMES!

"Now, the EDTA going through the stomach and intestine? It is not being eliminated in the urine, but in the feces, so if you really wanted to do the proper test you would check a 'stool sample' before and after starting the oral EDTA.

"You can see now that it is a complex question to try to compare intravenous with oral chelation. "If a person is taking the recommended dose of Super Life Glow [Karl Loren's product], he is getting 1,800 mg of daily chelating materials, of which 500 mg is EDTA.

"If a person is taking an IV treatment, he would be getting between 2,000 and 3,000 mg of EDTA. The EDTA would NOT be active for very long when taken intravenously, and would be active longer when taken orally.

"There is another issue. Intravenous EDTA would be all working within the blood stream, and generally its ONLY action would be to remove metals.

"Cystine and NAC, however, would not be active ONLY as binding materials. These are natural amino acids and the body may well have other uses for them besides chelating metals. It would not be very possible to know how much Cysteine, for instance, would be used to remove metals and how much would be used for other purposes in the body.

"Is this a complex question? Or not?

"Finally, perhaps the best way of comparing is to simply look at results of use, rather than the mechanics of action.

"EDTA taken intravenously seems faster than oral chelation. People will often get dramatic changes in their body after only three or four IV treatments. These dramatic changes usually take 30 days with oral chelation.

"My personal belief on this is that if you have an urgent need for fast action, IV chelation would be the best way to go.

"But, after about 30 days, or perhaps 60, I think the daily oral chelation would be at least as effective, and probably more effective, than a series of 30 treatments of IV EDTA.

"I have a complete analysis of one of the most recent approaches to chelation — using EDTA in a suppository. It would be more effective through the mouth, since it would stay active longer, but the suppositories are being hyped as prescription only, provided only by doctors, and costing as much as $50 for one suppository containing 750 mg of EDTA.

"There are also many examples of different combinations of the three different oral chelation formulas. . . .

"One more thing.

"Mercury is a common toxic metal in the body. It is generally accepted that EDTA, taken intravenously, does NOT remove mercury. However, Cysteine and N Acetyl Cysteine do remove mercury. So, intravenous EDTA is not useful in removing one of the most dangerous of all toxic metals we have in our bodies, while oral chelation does remove mercury.

"There are some interesting studies, not well known or validated, that show that oral EDTA may, in fact remove mercury, into the feces. This would make the oral chelation approach even more valuable than the intravenous approach." (See Karl Loren: at http://www.chelationtherapyonline.com/)

Calcium Binding Theory

A proper diet can also act as a chelator. "The proper program of low-fat, high-complex-carbohydrate diet and aerobic exercise actually is partially a natural process of chelation therapy.[39]" Specific foods and combinations of foods can, then, act as partial chelators. The extent and distribution of these foods would be too lengthy for this book. However, as an example, specific studies have been completed on the chelating effects of garlic which show that garlic has a chelating effect on those suffering excessive lipid deposits. Benjamin Lau, M.D., Ph.D., who has accomplished a great deal of research on garlic, shows that the ratio of Low Density Lipids to Very Low Density Lipids decreased in a study over a period of six months using a particular form of aged garlic, 1 gram per day. At the same time, with the same ingredients and same dosage, Cholesterol also decreased. In both instances during an initial 60 day period, the measurable levels of lipids increased, which was interpreted as an initial sloughing off of the excessive lipid deposits, after which a continuous decrease was discovered[46].

Gradually, free radicals affect tissues so that localized accumulations of lipid-containing (oil/fat) material (atheromas) within or beneath the intima (lining of vessels) surfaces of blood vessels clog up the 100,000 miles of capillaries, veins and arteries. Exposure to pollutants over a lifetime from food, air, water and drugs collect in various tissues throughout the body, in various ways. When EDTA chelates out many of these pollutants we find that we can now handle life better than before and we are healthier.

When EDTA binds with calcium, the consequence is the break-up of the plaque hindering the flow of blood in the arterial system. Probably, for many people, plaque formation in the arterial system begins sometime after birth about ages 4, 5 and 6 and continues onward until more than 50% of the system is plugged, and blood has a difficult time flowing and thence disease conditions become evident. Military records show on autopsies from Korean and Vietnam conflicts that many United States[28] soldiers aged 18-25 had coronary artery disease[64]. Even two of the three pioneer astronauts who died in the notorious oxygen fire prior to take-off — these men picked for their excellent physical condition — showed signs of atherosclerosis on autopsy.

There is a margin of safety built into every organ, and the circulatory system can compensate for increased demands for many years, until its flexibility and capacity is decreased to a critical limit.

In the calcium binding theory, calcium acts like a cement-binder in that it binds fatty substances together, probably over a scar tissue, and forms the plaque linings that cause the arterial system to decrease in flow volume. By Chelating out the calcium binder the plaque dissolves and increases the diameter of the artery while also increasing the artery's flexibility.

When a fluid flows through a pipe or tube, the rate of flow depends on a number of factors, including the pipe's length, its radius, the fluid's viscosity and the time of flow. All other factors staying constant, a very small decrease or increase in the radius of the tube decreases or increases the rate of flow, respectively, by a factor of the power of three. Since a smaller vascular opening also requires higher blood pressure to pump the blood through more work is placed on the heart and overall vascular system. With increased clogging of the circulatory system, therefore, our blood pressure increases while the quantity or volume of blood flow decreases drastically[65]. Since the human vascular system is not rigid, like metal pipes, the model of cross-sectional diameter and fluid flow can be over-simplified,

As the arteries may also stretch with higher pressure, therefore compensating to some extent for a smaller diameter of flow opening. However "perfusion scans have demonstrated increased brain blood flow after Chelation treatment . . . Doppler ultrasound studies in sample groups of up to 30 patients have demonstrated some cases of complete patency [the condition of being wide open] of carotid arteries following treatment . . . [and] there is a 28% improvement or enlargement of the lumen [inner lining] diameter . . . improvement in brachial-ankle blood pressure ratios . . .[39]" according to Zigurts Strauts, M.D. A 10% increase in vascular diameter of the arteries is enough to double the blood flow." As atherosclerosis progresses, and the pipes — the capillaries, arteries and veins — decrease in size, each cell of our body also receives considerably less nourishment than before partial clogging, as the amount of nourishment lessens with the decrease of blood flow. There is literally less opportunity to bring molecular food particles and oxygen to each cell. With less food and oxygen at each cell, the cell has less capacity to function. Less functioning of each cell means less ability to resist disease and stress, and less ability to repair damage already done. That, of course, means increased opportunity for every kind of disease.[28]

Perhaps two-time Nobel winner, Linus Pauling, Ph.D. has again scored with his theory of damage to the interior of the artery being the beginning of its clogging.

The Nitric Oxide Theory

Gary Gordon, D.O., M.D. says, "Chelation therapy has significantly helped more than one million people enjoy a higher level of health. Yet for many it clearly is not reversing plaque, although most patients see significant clinical improvement when treated with EDTA. I believe this is due, among other things, to enhanced NITRIC OXIDE produced in the body by our endothelium that simply functions far better when all lead and other toxic metals are removed. When this simple idea is understood we can make EDTA chelation a standard part of medicine. The nitric oxide benefit is already published and we can now help virtually everyone by giving up on the complex, and nearly impossible-to-prove, idea of reversing plaque.

"There are over 32,000 published articles on Nitric Oxide. These explain why chelation can enhance blood flow, even without reversing plaque, and this research clearly proves that almost every other benefit that has been reported in patients receiving the standard 1-1/2 to 3 hour chelation therapy can now be fully explained simply by the increased production of Nitric Oxide. I believe once this need to improve function of tissues through heavy metal detoxification is understood by everyone, we can then immediately extend most of the benefits we ascribe to EDTA therapy to everyone living on our metal toxic planet, affordably and conveniently, by switching to CALCIUM EDTA given orally everyday and further enhanced by periodic parenteral administration for deeper cleansing." (See http:// gordonresearch.com/)

How Are Treatments Given?

According to the first theoretical model, the chemical EDTA, an amino acid, acts like a magnet for positively charged calcium and other metal ions. The chemical EDTA "claws" onto the metallic ions and converts them to a chemical that is solvent, safe and easily washed through urine. While EDTA to some extent also flushes out beneficial compounds and elements, such as zinc and Vitamin B_6, these beneficial substances are replaced during the chelating process. A mixture of EDTA and vitamins and

minerals is placed in an intravenous solution, and the patient takes an intravenous drip for about 1-

1/2 to 3-1/2 hours in a doctor's out-patient room. New studies have shown that the same good effects

can be achieved in half the time, with a smaller volume of fluids. The patient usually sits beside others who watch television or read or simply visit with one another.

According to physicians who routinely use Chelation Therapy with their patients, it takes about 20 to 22 treatments for first results to make themselves known to the patient. Depending on severity of the

patient's overall problems, s/he may need 30, 40, . . . , 100 treatments given, usually, at the rate of about three per week which, according to some physicians, is an optimum frequency of treatment. Other physicians may vary the frequency of treatment, depending upon the patient's condition. Evaluation of the patient should be made at 3, 6 and 12 month intervals[66].

For the treatment to be maximally effective, good dietary habits and appropriate exercise are important. Alcohol, drugs (including many prescription drugs) and smoking will reverse the whole process, again causing free-radical damage that leads to atherosclerosis and subsequent disease problems that occur as a secondary condition of the inability of cells to receive their proper nourishment. Physicians who provide patients with EDTA Chelation Therapy will also counsel on the negative effects of bad diet and consumption of alcohol, drugs and smoking. They will advise appropriate diets that will either assist in the chelating process or will, by themselves, provide the body with natural chelating mechanisms. EDTA should not be used during pregnancy[66].

Chelation Therapy should normally be postponed until active liver diseases are properly treated or resolved unless there is no other choice available[66].

Usually a physician will supplement EDTA treatment with proper diet counseling and antioxidants which are synergistic with the benefits of EDTA. These are Vitamins C, E, beta carotene, selenium, glutathione and a spectrum of B complex vitamins. Iron and copper are free radical catalysts and excesses may counteract the benefits of chelation therapy[66].

EDTA Safety

Any drug can be dangerous under the right conditions, to the wrong person. Even milk can be exceptionally dangerous to one who is allergic to it. According to the manner in which drug safety is determined EDTA is about 3-1/2 times safer or less toxic than taking aspirin[36]. This measure is taken from a standard known as the LD-50, the **L**ethal **D**osage at which 50% of experimental animals will die in a specified period. "More than 1,000,000 patients have been treated in the United States alone, without a single reported incident of renal failure or death since 1960[48]."

As with any treatment, EDTA can be misused by those who do not follow a proper treatment protocol, and it is recommended that physicians use the protocol developed by The American College for Advancement in Medicine[28]. This pioneer organization has long ago established certification and standards of practices including appropriate training and education for all those physicians who wish to chelate patients.

Eliminating Pollutants and Damaging Metallic Ions

Anything you can do to better nourish (and oxygenate) individual cells you should do to relieve the burdens that you already carry. Anything you can do to avoid pollutants in water, food, and air you should do. One example, of a recently hidden negative is the use of chlorine in drinking water as a disinfectant. The "Environmental Protection Agency study showed that drinking highly chlorinated water 'subtly but noticeably shifted' a mouse's transport of cholesterol from high-density lipoproteins (the 'good' lipoproteins) in the blood to the 'bad' low-density lipoproteins, which foster atherosclerosis." J.

Peter Bercz, who headed the study, reported that hypochlorite, a very reactive by-product of standard water chlorination, "can also destroy polyunsaturated fatty acids . . . , including those essential to health[56]." Multiply this single effect of a standard, assumed-to-be-safe disinfectant of water, by the thousands of impurities found in air and food. Pure food, water and air are extremely important! But more — EDTA will also help you to eliminate many of these pollutants that are acquired over a lifetime, the same that contribute in so many ways to your overall condition. In addition, by stimulating a gland called the parathyroid, your body will reverse the flow of calcium to harden bones and teeth, thereby reversing Osteoporosis.

The poisonous, ineffective — damaging — fluorine dumped in our water is a subject requiring a lot more pages than this book! Avoid fluorine like poison, which it is!

Where To Get Help

There's been a great deal more research and clinical work using chelation therapy since this article was written. Alternative/complementary medicine, unlike allopathic practices, never stands still. There are also now a large number of physicians throughout the world who routinely offer Chelation Therapy to their patients. The best source for finding a physician in your area is the American College of Advancement in Medicine (ACAM), American College for Advancement in Medicine 380 Ice Center Lane, Suite C Bozeman, MT 59718; http://www.acam.org/? Its members consisting of physicians, scientists and health professionals meet semiannually where professional papers and new discoveries are presented by others. One can get acquainted with their latest research and discoveries latest recommended treatment protocol. This organization will also refer you to good sources of valid materials as well as provide sources of rebut against those who unwittingly or in ignorance seek to halt this great, new therapy.

Allergies and Biodetoxification

Somewhere back in the 1940s allopathic doctors discovered a possible treatment for pollen allergies, such as ragweed. They'd prepare a number of pollen allergens in individual small vials with individualized concentrations and, using a very small needle, they'd introduce these allergens just beneath the skin. They'd wait a few minutes and then measure the size of the allergic welt produced by each minor injection. The greater the diameter of the welt the more sensitive was the person to that particular allergen. Then, over a period of weeks, that particular allergen was injected in stronger and stronger dosages. This process worked very fine provided a sufficiently wide range of possible allergens was tried to cover the pollens found in the patient's immediate environment. Usually the desensitization process had to be completed before the allergen to which the patient was sensitive began filling her/his environment from plant pollination. External allergies can be discovered by the detective work of mixing together suspected allergens — pollen grains, house dust, cat hair, protein particles, et. al. — and after preparing the solution properly, inserting the extract just beneath the skin, where the size and severity of welts determines whether or not an individual is allergic to a particular substance.

Often this process worked well but it took a great deal of the physician's time, and so office helpers were trained. When it didn't work it was because the correct allergens were ignored or because the technician simply wasn't as careful as her/his boss.

The big mistake made by the so-called establishment physician was to extend these trials to food allergies. The method simply will not work for food allergies, as you will learn. When similar tests were developed for foods, or exposure to the increasing number of environmental chemicals, there was, at best, inconsistent results. Even today people will be given the skin-patch test which has been shown to be negative as proof that they are not allergic to the food the patch was supposed to test against. Food patch tests are extremely unreliable when making the determination for a food allergic reaction.

Food allergies contribute to many diseases, including the one hundred or so collagen tissue diseases often called

"Rheumatoid Diseases" as well as to Diabetes Type II. Food allergies can mimic the symptoms of many diseases.

Food allergies are now classified in alternative medicine under the heading of Clinical or Environmental Ecology where the environmental causes of allergic symptoms are unraveled.

Certain allergic symptoms have sources that are well known and easily found, such as those causing "hay fever" which springs from pollen or ragweed, pigweed, grass pollen, tree pollen and so on. This is an "external" allergy, as opposed to an "internal" allergy that springs from reactions to substances inside the body. There also seems to be a clinical distinction between a physical response to an allergen and

chemical sensitivity. For example breaking out in a rash due to chlorine — or some of its breakdown products — from water can be a chemical sensitivity rather than breaking out in skin hives from eating a banana which is a food allergy. This may be quibbling because, in the long view, both reactions are due to some chemical that the individual's body has not learned to handle.

Other external allergen sources can be almost anything: gases, fluids, etc. Strictly speaking, these are not allergies, but chemical sensitivities. Some people develop an "allergy" to something as common as the cooking gas from the cook stove. They cannot live near or by such sources without being sick.

People range from very, very sensitive to not sensitive at all, in a gradient scale. People vary considerably as to what they are allergic to.

The interesting — and distressing — part about allergies is that foods which were perfectly safe for much of our lives suddenly become intolerable — for no obvious reasons.

Since Theron Randolph, M.D. and four others organized the Society for Clinical Ecology in 1965 there has been a quiet revolution on how we view and test for food and other chemical sensitivities. By

1980 this society attracted 250 members. Dr. Randolph inherited some of his knowledge, and a great deal was his own major contribution to modern medicine.

There are claims, of course, that solving the food allergy problem will also solve the Rheumatoid Arthritis — or other Rheumatoid Disease — problem. Some of these claims may be correct and some may be, and most likely are, based on a mixture of three problems: Candidiasis, food allergies, and Rheumatoid Disease. More than likely, as we've suggested in other articles, Rheumatoid Disease and Candidiasis go hand in hand, and then an increasing number of food allergies begin to also take over our health condition. "Candidiasis" caused by an overgrowth of organisms of opportunity in the intestinal tract will be discussed in the next chapter.

On the other hand it's clear that Diabetes Type II is caused by some kind of allergic response which causes the beta cells in the pancreas to swell thus preventing insulin to be released in the blood stream.

And, as stated earlier, food allergies can, by themselves, mimic many diseases.

According to Paul Reilly, N.D. of Tacoma, WA, "Diet affects bowel flora and Gastro-Intestinal tract permeability. Both of these factors can, in turn, affect the amount of endotoxins (bacterial toxins released from dying bacteria) absorbed. In addition to their . . . role in stimulating B cell mitogenesis, endotoxins are potent activators of the alternate complement pathway, which promotes inflammatory processes. The Kupfer cells of the liver are integral in elimination of circulating immune complexes as well as antigens absorbed intact from the gut. <u>If the liver is not functioning optimally, due to endotoxin damage, these undegraded antigens may be released into the systemic circulation where they can activate further complement and release inflammation[69]</u>."

Allergy reactions also contribute to free-radical pathology, and that extra burden on the body can contribute to arthritic symptoms as well. After all, free-radical pathology, and subsequent damage, is what arthritis is all about. Cleaning up or preventing the development of extra free-radicals, even temporarily, should give some relief, as seems to happen when using EDTA Chelation Therapy, DMSO Intravenous Therapy, or other similar means.

A most important publication to read and understand if you suspect that you're a candidate for multiple allergens from foods and other sources is *An Alternative Approach to Allergies*, by Theron

Randolph, M.D. and Ralph Moss, Ph.D.[68]

Allergies, surprisingly enough, are also addictions, or at least there is sufficient commonality between the phenomena of food and some other allergies and addictions so as to suspect an actual biological link.

Warren Levin, M.D.[70] has summarized very nicely the relationship between allergies and addictions

of foods and chemicals."A new concept to the medical profession, but one of great importance to the healing arts, is food allergy/addiction. You will notice that I do not speak of allergy or addiction or of

allergy and addiction, but rather of a single entity—allergy/ addiction. These two different aspects are as inseparable as heads and tails on a coin. Depending on which aspect is facing you, one or the other side may be more obvious but the obverse is always there.

"Most of us are acquainted with the obvious food allergy reaction. The patient who breaks out from strawberries or swells up from shellfish or who gets asthma from peanuts is well known and recognized by the doctor or layman. However this type of acute reaction represents a very small percentage of all food allergy/addiction reactions.

"The acute reaction occurs from exposure to a food which is not eaten regularly. The reaction may affect one or several organs or systems, but tends to affect the same systems in a particular patient with each repeated exposure. In other words, any organ in the body is capable of responding as the shock organ. If the nose reacts you get hay fever. If the lungs react, asthma. If the skin is the shock organ you get eczema or hives. If the intestinal tract is the responding organ you get diarrhea or constipation or nausea and vomiting or gas or a combination.

"Allergy Causes Mental Symptoms

"One of the most important shock organs that can respond to the allergic insult is the brain. The brain can show localized areas of allergic reaction similar to hives on the skin. Since the changes in the circulation, the localized swelling, the increased pressure of this allergic reaction are all taking place in the unyielding confines of the skull, the symptoms and signs of brain allergy can be severe or mild and manifest themselves as any physical complaint. The most common ones are headaches, fatigue, uncontrollable sleepiness at inappropriate times, inability to concentrate, memory lapse, incoordination, actual hallucination, changes in perception from any of the five senses — taste, smell, touch, sight and hearing. There can even be loss of consciousness and convulsions. The most important thing to understand about cerebral allergic symptoms (and I should say that cerebral refers to the most complicated portion of the human brain) is that these allergic symptoms can frequently mimic exactly the symptoms that have classically been attributed to nervous breakdown, neurosis or psychosis. In other words the diagnosis that "it's all in your mind" may really mean that "it's all in your brain" and caused by an allergic reaction

in the brain.

"The most obvious example of a food addict is the alcoholic. Suppose we look at the history of an alcoholic from the point of view of allergy/addiction. The first drink is almost always the social phenomenon. The drug affect of alcohol is experienced as pleasant and unwinding, the relaxation effect. This may be repeated socially at irregular intervals for years, without any addiction developing. Then perhaps after a tough day at the office the businessman may try a martini before supper to obtain the same relaxation (still from the drug affect of alcohol.) When this becomes a habit the stage is set for addiction. Food addiction develops slowly from frequent repeated exposures to a potentially addicting substance. "It is at this point that the addiction phenomenon becomes manifest by its major clinical sign — the withdrawal phenomenon. If you are addicted to something you feel better when you take it and after a period of being without it you begin to feel worse. Depending on the severity of the addiction it may be very mild and difficult to recognize, and express itself just as craving for the substance to which you're addicted. Some people just *know* that they are going to feel better if they have a cup of coffee, and other people just know they can't get started unless they have their drink of orange juice, and other people don't even recognize it — they just think that it's perfectly logical to have bread with every meal and they don't consider a meal complete without a piece of bread. What they don't realize is that the craving is to satisfy an addiction.

"Withdrawal Symptoms Lead to Addiction

"So let's look at our alcoholic again. He's been taking a martini now regularly when he comes home from work to unwind, and very subtly and gradually he becomes addicted. Every day by supper time his

addiction is beginning to have its affect, and he relieves it by taking his customary drink. However when addiction becomes progressive the length of time that the offending substance relieves symptoms becomes less and less, and soon our harried businessman notices that somewhere around three-thirty or four o'clock he is really beginning to feel frazzled. However if he keeps a little bottle in the drawer and takes a nip about three or three-thirty he can avoid that down feeling and of course it's an easy thing to do and that's only two drinks a day, and another alcoholic is on the way.

"The addiction increases, the withdrawal period becomes sooner and now we find that in order for him to function well he's got to have a drink when he goes out with the boys at lunchtime. If he is intelligent he may skip the mid-afternoon nip from the drawer because he does not need that anymore but if he is a slave to habit he will continue to have that drink as well as the one before supper.

"It's important to notice at this time that the patient is functioning better *with* the alcohol than he does without it, even though alcohol is a total depressant to the nervous system, interferes with reflex time and in general produces less efficient functioning. In the person with an alcohol problem the non-alcoholic state is no longer normal. It is a state of withdrawal from an addicting substance and the depression and malfunction that accompanies withdrawal is worse than the state in which the stimulation of the addicting substance is in effect.

"Eventually, we get to the point where the patient is drinking every hour or two during the day to avoid the withdrawal syndrome, and he is functioning much below par but he does function as long as he continues to take his alcohol. However, now we see where the patient when he goes to bed at night, is going to go through an eight hour period and when he wakes up in the morning he's going to be in severe withdrawal. This of course is the classical evidence of addiction to alcohol — the patient who wakes up in the morning hung-over, nervous, irritable, and all he has to do is take a tiny sip of his favorite alcohol and he relieves withdrawal symptoms temporarily.

"It is obvious to most people except the alcoholic that the best course of action is to go 'cold turkey,' to suffer through the withdrawal syndrome, to detoxify and then to avoid the offending addicting allergic substance so that optimum body function can be obtained.

"In general we know that this detoxification or desensitization or cold turkey phenomenon takes about five days for food substances. What has been further recognized is that once a patient has gone through this cold turkey phenomenon and eliminated the allergic addicting substance completely, his body then no longer craves it and actually at that point becomes acutely reactive in an allergic way to the next exposure. This is extremely important in the diagnosis of food allergy/addiction.

"It is important to remember that any food can be addicting. The best foods — wheat germ, liver, yeast, meat, fish, fruit, vegetables — are capable of inducing allergy/addiction just as well as the junk foods and alcohol. However it seems the more quickly a given food is absorbed from the intestinal tract; the more likely it is to produce the allergy/addiction response.

"Fastest Absorbed Foods Are Most Addictive

"Next in line to alcohol for speedy absorption from the intestinal tract are the refined carbohydrates like white sugar, white flour, and corn syrup. In nature's foods the absorption of carbohydrates is slowed down by the presence of indigestible fiber, protein and oil. The refining process eliminates these factors which retard absorption and the result is increased incidence of allergy/addiction. The combination of these refined foods with alcohol is disastrous to the susceptible patient.

"Following the refined carbohydrates in speed of absorption are the natural carbohydrates, fruits, starchy vegetables and cereals, then the proteins — meat, fish, poultry and eggs and finally the slowest of all — fats and oils. It is for this reason that many severely food sensitive patients are able to tolerate foods that are fried in oils Chinese style using the classical Chinese wok technique.

"For anyone with multiple food allergies this method of food preparation is highly recommended. "The problem of identifying food allergy/addiction then becomes primarily dependent upon the

recognition of the possibility. It's the old story in medicine — if a doctor doesn't think of the diagnosis during his contemplation of the patient he will never make a diagnosis. Once the possibility has been considered however, demonstration or confirmation of the correct diagnosis and treatment is straightforward. For in this case the diagnostic procedure is therapeutic — that is, eliminating the offending substance from the diet will both demonstrate the allergy and relieve the patient. Many patients are skeptical even when they feel better after having eliminated their offending substances. For the skeptics confirmation is again an easy and straightforward procedure — one just says, "OK, try that food all by itself and see what happens." Despite the fact that this procedure sounds so easy it is only easy in those

situations in which the patient is allergic to one or a very few substances.

"Unfortunately, many patients have multiple allergies of varying degrees to many if not most of the foods that they eat. In such a situation eliminating a single food may not produce the relief that is sought and the withdrawal symptoms are merely super-imposed on the general depression and low functioning level, so that the patient feels worse and does not get relief at the end of the five day elimination.

"Fasting Unmasks Allergies

"It is in recognition of this particularly complex problem that the technique of total fasting has been to note that after many years of divergent pathways to health a number of different disciplines are finding that they have much in common. The religious ascetic frequently fasted to cleanse his body of impurity while he meditated, and noted that he was healthier in mind and body when he was through. The nutritionally oriented 'health nuts' and some of the old time doctors and naturopathic physicians have advocated fasting as therapeutic and detoxifying. Although the techniques of the various fasts have been different, the general concept is the same when viewed from the allergy/addiction point of view. By eliminating all the offending allergic substances the body does begin to function at a more optimum level.

"Needless to say, before starting on this procedure one should have the check-up and approval of his or her physician to make sure that the rare contraindications to fasting such as adrenal cortical

insufficiency or Addison's disease and other debilitating illnesses are not present.

"OK, so you're checked out and ready to start the fast. Just what does it mean to go on a total fast? Well it means exactly that, you are not going to eat anything, you are not going to put anything into your mouth except pure water, distilled water from glass bottles. The only thing that you drink is pure water without any mineral content — no tea or coffee made from pure water — there will be no smoking either, smoking is one of the commonest food allergy/addictions — and that basically constitutes the fasting procedure. "The total period of fasting should be not less than 4-1/2 days. Some people continue to fast longer

If they are tolerating it well and feel that they have not completely eliminated their toxic load. [It may take 5 days to clean all foods from the intestinal tract: Ed.] In general one should go into a fast expecting to feel worse before feeling better. The healthier the patient the less withdrawal reaction will be noticed. The more allergies and the unhealthier the patient, the more severe would we expect the reaction to be. Usually if the patient's problem is primarily food allergy, the patient is feeling much better by the afternoon of the fifth day.

"At this point we start refeeding the patient with the idea of avoiding a demonstration of an allergic reaction or the development of an addiction. That means the following rules are to be followed:

"1. Initially after the fast eat only one pure food at each feeding.

"2. The first few foods eaten should be foods that are not suspected of allergy or addicting potential to the patient. That means in general foods that are not in the usual daily routine diet. In some cases one must resort to exotic foods such as venison, bear or buffalo meat, kohlrabi, endive and rutabaga as vegetables. Goat's milk products are frequently acceptable. Remember that this is only in the initial phase of eating after the fast and eventually ordinary foods should be utilized for all but the worst cases. "3. If possible the first time a food is eaten after the fast it should be a fresh organic food known to be

free of pesticides, preservatives or any processing. It is amazing how many people think that they are

allergic to apples only to find that it is the chemical spray at fault. Or an allergy to oranges turns out to be due to the artificial color and not orange itself. If there is no reaction to the organic product, the next exposure could be from the ordinary source of supply whether fresh, frozen or canned. I must add to keep my conscience clear as a nutritionist, that from my point of view everything we eat should be fresh and free of processing except as processed in our own kitchen.

"4. Everything that is taken by mouth must be cleared of suspicion by individual tests. That means the first time you drink the tap water it must be all by itself. It is amazing how many patients are sensitive to the chlorine and fluorine and other pollutants in our water supply. It also means that every vitamin, mineral or food supplement as well as any medication must be independently judged by taking it and it alone and observing the effects. One of the biggest problems in the so-called neurotic patient is allergy/ addiction to tranquilizers. In some cases to the medication itself, in other cases fillers in the capsule and frequently to the artificial coloring. However, you must beware of discontinuing any medication for the fast without your physician's knowledge even though any prescription can be a factor just as any food or food supplement can. Ideally nothing should be taken during the fast except distilled water and the time that it is eaten. In column B keep a record of how you feel. Any change for the better or worse should be recorded with the time of the occurrence. In addition keep a record of your pulse rate for one minute period before you eat each feeding and every ten to fifteen minutes for an hour after each feeding. A change up or down of 12 or more beats a minute is suggestive of food allergy.

"6. Continue eating single foods at each feeding until you have found a number of foods that do not produce reaction. After a few days of unusual foods start testing the most likely foods, the ones you eat regularly. Remember not to test complex foods like bread. This would be getting wheat, yeast, egg, shortening all at once. Test each ingredient separately. Foods for testing can be raw or cooked without any condiments or seasonings except for sea salt which may be used. Boiling, steaming, broiling and baking are the preferred cooking methods using the same water as for the fast.

"Preservatives

"One of the major problems that have beset mankind from its earliest efforts at civilization has been that of spoilage of food. Over the century the various tribes and races developed their own techniques for preventing food from going bad. Salting of meat, drying of grains, smoking of various foods, pickling in various ways and preserving in specially controlled temperatures and light are all included in some of the ingenious ways early man took care of this problem. However modern technology has come into the picture and with the ability to synthesize chemicals of great complexity, and in many cases to design a chemical to perform a certain function, food technology has become a billion dollar business and a very competitive one. From the original purpose of preventing spoilage we now have emerged into a cutthroat chemical competition to make the most brilliant colors, the most powerful tastes, the most artificial consistencies by modifying or in some cases imitating foods with chemical conglomerations.

"The average child today eats a fresh strawberry and says "Oh, it doesn't have any taste," because he is so used to the intense artificial strawberry taste that he gets in anything he associates with strawberries; and the color of real strawberry is very pale in comparison with the garish pink of strawberry ice cream which is such a load of chemicals that I think it is a travesty to refer to it as ice cream. We are making people in this way get further and further away from natural food and dependent more and more on artificial colors, flavoring and the large numbers of preservatives. The important thing to realize is that all of these chemicals are frequent producers of allergic reaction and many people with long standing histories of erratic behavior, nervous breakdowns, hyper-active children are merely showing the results of the chemical sensitivity of the brain. It is certainly true that people can become allergic to the purest of foods from the harvest of nature. However, when people have these sensitivities they are much easier to handle when one is merely trying to avoid a food than when one has to consider the chemical problem as well.

"The log that you've meticulously constructed will often show two kinds of allergies. One where the allergen has caused a bodily reaction immediately and the second that manifests in about 3 days. That's the reason for the log.

"As there are two kinds of allergies, one that will strike shortly after eating the substance, and a second that strikes three days later, many physicians recommend a blood test from a laboratory that

specializes in food allergy tests from blood samples[71]. These blood tests, when performed by a specialist laboratory can reduce the need for constructing a day-to-day log of your eating habits and allergenic responses."

In an example of a chemical sensitivity triggered by a food, Ed Wendlocher described his problem and pursued its cause to the end, now helping others through his book *Inflammation Nation*[72]

Ed Wendlocher, founder and president of the Arthritis Help Centers, Inc.,[72] suffered from arthritis for many years until he discovered his sensitivity to various foods. He promoted clinical studies that resulted in several booklets, including *Pain Foods*! After careful studies over many years it was learned that many taste enhancers, such as capsaicinoids, were exempted by the food labeling act and were also found in small quantities in many ordinary foods. These, it was discovered, caused many people, including Ed Wendlocher himself, to suffer from the classical phenomena of "arthritis."

Now the mechanism is revealed through further academic research that capsaicinoids do, indeed, play a serious role in creating inflammation, tissue damage and "arthritis!"

We highly recommend obtaining the Arthritis Help Center book *Inflammation Nation*[72] describing

foods that may be causing arthritic problems.

Ed Wendlocher says, "Harvard Medical School researchers have now found that the receptor activated by chemicals in 'hot' chili peppers is also responsible for the ongoing, burning pain associated with inflammation, tissue damage and arthritis!"

"The chemicals in the 'hot' chili peppers that cause them to be 'hot' are the capsaicinoids. Capsaicinoids are strong irritants that act directly on the pain receptors in your skin and mucous membranes. The strongest capsaicinoids are capsaicin and dihydrocapsaicin. Capsaicin is so strong that a single drop diluted in one million drops of water will still warm your tongue. Like dihydrocapsaicm, it delivers a sting all over your mouth. A third capsaicinoid, nordihydrocapsaicin, produces a warmer, mellower sensation in the front of your mouth and palate. A fourth, homodihydrocapsaicin, packs a delayed punch, delivering a stinging, numbing burn to the back of your throat.

"Until now, capsaicin has been reported to primarily have beneficial effects on the body. It is best known as an effective 'pain relief' substance when applied topically to the skin where it destroys certain nerve cells and prevents pain signals from reaching the brain. However, increased research of capsaicin is now uncovering that it also has significant detrimental effects on the body.

"Capsaicin is now confirmed to be a primary cause of the on-going, burning pain associated with inflammation, tissue damage and arthritis! Capsaicin is a strong irritant. Applied to the skin, it causes the small blood vessels under the skin to dilate; increasing the flow of blood to the area and making the skin feel warm. It stimulates nerve endings in your mouth normally stimulated by a rising body temperature, sending impulses to your brain that release endorphins giving you a false sense of well-being. Eating 'hot' chili peppers may upset your stomach, irritate the lining of your stomach, irritate your bladder so that you have to urinate more frequently or even make your urination painful.

"The 'hot' chili pepper plants are 'cousins' of tobacco [and tomatoes] being in the same Solanaceae plant family. The 'hot' chili peppers contain many of the same natural toxins as tobacco. By comparing the established LD-50 values (measures of toxicity), we see that the capsaicin in 'hot' chili peppers is in the same league as a dangerous toxin as is nicotine in cigarette smoke.

"Capsaicin is now used commercially as a pesticide on fruits and vegetables as it both kills insects and repels animals from crops. Again, based on LD-50 values, it is one of the more dangerous toxic pesticides in use today!

"'Hot' chili pepper, also known as cayenne pepper, is made from the seeds and pods of Capsicum peppers, a species completely different from *Piper nigrum*, the plant whose fruit is used as black pepper (the one in the shaker on your table). The Capsicum peppers are native to Mexico, Central America, the West Indies and much of South America, but similar varieties are also native to the Far East. They may be long and thin like the cayenne pepper, large and firm like the Anaheim, cone shaped like the jalapeno or small and cherry shaped.

Tabasco peppers, used to make a popular hot sauce, are a variety of

'hot' peppers known as *Capsicum frutescens*. Ground red pepper labeled cayenne pepper or simply red pepper is made by grinding the smaller, more pungent Capsicums. The term "red pepper" may also be used to describe ground red pepper milder than, cayenne. Crushed red pepper, the spice you find in pizza parlors, is made from the seeds of the 'hot' varieties of *Capsicum annuum* and *Capsicum frutescens*. Chili powder is a blend of red pepper with other herbs and spices.

"Recent studies completed in association with scientists at a major university show that persons with arthritis can significantly reduce their pain, swelling and stiffness by conscientiously avoiding the foods containing the 'hot' chili peppers and certain other food ingredients!

"The problem: 'hot' chili ingredients are not easy to avoid as they are rarely shown on the food label by that name. They are usually shown on the label as spices, spice extracts, flavorings, natural flavorings or seasonings; or added as colorings or preservatives and not shown at all!"

Bio-detoxification

In 1950 American science fiction readers were suddenly presented with a new "science of the mind". *The Analog Science Fact and Fiction magazine* editor, John W. Campbell, Jr., was a most remarkable writer, editor, critic of scientists and standard bearer for the proper use and understanding of the scientific method. He developed almost single-handedly the modern field of science fiction, exploiting chiefly "hard science fiction" where an interesting story must be told within the framework of real or possible science. Campbell developed several generations of writers, chiefly with his ability to creatively conceive of new permutations and possibilities of that perception we call reality or possible reality.

While John W. Campbell was truly a genius in his own right, and while he trained many writers who are now revered writers in their own right, a small handful he did not train — Robert Heinlein, Theodore Sturgeon, A.E. van Vogt. . . . One such was a red-haired, flamboyant geniuses' genius by name of Lafayette Ron Hubbard originally from the state of Montana, and one who reputedly could sing any part of four-part harmony.

Campbell started another magazine titled *Unknown* where aged fairy-tales were retold in modern vein.

L. Ron Hubbard wrote some of the enduring classics in both genre in both magazines, the former consisting of "hard" science fiction, and the latter of the mold of Arabian Nights but adapted to the modern world.

Now this may seem like a strange introduction for application of medical techniques, but wait. You'll see it all ties together.

In 1950 John W. Campbell, Jr. announced that *Analog* would present the world's first introduction to a "science of the mind" called *Dianetics*®[73].

Before you balk, keep in mind that the first description of equi-orbit satellites for communication purposes was also found between *The Analog Science Fact and Fiction* pulp pages, conceived by Arthur C. Clarke, a brilliant science fiction writer in his own right, and president of Sri Lanka University of Ceylon. You may have seen his movie *2001: A Space Odyssey*. Further, that many innovative ideas first

found their appearance in Campbell's science fiction magazine. Consider, also, that the brilliant writer and Ph.D. in biochemistry, Isaac Asimov, cut his teeth on Campbell's advice. In case you are not aware of it, Isaac Asimov had more than 366 books to his credit, about half divided between science fiction and half to interpretation of every field of science for the layman. He also retained the title of full Professor at Boston University of Medicine where he was employed before he became a world-class writer and Grandmaster of Science Fiction. His books can be found in every library in the world, from grade school through graduate school[73, 74].

Campbell introduced Hubbard's Dianetics on his reading public that consisted of a very high percentage of engineers, scientists and teachers. L. Ron Hubbard's *Dianetics: The Modern Science of Mental Health*[75] was held in disdain at the time of its birth, being handily scoffed at and ridiculed by every psychologist, psychiatrist and medical Authority of the day. But, without any advertising whatsoever, or promotional book reviews, the first book of *Dianetics*®[75] sold through word of mouth a million dollars worth in one year. These funds were immediately put to use by a foursome Campbell, Hubbard, an electronics engineer named Don Rogers and a Medical Doctor who specialized in psychosomatic medicine, Joseph Winter, M.D. — to establish Hubbard Dianetic Research Foundations across the nation.

One of us had the good fortune to attend one of these early research centers in Elizabeth, New Jersey in 1951.

Hubbard had had the audacity to question medical practices, including the psychiatric practices of destroying a man's mind by electric-shock in order to bring about tractability. He also brazenly announced that the mind, and his new knowledge, was the key to ridding the world of all non-physically based insane behavior and psychosomatic illnesses. Considering that even today medical practitioners estimate that perhaps 70% of all human sicknesses as being psychosomatic, or carrying a psychosomatic component, Hubbard was defining a mighty large territory in his claims.

No man should be so daring when challenging medical Authority!

Much history passed by after those early days, and Hubbard, though constantly besieged by Authority from every side, and though ridiculed by various news media, boldly continued his developments into what is now known as the "technology" of The Church of Scientology. The word DIANETICS®[73]" and the word "SCIENTOLOGY®[73]" are registered, under the Religious Technology Center[73].

Do you remember the sixties and the drug-scene hippie era?

Hubbard set out in the late sixties to solve the drug addiction problem. There is no written history that I am aware of that describes Hubbard's trials and errors in finally solving this most perplexing problem. We wish we knew of such an historical account. It must be interesting. We would pass it on to you.

Hubbard developed/discovered a way of detoxifying lipids, or fats in cells that contain very minute amounts of chemical pollutants. He found that he could rid the body of these "triggering" chemicals, and by so doing, the drug addiction was gone as a physical entity. His DIANETICS® and SCIENTOLOGY® processes, he felt, could solve the psychic component.

His sweat box technique was picked up by several medical groups in California where it was used successfully for the purposes intended. However, one of the main medical groups, headed by Zane Gard, M.D., was closed by action of the California licensing board, and, presumably, also the influence of the patented drug dominated FDA[8]. (Some of Dr. Gard's amazing curative results can be read at the website *http://www.arthritistrust.org,* "Research" button, then "Research and Letters" button, then find "Gard" alphabetically along left hand margin.)

The process remains available throughout the world at every Church of Scientology location, including its CELEBRITY CENTRES®, where the service is provided under the name of "THE PURIFICATION RUNDOWN®," for spiritual cleanser.

By now if you've developed the idea that very little in establishment medicine will solve your health problem you're probably right. You should also begin to understand that there are many alternatives successfully employed by physicians not all of which stem from academic university atmospheres.

You should also feel that one ought to hold no barriers to the search for wellness, but take it where it works and reject it where it does not work, whether found in traditional medicine or not.

The body must maintain wellness functions, such as adequate blood circulation, which is the means to nourish each cell so that cells can properly function. To insure this, we arrived at EDTA Chelation Therapy. The body must rid itself of excessive free-radicals generated via various natural processes. It was built to do so by exercise, as lactic acid formed during exercise is a natural chelator. In the absence of a healthy body with a healthy metabolism the natural ridding of excess free-radicals seems inherently impossible. To solve that problem also leads to EDTA Chelation Therapy and to food allergy challenges, as well as good nutritional habits.

Of all the various health processes — nutritional, exercise, medicinal, chelation therapy, etc. — none of these can solve the problem of alcohol and drug addiction — or the problem of residual poisons accumulated over a life-time that are stored in the fatty parts of our cells. These triggering metabolites cause many different sorts of "impossible-to-solve" medical problems. Dr. Gard, using Hubbard's sauna approach was solving many until his license was revoked by the ignorant and uncaring.

We learned of the problem of residual toxins stored in fatty part of cells at a professional medical meeting of the American College of Advancement in Medicines[76], advocates and researchers of Chelation Therapy and other advanced medical regimens.

Whereas EDTA Chelation Therapy solved many hitherto intransigent medical problems related to peripheral circulation, there was a whole class of problems that it would not solve. It seems that residual chemicals that reside in the fatty parts of our cells can come from taking drugs, including medicines, or hard drugs from the street, or from anesthesia during surgery. Some come from soil and air pollutants, such as found in pesticides and herbicides (remember Agent Orange), consisting of various organic poisons called PCBs, Hexa PCB, PBB, Heptachlor Epoxide, Dieldrin, and so on. Agent Orange is a good example of a chemical that, during its manufacturing processes, collects very small amounts of a dangerous, cancer-forming chemical called Dioxin that can also create birth defects. This chemical in turn creates for the human effects far beyond its apparent volume and creates the damaging effects for years ahead, perhaps for the individual's lifetime.

Residuals from drugs deliberately taken such as morphine, cocaine, heroin, tobacco, and alcohol are also found in the fatty parts of cells.

Consider that the brain consists mainly of fatty (lipids) cells! And that "lipids" are also found everywhere throughout the body!

These residual chemicals as stored act as triggers creating large behavior manifestations that simulate every kind of mental, emotional and physical illness.

The very fact that you "like" the habituation with a particular drug or food, for example, is an illustration of the triggering action of a chemical that leads you to massive behavioral changes that you would not otherwise make. Try to get tobacco-addicted peopled off from their cigarette, for example. Listen to their many different and inventive rationalizations.

Or witness the massive behavioral changes that the small residual chemicals create for the tobaccoaddicted: They stop at the store to buy cigarettes, fumble in purse or wallet for money, carry out the package, start the car, open the package, take out a cigarette and lighter, light the cigarette and inhale deeply blowing smoke out. They put ashes in a tray, and eventually crush the cigarette there, too. This cycle is repeated over and over in some variation — all caused by an illusion called "I want" or "I feel more comfortable with" which is subjectively felt as a desire, and that desire and behavior pattern stems from small triggering chemical elements that reside in fatty parts of cells.

I cited the example of tobacco smokers because the addiction is so common, familiar to all, and easily amendable to observation. But all of the other drugs and chemicals named, and more, will create similar unconscious behavior manifestations which we are prone to "explain" i.e. rationalize away, after the fact.

By satisfying our subjective "desire" for the chemical involved, our body restores a balance of freeradical pathology that leads to the activation of the consumption in the first instance. This is known as a "homeostasis," a restoration of the same state, however unhealthy.

Free-radical pathology, unchecked, leads to extra burdens for patients and contributes to their pain and disease. Removing the extra burdens means more bodily systems and organs capable of fighting the great fight.

When we first heard physicians discussing the shortfalls of using EDTA therapy to solve this particular problem — as Chelation Therapy "only" solves problems of peripheral circulation and Osteoporosis — we began to pay attention to possible solutions. Within half a year we learned that L. Ron Hubbard had probably solved the problem back in the late sixties and early seventies under the title of "THE PURIFICATION RUNDOWN."

We sought for some objective evidence of the results of his invention, which was supplied to us by a friend in the form of a published scientific paper written by doctors David W. Schnare, Max Ben and Megan G. Shields[76].

While I know that scientific jargon is not easy on the eyes or ears for the uninitiated, I think that the scientists' summary of their report is sufficiently revealing to risk its enclosure, which follows:

"With human exposure to environmental contaminants inevitable despite the best application of environmental laws and protection technologies, interest has grown in the potential to reduce the levels of contamination carried in the human host. This study demonstrates the promise of a comprehensive treatment for reduction of body burdens of polyclorinated and polybrominated biphenyls (PCB and PBB) and chlorinated pesticides. Adipose tissue concentrations were determined for seven individuals accidentally exposed to PBB. These patients underwent the detoxification treatment developed by Hubbard to eliminate fat-stored foreign compounds. Of the 16 organohalides examined, 13 were present in lower concentrations at post-treatment sampling. Seven of the 13 reductions were statistically significant; reductions ranged from 3.5 to 47.2 percent, with a mean reduction among the 16 chemicals of 21.3 percent (s.d.17.1 percent).To determine whether reductions reflected movement to other body compartments or actual burden reduction, a post-treatment follow-up sample was taken four months later. Follow-up analysis showed a reduction in all 16 chemicals averaging 42.4 percent (s.d. 17.1 percent) and ranging from 10.1 to 65.9 percent. Ten of the 16 reductions were statistically significant. Future research stemming from this study should include further investigation of mobilization and excretion of xenobiotics in humans[76]."

The California Firefighter[77] contains information of great interest, because it illustrates how these minute triggering elements, when stored in cellular lipids, can affect our lives grossly.

Those exposed to toxic poisons, such as firefighters, will work normally day to day, when "suddenly" a chronic ailment, disability or disease emerges which, if not fatal, can drastically degrade the quality of living.

The Foundation for Advancement in Science and Education[78] (FASE) began studying the toxic bio-accumulation and storage of chemicals in the body and how to reduce the body's burden of stored chemicals. These environmental contaminants can cause perceptual, learning and emotional problems for years following exposure by ingestion, inhaling, through the skin, or other means.

As reported, participants in the FASE study were put through the Hubbard regimen. Upon completion of the program, the Michigan participants revealed significant reductions of all chemicals originally found in their bodies, including PBBs and PCBs. Even more noteworthy were the results of a four-month follow-up examination which demonstrated that the contaminant levels had continued to go down after completion of the program. Dr. David E. Root, an occupational health specialist in Sacramento, CA was Medical Director of the Sacramento Detox Center where many of these tests were conducted.

Of particular interest is the case of Michael Del Puppo, a California police officer who had liquid Phencyclidine (PCP or "angel dust") thrown into his face in the line of duty a number of years ago. He suffered from severe headaches, memory problems, irritability and fatigue for three years prior to undergoing detoxification at the Los Angeles Detox Center.

Zane Gard[79], who now practices in Mexico (last we learned), has written up numerous case histories of otherwise intransigent cases. He, his wife and daughter were exposed to Agent Orange, and sought a method of eliminating the poison and its effects, which led them to Hubbard's method that Dr. Zane Gard later incorporated into a specialty medical practice. (Go to http://www.arthritistrust.org, then punch the "Research" button then the "Research and Letters" button to find and read about Dr. Gard's amazing results.)

Hubbard's technique is this: Near a sauna he specified about 20 minutes of physical exercise to get blood circulation flowing adequately. Then each participant enters the sauna which has a temperature between 140 and 180 degrees (F) for about 3-1/2 hours daily and each day for about three to four weeks. Dry sauna is preferred, but you may use a steam or wet sauna if you wish.

The object is to create continuous and copious sweat. It is the sweat elimination system that permits the body to rid itself of deadly toxins stored in the fatty parts of cells.

You're free to leave the sauna anytime to take a shower, rest in cool air, or to eat lunch — and then return. If you leave simply to escape the heat and sweat you're cheating yourself, as you'll simply have to endure for a longer number of days until the chore is completed.

The body cannot sweat so long and so copiously without replacing minerals and fluids. Hubbard developed an adjusted mineral intake, identifying necessary salts and liquids, including the replacement of "good fats" for the "bad fats" that you wish to sweat out along with stored toxins. In the Hubbardian procedure a monitor checks your stated results each day. From the amount of niacin required to bring about a niacin flush they also determine the appropriate dosage of replacement vitamins, minerals and fatty acids for the next day.

Before trying this procedure, we'd heard stories of many different and diverse strange phenomena. We'd heard that one experienced (or re-experienced) anesthesia, sunburns (appearing exactly as seen on the beach, swim suit straps and all), hallucinatory images and sensations, and so on. These are what Hubbard called "restimulations of past experiences" from when the drug, radiation or environmental pollution was first encountered.

At first one of us found it extremely difficult to force himself through the rigorous sweat ordeal, and especially the heat, wanting to give himself every excuse — rationalization — for not being there. "I would 'dope off' in a deep lethargy. Then, as the days passed and I found it easier to exist in the hotbox, I found different sensations occurring. One day I tasted and smelled and had every sensation of again being drugged with nitrogen oxide — laughing gas — which stemmed from only one place. I'd had teeth pulled in a dentist's chair in the nineteen forties.

"Another time I re-experienced the sickening smell of ether, this from an adenoid surgery in the doctor's office in the thirties.

"Most difficult to explain was another experience after my day of sweating and about two weeks into the detoxification. I was home lying on the bed watching television and I perceived that my body, longitudinally through my forehead, nose, chest and crotch, was split by two temperatures. My left side was extremely hot to touch and the right side quite normal. I'd had two operations on the left side but I know not why the relationship in splitting the body so neatly, unless it was related to the lymph system, which seems to anatomically split along these lines. This experience lasted for three hours.

"Apparently in a way that I do not yet understand, radiation of various kinds is also stored in these lipids, as witness the phenomena of old sunburn reappearing."

Hubbard discovered that on completion of the sauna experience most physical addictions disappeared leaving only the psychic component that led to the addiction in the first place. This component he proposed to handle by the technology administered by the church, which is another subject in itself.

The essential difference between Hubbard's program and those of medical centers, where the program been accepted by a small number of physicians, is that the medical centers provide periodic laboratory tests to ascertain the current levels of toxins in the lipids. Since there are nearly an infinite number of possible toxins one must be choosy about what is tested for or the costs can be excessive.

Hubbard's program relies more on experience coupled with one's own intuition as to when you are through. You can plan, however, on a minimum of about three and one half weeks which can often be scheduled at your convenience, such as after working hours.

I can't promise that you will obtain any observable benefit from this program, as I cannot know if you have stored environmental toxins or that you will release them successfully. If you do have such poisons affecting your various systems, and if you do release them successfully, you will surely be better able to fight off most diseases. Zane Gard, M.D. data referenced earlier assures you of benefits.

Other Biodetoxification Regimens

Many different regimens exist for cleansing the body, and each physician will have his/her own favorite. Our chapter on *Candidiasis* covers several other good mechanisms.

Candidiasis: Scourge of Modern Medicine

Introduction

Here is a systemic, damaging disease that has grown rapidly ever since the advent of modern antibiotics! It can simulate nearly every disease imaginable and therefore causes tons of misdiagnosis. Usually, the more it's treated with antibiotics the worse it gets. To make matters even worse, most allopathic doctors don't recognize it. Oh, they will name it as "candidiasis" if they spot a white fungus on the mouths of already over-pilled and immune-comprised oldsters; or on the lips of small babies without sufficient nourishment; or, as a "vaginal infection" in females. Even so, and especially in the latter case, they make the ultra-stupid mistake of calling it a localized infection when, in point of very strong fact, it is a systemic infection.

Read on, and we'll explain!

According to the *Candida Research and Information Foundation Newsletter*[80], "The numbers continue to grow of people of all ages presenting with what has become an all too familiar set of symptoms who are told by their doctors to see a psychiatrist, to grow up, to have an affair, to go get a job, or simply laughed out of the office . . . among the many stories. . . . there is indeed a problem — a serious problem . . . affecting the young and the elderly and all age groups in between."

The article, of course, is speaking of the wide-spread, modern disease known as Candidiasis and also known as monilia when found in the mouth.

The fact that the immunological system is not up to snuff in many sick folks has led medical research, through pharmaceutical companies, to search for a means of "modulating" the immunological system. This is hardly a logical reason for further damaging it by means of cytotoxic drugs, gold, penicillamine or long-term corticosteroids. Indeed, this is also not a scientific rationale for assuming that the cause of degenerative diseases is because of the obviously pill overloaded and weakened immuno-logical system.

Heavy use of antibiotics will knock out the "good guys" microflora in our intestinal tracts, and that fact in turn permits organisms of opportunity such as the ever-present yeast organism *Candida albicans* to take over. The disease that results, systemic Candidiasis, is not yet recognized by orthodox medical practitioners but its symptoms and effects should become ever more obvious to all. Whether or not the only cause for Chronic Fatigue Syndrome is *Candidias albicans* is not known, but that it is one of the major causes of the symptomology can be readily assumed based on improvement that follows when Candidiasis is treated against. Even less known by established medical practitioners is that "vaginal candidiasis does not occur naturally without concomitant of *Candida albicans* within the large bowel and that a cure is not likely as long as the vagina remains the only treatment target[81]." It bears repeating several times: a vaginal yeast infection is an outward sign of a system-wide invasion.

"Candida's presence, normally contained on skin, mucous membranes, or in the bowel, can be compromised by immunodeficient states usually induced by diabetes, pregnancy, or certain drugs. The latter include antibiotics, steroids, birth control pills, and chemotherapy. Thrush, common in infants before the full development of their immune systems, is frequent in immunocompromised individuals. "Chronic and often undetected, candidal infections are regularly associated with symptoms linked to every system of the body. Yeast cells (which are normally harmless and found within the intestinal tract) can be compromised by antibiotics, acid-base imbalances, nutritional deficiencies or parasites, so that they lose their protective cell-walls. Invading and distorting the intestinal wall with mycelia (rootlike projections), they disturb the absorptive capacity of the gut. Considered part of 'the leaky gut syndrome,' they allow multiple antigens and toxins to enter the blood stream and spread throughout the body. Food allergies, although seldom diagnosed, are tied to this aspect of gastrointestinal dysfunction. "The presence of Candida can increase the toxicity of staphylococcal infections by multiples of 100,000, thereby suggesting a strong association with toxic shock syndrome. The latter, one of the medical mysteries of the 1970's. . . . [82]"

According to James P. Carter, M.D., Dr. P.H, "Iwata in Japan discovered . . . that Candida species produce toxins . . . injecting Candida toxin into mice showed that it caused immuno-suppression, among other abnormalities. . . . In 1977, *JAMA* published the results of a study done at Michigan State University on college students who had recurrent vaginal Candidiasis. The authors pointed out that it was insufficient to treat only the vaginal infection. They also recommended changes in diet and lifestyle and suggested back then (1977), that the infection may have some effects on the immune system[83]."

Almost all desperately sick people, by virtue of their overloaded and weakened immune system, suffer also from Candidiasis, or "organisms of opportunity" similar to Candidiasis. Those who are presumed to already have a weakened immune system, and who are obviously suffering from Candidiasis, certainly don't need another factor to further stress their immune system!

Candidiasis also creates additional food allergies, over time.

Therefore, in addition to, say, symptoms caused by a particular disease like one of the one hundred rheumatoid diseases (so-called "self-immune" system diseases), victims also suffer from Candidiasis **and** food allergies, and both candidiasis and food allergies add their own symptoms to the brew. Victims of Candidias may also have symptoms that mimic those of other categorized diseases.

As the latter two conditions, Candidiasis and food allergies, often go unrecognized by traditional practitioners, all symptoms are blamed on some disease which has been nicely categorized by long-ago symptomologists who also declare the disease as "incurable."

All sick folks should consider as part of their overall "get well" program treatment against Candidiasis — or at least find a specialist who understands its systemic nature.

Candidiasis, a yeast/fungus organism that seems to be everywhere, was first defined (*The Missing Diagnosis*) as a set of manifesting symptoms or syndrome by Orian Truss, M.D. of Birmingham, Al[80].

William B. Crook, M.D. of Jackson, Tennessee popularized Truss's findings in his book, *The Yeast Connection*[85]. Other physicians have also added to the popularization, such as Morton Walker, D.P.M. and John Parks Trowbridge, M.D. [84], *The Yeast Syndrome*, Dennis W. Remington, M.D. and Barbara W. Higa, R.D., *Back to Health*[86].

Subsequent investigations by many physicians seems to have verified Truss's findings, and slowly but not fast enough, it is being accepted by the ultra-conservative medical establishment as a properly defined and diagnosed disease.

Candida albicans, which is found most everywhere, invades various parts of bodily tissues, resulting in localized infections. Common sites of infection are the mouth as in infant Thrush, gastrointestinal tract, vagina, urinary tract, prostate gland and skin and fingernails and toenails.

Under normal conditions our bodies are able to resist this invasion, as it does other germs. Whenever various substances weaken the immunological system, the yeast/fungus organism begins to spread, and in the spreading creates virtual havoc throughout the body parts and systems.

The yeast/fungus invasion may cripple the immune system so that it can no longer repel invaders. It can open the door to allergies to foods and to sensitivities to chemicals. It is believed that it invades the intestinal wall where toxins from microorganisms and protein molecules from your food enter the blood stream being there recognized by antibodies as a foreign antigen. Because proteins are derived from common DNA (gene molecule) structure, each time a new protein enters directly into the bloodstream, it, too, can become recognized as a foreign invader, and thus a "cross-reactivity" occurs, causing one to have increasingly more food allergies.

Yeast, remember, feeds on sugars and carbohydrates that easily convert to sugars. In turn, yeasts produce a series of chemical products as waste among which are acetaldehyde and ethanol. Ethanol daily inebriated. Acetaldehyde is produced as the alcohol is metabolized and is about six times more toxic to brain tissue than ethanol. Acetaldehyde is the metabolic product of ethanol and the part that provides your headache after drinking too much alcohol. These two chemicals from well-planted yeast — acetaldehyde and alcohol — are probably responsible for the following effects, according to Dr. Orian Truss[80]:

1. Cell membrane defects, damage to red and white blood cells and other problems.

2. Enzyme destruction. Enzymes are the key to breaking down foods in the body so that they can be utilized as nourishment.

3. Abnormal hormone response. Hormones regulate your bodily functions. Some of the symptoms caused by *Candida albicans* are these:

1. Allergic reactions.

2. Gastrointestinal problems: bloating and gas, diarrhea, abdominal pain, gastritis, gastric ulcers, constipation, and many others.

3. Respiratory system: sore throat, sore mouth, contribution to sinus infections, bronchial infections and pneumonia.

4. Cardiovascular system: palpitations, rapid pulse rate, pounding heart.

5. Genitourinary system: vaginitis, frequent urination, lack of bladder control, itchy rashes, etc.

6. Musculoskeletal system: muscle weakness, leg pains, muscle stiffness, slow coordination, and so on.

7. Central Nervous system: Headaches, poor brain function, poor short-term memory, fuzzy thinking and so on.

8. Fatigue is extremely common as impaired metabolism doesn't enable the body to get enough fuel and impaired enzyme functioning inhibits energy production.

9. Weight gain is common.

As can be observed by reviewing the above characteristic symptoms (which are not complete) many similar symptoms may "present" with a so-called intransigent disease. It is often difficult to discriminate between one cause and another as diseases operate on the same tissues, the same organs, producing similar symptoms, in similar ways.

Many diseases increase in intensity with a weakening of the immunological system. *Candida albicans* (and related species) spreads with a weakening of the immunological system.

Numerous intransigent diseases as well as Candidiasis seems to lead to food allergies and other kinds of allergies over time.

Both food allergies and Candidiasis produce similar symptoms in many bodily tissues. Both diseases are systemic in nature.

Candidiasis spreads with the use of almost any kind of surgery where antibiotics were used, or if you've been given antibiotics orally for any purpose you probably suffer from some degree of Candidiasis. Why? Because the antibiotics kill off the "good-guys" bacteria required in your intestinal tract for good nutrition, the yeast/fungus spreads taking the "good-guy's'" place, and it sends rootlets into the intestinal mucosa helping to age your total system. These "good guys," such as *Lactobacillus acidophilus*, need to be replaced.

Candidiasis is usually controlled through a combination of diet control and medicines some of which are prescription and some non-prescription. Usually the physician who suspects Candidiasis also attempts to strengthen the immunological system by one means or another.

It is important to replace the yeast in the intestinal tract with *Lactobacillus acidophilus* as well. Here is another reason to take it. *Lactobacillus acidophilus* helps digest food and especially milk sugar. Some varieties also synthesize vitamin B and some reduce serum cholesterol levels.

Candidiasis is a real syndrome, much controversystill exists. Allergists, immunologists, and gynecologists see this syndrome as a fictional one, probably because the manifestations are seen too often, the need for treatment too frequent, the testing for its presence and effect too inadequate, and because almost everyone suddenly has become an expert in its presence or absence. Most shocking, since many rheumatologists do not recognize Systemic Candidiasis as a problem, they often misdiagnose the condition as being that of Rheumatoid Arthritis or some other "incurable" disease, and they mistreat accordingly.

Paul A. Goldberg, M.P.H., D.C. says, "In 1977 I was a graduate assistant at the University of Texas Medical Center (School of Public Health) in Houston, TX. I had the opportunity to observe many cancer patients at the M.D. Anderson Tumor Institute there. Many (perhaps most) had candidiasis. The candidiasis was not the cause of their cancer — rather it was part of the lowered resistance that had likely contributed to the cancer itself. Most sick people have yeast overgrowth . . . but yeast overgrowth is not what makes so many people sick — rather it is their lowered resistance. So, as our population continues to develop more and more degenerative ailments, what do we do? As a culture, ultimately, in addition to treating the effects of our lifestyles (e.g. the yeast), at some point the way of life in this country led by so many folks has got to be changed in some very fundamental ways.

"Why do so many people with candidiasis never get well? Perhaps, as suggested, it is because of changing yeast forms, not strict enough diet, not enough time given to treatment, etc. — but it is also because the real resistance of the patient never has the chance to really increase.

"Rest, sleep, sunshine, peace of mind, a conducive healing environment, none of these things is provided. So — armed with only a few drugs, supplements, and diet, a few recover partially, but many stay ill[87]."

Testing for Candidiasis

Most "testing" for the presence of Candidiasis takes place by means of a questionnaire which the patient fills out and the questionnaire is then evaluated by either a physician or a medical technician. If a score of predetermined criteria is reached, one is at risk for having the syndrome, otherwise probably not.

Usually the questionnaire is based on some variation of detail of the following characteristics, as listed by Morton Walker, D.P.M. and John Parks Trowbridge, M.D.[84]:

1. Feeling lousy all over, even after having had many treatments;
2. Cause of rotten feeling can't be identified;
3. Patient has had repeated courses of antibiotics;
4. Subconscious preference for foods made with yeast — bread, beer, wine, alcohol, and certain cheeses;
5. Craving for sweets and other sugar-containing edibles;
6. Insistent desire for refined simple carbohydrates — candy, chocolate, cake, cookies, soda pop, junk foods;
7. Discovery that sweets and simple carbohydrates give a quick pick-up followed by a letdown;
8. Low blood sugar;
9. Usually high preference for alcoholic beverages;
10. Usage of birth control pills;
11. Usage of corticosteroids or other anti-inflammatory or immunosuppressive drugs;
12. Multiple pregnancies;

13. Abdominal pain, vaginal infections, PMS, menstrual irregularities, discomfort during sex, loss of libido and/or impotence;

14. Athlete's foot, jock itch, fungus infection of finger and/or toenails, fungus infection of skin;

15. Feel more tired on damp days or in moldy places such as basements, cellars or working in garden;

and

16. Discomfort in proximity of smoke, chemicals and/or perfumes.

Usually a high score on listing made from these characteristics is a very good indication of suffering from Candidiasis.

There are accredited laboratories that perform accurate, objective testing for the presence of the organism. Such tests may be done in two stages, the first called the Micro-ELISA technique that detects circulating levels of Candida antigens, Candida antibodies IgG, A and M, and immune complexes. In the second stage of the test, the patient's lymphocytes (white cells) are challenged with Candida to evaluate inhibition of lymphocyte multiplication by budding (blastogenesis). Most alternative/complementary doctors, though, can almost immediately spot a Candida problem from answers to the above or similar list.

Treatment for Candidiasis

There are a number of recommendations for the treatment of Candidiasis, most of them relying on diet, a particular fatty acid, or a substance damaging to the yeast organism but not to human cells.

The prescription drug, Ketoconazole, is used by some physicians.

Some use combinations of the above, coupled with mechanical or other means for cleaning out the intestinal tract.

The probable reason for so many approaches is because some physicians see improvements by one means and stay with that means, while others see improvement by other treatments and so favor that means. What most physicians do not recognize is that *Candida albicans* has six switching mechanisms[88], and seven viable forms, the last being a cell-wall deficient form[88, 89]. While it is well known among microbiologists, that microorganisms will change shape and function according to their surrounding environment (i.e., more acid or alkaline, et. al.), it is not very well known among establishment physicians; or, if it is known, it is handily ignored so far as development of appropriate treatments for form/ function changing organisms.

A person who is symptomatically infected with *Candida albicans* most likely has the organism spread throughout many different tissues in the body. As different tissues may very well provide differing environments for the organism, it follows that there will be many different forms of the organism throughout the body. For example, a cell wall deficient form not being recognized by the host's immune system will float around in the blood stream until it changes to one of the other six forms. The blood stream, then, would provide a constant foci of infection for the organism. If only the intestinal tract is treated — as many physicians do — then there will be a constant return of the organism after what appears to be a "cure" occurs.

The reason that *Candida albicans*, and other organisms of opportunity, have so many switching mechanisms is because they, like us, wish to survive, especially so as a species. They've spent many millions of years "learning" how to survive.

It is because of the seven viable forms taken up by *Candida albicans* that a particular treatment produces (1) extremely slow patient response or (2) no response at all.

Our conclusion has been that if Candidiasis is to be effectively and quickly treated, all forms of treatment should be used either at the same time, or in as quick a succession as medically possible. Some of these will be described in detail in what follows.

Ketoconazole (Nizoril)

"Carol Jessup, from the University of California at San Francisco, treated 1,100 Chronic Fatigue Syndrome (CFS) patients with the anti-fungal drug ketoconazole, and 84% of these patients showed significant improvement. All of her patients met the Centers for Disease Control's definition of CFS." According to one medical doctor[83], Candidiasis was adequately treated in those patients who tested positive by the above described test within three months by use of the prescription drug, Ketoconazole, without any diet being required. He felt that it was "ludicrous to assume that one can 'starve Candida out' by avoidance of sugar, yeast and moldy foods." This feeling is contrary to the practices of most alternative/complementary doctors.

The same physician reported that those who tested negative by the above test (about two-thirds of those who presumed they were affected by the disease according to their own questionnaire) actually suffered from other allergies, hypothyroidism, other infections, heavy metal toxicities (especially mercury) and various types of functional non-specific disorders.

His conservative conclusion was that there are probably some patients with intractable problems who should at least be tested for Candidiasis and if found positive, given a trial therapy such as Ketoconazole.

According to Raymond Keith Brown, M.D., additional "conventional treatment for candidal infection primarily involves antifungal agents such as clotrimazole, administered locally for thrush and esophageal involvements, nystatin for bowel therapy, and . . . , Fluconazole, and Itraconazole, for systemic infections. To avoid the side effects of these agents, many practitioners use natural substances, herbals, homeopathy, and acupuncture as possible alternatives[82]."

Some physicians will place their suspected Candidiasis candidates on rather extensive, stringent diets sometimes lasting for a year or more along with various medicines both prescription and nonprescription. Usually the diet approach coupled with certain fatty acids that damage the yeast organism, but are harmless to human tissue, is used often in conjunction with nystatin, also a substance that is harmless to human tissue.

Candidiasis problem and its treatment comes from a paper written for his patients by Gus J. Prosch, Jr., M.D.[91] a most complete description of the Chronic Systemic

Gus J. Prosch, Jr., M.D. Candidiasis Approach

Chronic Systemic Candidiasis

The Fungus Among Us

Every human being from the day of birth lives in a sea of bacteria. Infectious germs known as microbes swim throughout our bodies at all times. These microbes can live in our throat, mouth, nose, gums, gastro-intestinal tract, blood, bladder, vagina, and numerous other body tissues. These microorganisms which may be bacteria, viruses, fungi, or parasites, are as much a part of every human being as foods and chemicals. Figuratively speaking, they are constantly trying to "eat us alive." In some people they succeed and death follows. Even if we die of causes other than infection, they eventually eat our physical remains. Only healthy cells, organs and tissues within our bodies can effectively defend against infectious microbes.

Microorganisms, whether they are viruses, fungi, bacteria or parasites do not usually cause illness until an individual's host resistance declines. "Host resistance" is a technical term that doctors use to describe the complicated mechanisms by which our bodies fight off infections.

One of the most important defense mechanisms is the destruction of invading germs by our white blood cells, known as leukocytes. These special blood cells actually eat the germs and make them harmless. However, before these white blood cells can even be manufactured in the body, there must be an optimum supply of vitamins, minerals, amino acids and fatty acids. Many of these nutritional supplements, as well as adequate trace minerals, must be available in our bodies in order for these white blood cells to be manufactured properly. If even a single amino acid or fatty acid is deficient or absent from the body, leukocyte production is decreased and may even stop. When this happens, host resistance within the body is diminished and an individual becomes more susceptible to infections of all kinds.

There is another "host resistance" defense mechanism that we need to fight off these microbes, as well as any foreign substance that enters our body. These substances are called antibodies. When our bodies are receiving optimal nutritional support, specialized protein substances known as antibodies are produced. They are also produced by the white blood cells and these substances are constructed from chains of amino acids (proteins).

Antibodies attack the invading germs and render them susceptible to destruction by other white blood cells. Any germ that enters the body always stimulates antibody production that is specifically targeted against that particular type of microbe and no other. Once the body has made these specific antibodies, the lymph cells (another type of white blood cell) can then reproduce them any time they are needed, provided there are optimum levels of amino acids, vitamins, fatty acids, minerals and trace elements, along with enzymes from which they can be constructed. Therefore, if your antibodies against the tetanus or lock jaw germs (the reason for tetanus vaccinations), for example, have been sensitized, you will more than likely remain free of tetanus even if you are exposed to the tetanus germ. In such a case, your "host resistance," which has been maintained by proper nutritional support, will be functioning properly.

It is important to understand, therefore, that in the real world in which we live, infectious illness occurs not because germs arbitrarily decide to attack our bodies, but illness from germs occurs because our nutritionally deficient, debilitated bodies permit these microbes to set up residence. In short, an opportunist germ is an infectious agent that produces disease only when the circumstances in our body are favorable.

Nutritional deficiencies can severely impair the integrity of a healthy immune system. There are, however, other factors that are also critically involved in resistance to infection. The eating of large amounts of sugar or sugar containing foods, for example, paralyzes the phagocytic capacity (the eating up of germs) by our white blood cells.

Therefore, when you do not get your proper rest and/or exercise, resistance to infectious invasion decreases and it becomes easier for you or anyone to become infected with different germs.

Similarly, severe stress, such as the loss of a loved one, exposure to various chemical irritations, anxiety, chronic food-chemical allergies, and even chronic constipation or diarrhea, are other factors that can influence your resistance to infections. Yet at the top of all these possible causes of poor health, specific nutrient deficiencies must be corrected before you can "get well."

Traditionally, the standard medical treatment for any bacterial infection consists of the administration of some form of antibiotic. Chronic Candidiasis is not like a streptococcus infection that, with the appropriate antibiotic care, one can expect eradication of the organisms from the body for several years.

Typically, with most physicians today, very little or no advice is given to the patient concerning nutritional support for weakened resistance. And, although traditional treatment generally involves drugs and chemicals that may relieve symptomatic disorders, the use of drugs does not cure the underlying nutritional-metabolic deficiencies which are usually the fundamental cause of the illness in the first place.

Antibiotics are very helpful and necessary in treating certain kinds of infectious illnesses. We must never forget, however, that if the nutritional root cause of infectious disease is not treated, illness after illness may continue to occur and often become worse as time goes on.

We must also never forget that typical antibiotic medical treatment aimed at the symptomatic relief of infectious flare-ups does in fact sometimes produce serious side effects in the form of fungal disorders as well as suppression of the immune system itself.

What is Chronic Systemic Candidiasis

Candida albicans, a form of yeast, is present in all of us not long after birth. It lives in our intestinal tract and is a yeast-like organism which in the infective phase produces a condition called "Thrush" or "Candidiasis."

Most medical practitioners feel that in the absence of the overt or obvious signs of Candidiasis, which is the acute infection stage of *Candida albicans*, there is no concern about this organism; and because of this, chronic Candida overgrowth has not been well recognized. Normally symbiotic bacteria (good germs), proper gastro-intestinal pH (acid and alkalinity balance) and the body's immune system keeps *Candida albicans* in check.

Candida albicans is also called an opportunistic organism, because when a human becomes severely debilitated or nutritionally deficient, or if the immune system is compromised, or if the normal defenses (skin, decreased white blood cells, etc.) are bridged, then Candida can invade the deeper tissues as well as the blood stream. Before today's modern technological advances most physicians did not believe that Candida could invade the body tissues. However, with the AIDS epidemic worsening, autopsies on patients dying from AIDS (their immune system is totally destroyed) are showing invasion of this Candida germ in the brain, lungs and other body tissues. Because of this finding, many physicians are taking a second look at the Candida problem and they realize that the germ can invade body tissues and cause systemic disease and many are trying to learn more about how to treat this condition.

Most physicians now recognize that *Candida albicans* can grow out of control in the nurturing environment of the mucosal (lining of the intestine) surfaces. Rapid and sustained *Candida albicans* overgrowth can lead to the pathogenic and often debilitating condition known as "Polysystemic Chronic Candidiasis." This is the fungus form of the disease. This new form of Candidiasis demands recognition and treatment. Many patients with this new form have had their symptoms for several years (chronic) and the symptoms usually involve multiple organ systems (Polysystemic). Because the syndrome produces so many symptoms involving multiple organ systems, it has been labeled Polysystemic Chronic Candidiasis.

Candia albicans is capable of changing its anatomy and physiology as it grows in the intestines. If its growth is mild and not overwhelming it remains a symbiotic (living naturally in the body), sugarfermenting organism that may manifest itself in such common conditions as oral thrush or vaginitis. However, if left unchallenged, *Candida albicans* converts into an invasive mycellial fungal form whose rhizoids (finger-like projections) penetrate the gastro-intestinal mucosa causing many types of disease symptoms.

When the mucosa is penetrated by these rhizoids, the absorption of vitamins, minerals, amino acids and fatty acids can be seriously compromised and will further lead to many additional nutritional deficiencies. This breakdown and penetration of the mucosa results in the release of *Candida albicans'* metabolic toxins into the blood stream, along with intestinal substances, including undigested cellular proteins. The results of such far-reaching toxic and antigenic assaults can lead to tissue damage and systemic effects that constitute Polysystemic Chronic Candidiasis.

C. Orian Truss, M.D.[80] told how a yeast-free special diet and anti-fungus medication helped many of his sick patients to get well. His findings have helped me to help hundreds of patients to health and happiness. He said that the Candida organism can increase its numbers during periods of stress or lowered immune potential of the individual.

It is well known that the use of antibiotics for a long period of time can increase the Candida population in the intestinal tract as well as the regular use of oral contraceptive medications and other drugs.

The yeast-like state is non-invasive but when it changes to the fungus form, it is invasive into the body. Penetration of the gastro-intestinal mucosa can break down the boundary between the intestinal tract and the rest of the circulation and allows introduction into the blood stream of many substances which may be antigenic. This may explain why many individuals who have chronic Candida overgrowth commonly show a wide variety of food and environmental allergies. The incompletely digested dietary proteins can then travel into the blood stream and exert a powerful allergic assault on the immune system which is seen as allergy, even producing a wide variety of effects such as cerebral allergy with depression, mood swings and irritability being a result.

Dr. Truss found that the classic test for *Candida albicans* overgrowth, a stool culture, does not always pin-point the chronic infection problem. His experience suggests that a clinical trial of an anti-Candida program is best administered when there are symptoms suggesting Candida overgrowth. Relying upon stool culture information alone to assess the problem many times leads to a missed diagnosis.

In my practice, I also use a simple urine test known as the "Indican Test" to help me in diagnosing this condition. It has been shown that when the yeast overgrowth plugs up the villi of the intestinal mucosa, a gas known as Indole is formed and this gas is absorbed into the blood stream and carried out through the kidneys. Measuring this Indole in the urine gives me a fairly good indication that a person may be suffering from an overgrowth of Candida. This is not a specific test, and is not reliable to determine a patient's response to therapy.

When the Candida yeast germ changes to a fungus form it definitely weakens our immune system. Our immune system is also affected adversely by heavy exposure to molds in the air and by exposure to chemicals, especially when this exposure is heavy or continuous. These chemicals may include gasoline, diesel fumes and other petro chemicals, formaldehyde, perfumes, cleaning fluids, insecticides, tobacco, and other indoor and outdoor pollutants.

When your resistance is lessened, you may feel bad "all over" and develop respiratory, digestive and other symptoms, including fatigue, nervousness, depression, muscle aches and genitourinary symptoms, and you are apt to develop sensitivity to additional foods and to numerous chemicals in your environment. Such allergies cause the membranes of your nose, throat, ear, bladder and intestinal tract to swell and you tend to develop nose, throat, sinus, ear, bronchial, bladder and other infections.

Because you develop such infections, you're apt to be given a "broad spectrum" antibiotic by a physician who really does not understand the Candida problem. Such antibiotics promote the growth of Candida and your illness may continue until the cycle is interrupted by a comprehensive program designed to decrease the growth of *Candida albicans* and increase your resistance.

Since the immune system is involved in fighting Candida and other infections, as well as allergies, I have noticed that in many patients, as the fungus overgrowth becomes worse, a patient's allergies become worse, and thus a vicious cycle begins; and the only way to break the cycle is to get the fungus overgrowth treated, which allows the immune system to better fight the allergies. Therefore, when a patient begins treatment for this Candida problem the allergies usually begin to get better even though it is a slow process.

Not to diagnose and treat *Candida albicans* is a serious error because I've found that it causes more misery among women and men than all other diseases combined. In fact, I call the condition the great mimetic, because it can mimic almost any disease, from eye infections or allergy to colitis, cystitis, gastritis, brain tumor, multiple sclerosis, [arthritis] and even insanity.

Symptoms

Symptoms may result when the yeast *Candida albicans* succeeds in penetrating the tissues. Some of these symptoms result from allergic reactions to yeast products entering the blood stream from the sites of tissue invasion, while others may be due to toxic mechanisms (non-allergenic).

Finally, in the intestinal tract and vagina, the toxins originate, at least in part, from the sites of tissue invasions by this fungus. The yeast toxins affect your immune system, nervous system and endocrine (glandular) system. Moreover, these systems are all connected.

Therefore, fungus toxins play a role in causing allergies, vaginal, bladder, prostate and other infections, as well as fatigue, headache, depression and other nervous symptoms.

Yeast toxins also play an important role in causing loss of sexual interest, impotency, premenstrual tension, menstrual irregularities, infertility, pelvic pain and other disturbances of hormone function.

Every part of your body is connected to every other part so that when fungus toxins affect one part of the body, they are also causing change in other parts. Therefore, many varied symptoms may occur in men and women, depending on which system or which body organs and tissues are affected.

In women, I've found that the most common symptoms include fatigue, headache, depression, bloating in the abdomen, vaginitis, sex and menstrual problems, memory loss and a feeling of cobwebs in their thinking. I also see quite often as symptoms of the fungus infection, muscle and joint pains, numbness and tingling in various parts of the body, as well as nasal congestion, irritability, crying spells, and hives or itching.

Occasionally I see patients who have chronic constipation and/or diarrhea, along with PreMenstrual Syndrome (PMS), infertility and Mitral Valve Prolapse. In fact, I've noticed that over 80 percent of the women who have been diagnosed as having Mitral Valve Prolapse suffer from this overgrowth of *Candida albicans*.

I've also noticed that women develop the fungus connected health disorders more frequently than men. This is probably due to hormonal changes associated with the normal menstrual cycle, because the changes promote fungus growth as does birth-control pills and pregnancy.

In women, the anatomical characteristics of a woman's genitalia make her more susceptible to vaginitis and urinary tract infections.

Women also visit physicians more often than men. Accordingly, they are more apt to receive antibiotics for respiratory, skin, urinary and other complaints.

In men, the most common symptoms I see are fatigue, depression, headache, irritability, memory loss, along with impotency and impaired sexual drive, bloating and abdominal pain.

I often see men who also have jock itch and athlete's feet, along with prostatitis, nasal congestion, skin problems, hives and itching.

Men can also have bouts of severe constipation and/or diarrhea and I have noticed that over ninety percent of patients, who have been diagnosed with Irritable Bowel Syndrome or spastic colon, suffer to a degree from this fungus overgrowth of Candida. This condition is more prevalent in men who take repeated courses of antibiotics or who consume lots of sweets, breads and alcohol.

I become suspicious of this condition in any patient who is bothered with recurrent digestive problems, food and inhalant allergies, and especially those who are bothered by fatigue, depression and nervousness. I do not, however, think that the disease is transmitted back and forth from husband to wife, but I have not been able to prove this.

When children receive repeated antibiotics, the friendly germs are wiped out and the yeast multiplies and changes into the fungus form. The toxins are produced which may affect the immune system, nervous system, respiratory system and skin. So children may also develop yeast-connected or fungus-connected health problems including diarrhea (and other digestive disorders), skin rashes, constant colds, recurring ear disorders and unusual susceptibility to chemical fumes and odors.

Among the most frequently seen fungus related disorders in children are those affecting the nervous system. Common symptoms include irritability, hyperactivity, short attention span and behavior and learning problems. Moreover, the nervous system problems in some autistic children are fungus connected[7].

Treatment

Successful treatment of Candida fungus overgrowth must follow a four-pronged attack to be effective. All four modalities of treatment must be strictly adhered to; otherwise treatment will not be effective.

I cannot emphasize this point too strongly and repeat **that you must follow the treatment plan exactly in order to get the best results of therapy. If you want to get well, you must follow these four steps of treatment and if you neglect any one of these four important steps, your treatment will be either prolonged or unsuccessful when these instructions are not carried out.**

These four steps include (a) killing the fungus overgrowth with proper diet (starving out the fungus) and medication (killing the fungus), (b) nutritional supplementation and correction of vital nutrients to build the immune system, (c) establishing a normal good bacterial flora in the intestine by supplementing *Lactobacillus acidophilus* (good intestinal germs), and (d) avoiding antibiotics, hormones, steroids and allergic foods. Of course there are other things a patient may do to speed up the healing process such as receiving proper rest, developing an exercise routine and sometimes adding garlic, aloe vera, Pau D'Arco tea and other helps.

A. Diet and Yeast Killing Medication.

The purpose of the strict diet is to limit the type of foods that feed the fungus. These foods will be discussed in a later section under Diet.

There are numerous medications that can be used to help eradicate the fungus. Some doctors use primarily nystatin powder and this is an excellent medication for treating the fungus overgrowth. I don't routinely start my patients on this medication because it is quite expensive and usually patients have to be treated for years instead of months.

I use a number of medications to treat the fungus overgrowth and some of these are more effective than others: caprylic Acid, tannic stearates and albuminates, fatty acids and even extracts from certain plants and vegetables, as well as some homeopathic remedies.

In addition, I have been recently introduced to vaginal prescription medications, but these are extremely expensive and I prefer treating my patients in a natural way without the use of drugs and chemicals that could be dangerous to some patients.

With any drug or medication, however, ***it must be emphasized that the worst thing a patient can do is to stop the treatment before therapy is completed, no matter what medication is given.*** A common problem that I have experienced many times is that patients try to "play doctor" with their treatment and after a couple of months of therapy, they begin to feel so much better that they think they are well and stop the treatment. It is impossible to get this fungus overgrowth under control until at least three or four months of therapy, and when patients discontinue the treatment, the remaining fungus that have not been destroyed will simply grow back and very often will build up a resistance to the medication that had been taken to kill the fungus overgrowth.

Patients who fall into this trap are always regretful so I insist on emphasizing to the patient that they should never stop the treatment on their own without consulting me first.

b. Vitamin, Mineral, Fatty Acid and Other Nutritional Supplements.

In order to build a patient's immune system, we must correct any vitamin, mineral and fatty acid deficiencies because all patients who have the fungus overgrowth are suffering from some or many nutritional deficiencies. Some doctors have developed a special vitamin-mineral supplement that is made available for patients that are yeast free, sugar free and is prepared in a special manner to get the best results.

I also must be sure all fatty acid deficiencies are corrected and I make sure this is accomplished by furnishing patients with supplements of the correct, necessary type of fatty acids.

I also instruct the patient in the proper eating habits to make sure that they do not develop further deficiencies of these vital elements in the future.

I also have to be sure that certain amino acid deficiencies are corrected and this is done by supplementing certain amino acids in the vitamin/mineral supplement as well as making sure that the patient is following the proper diet.

The above measures are absolutely necessary to ensure that the immune system is functioning properly, and to also ensure that the patient gets well as soon as possible.

c. Establishing a Normal Gut Flora.

To build up the good germs in our gastrointestines, I routinely prescribe a special form of *Lactobacillus acidophilus*. There are literally dozens of different types of acidophilus on the market today and the majority of them simply do not work. I've searched the entire United States for available types of acidophilus and I now routinely make available to the patient the type that I am confident is the very best available.

The type I use is a powdered form (absolutely essential), and it must be refrigerated, and it contains at least ten billion good germs per one-fourth teaspoon which equals one gram.

I've chosen this product because of its potency, good quality and effectiveness. Although the claims and labels on many types of acidophilus look the same, there are many strains that are not effective and have low potency and low bacteriologic count due to storage and handling. The type I use has proven that it works and is effective.

Acidophilus in capsule form is not effective because we must build up the good germs in the mouth and throat. Capsules simply bypass these areas.

The proper manner to take the acidophilus is to take one-fourth teaspoon four times daily, mixed in a small amount of water and swished a few seconds in the mouth and then swallowed.

The main bottle should be refrigerated.

A good way to take the acidophilus when away from home is to get a small empty pill bottle or vial and after taking the morning dose, place one-fourth teaspoon of the powdered acidophilus in the vial. This should be carried with you, and at lunch time the powder can be dropped into a small amount of water and swished in the mouth and swallowed.

d. Avoidance Recommendations.

Patients are advised to avoid antibiotics in any form as well as hormones, steroids and foods that they are allergic to.

Quite often, some patients will get a secondary infection from some type of germ such as a sore throat and call me to find out whether they should take an antibiotic or not. If the patient lives in close proximity to the Clinic, I recommend that instead of taking an antibiotic, they come to the Clinic where I can give them an intravenous infusion that will kill most any germ, and thereby the patient does not have to take an antibiotic. (See following chapter or *Three Years HCl Therapy* booklet as found at our website http:/

/www.arthritistrust.org.)

Some patients are prescribed an antibiotic by their Dentist when they have dental work done, and I prefer that when this event happens, that these patients come to the Clinic for an intravenous infusion. (See following chapter or *Three Years HCl Therapy* booklet as found at our website http://www.arthritistrust.org.)

Of course, sometimes patients live a great distance from our Clinic and are unable to come in for this injection. In such situations where they may have to take an antibiotic anyhow, I recommend that they take at least one-half teaspoon of acidophilus every time they take an antibiotic pill and also recommend that these patients take at least eight thousand to ten thousand milligrams of Vitamin C in divided doses each day. This will help to stimulate the immune system as well as to build up good germs that the antibiotic would be killing.

As far as hormones, or steroids are concerned, I prefer that patients not take the substances, but sometimes patients must continue taking these medications, and I have found that we can usually get the patient's fungus overgrowth under control even though taking these medications, but it does take longer.

Should the patient have any questions concerning this item, I ask them to discuss it with me during their visit.

Discussion

The most striking characteristic of the clinical picture of Polysystemic Chronic Candidiasis is its complexity. The erratic function in many organs is evidenced by appropriate symptoms. Particularly, those originating in the central nervous system, the GI, and GU tracts, endocrine glands, skin, mucous membranes, muscles and joints, and respiratory system.

To those hearing of Candidiasis for the first time, this very complexity of its manifestation is perhaps the most single obstacle to acceptance of the concept that Polysystemic Chronic Candidiasis may be responsible for chronic illness. The objection voiced most often is that nothing could cause such multi-system illness. This reaction is understandable if human illness is viewed primarily in terms of individual organs and systems, and categorized as heart trouble, liver disease, kidney disease, stomach trouble, etc.

There are several other problems which occur at a frequency greater than expected in the general population to those suffering from Polysystemic Chronic Candidiasis.

The first of these is mitral valve prolapse with dysautonomia (a broad term that describes any disease or malfunction of the autonomic nervous system). The medical history usually reveals that the symptoms on which these diagnoses were based had their beginning after typical symptoms of mold sensitivity had been present for several years. If we assume that these conditions are being diagnosed with reasonable accuracy, there has been a sharp increase in their incidence and it has paralleled the similar increase that has occurred in chronic fungus infections since the advent of broad spectrum antibiotics, birth control pills and steroid hormones.

As for the overgrowth of the fungus form of the Candida, we do know that a chemical called acetaldehyde is formed and this can have an effect on collagen (connective tissue) metabolism. This, I'm sure, is in some way related to the mitral valve prolapse problems and it may also be related to an increase of a condition called Carpal Tunnel Syndrome, which I'm seeing more frequently.

I'm also finding that many patients exhibit extreme intolerance to formaldehyde. Many companies in the home construction business are using formaldehyde in glues for plywood and paneling boards, etc. and this problem seems to be getting worse.

Occasionally patients date the onset of their Candidiasis to heavy formaldehyde exposure. Along with this, allergic reactions to products of *Candida albicans* occur frequently due to the antigens of this fungus. Allergic rhinitis and asthma are not uncommon and chronic idiopathic urticaria (hives) is frequently due to the antigens of this fungus.

Allergy to pollen, other inhalants and foods may appear in quick succession soon after the onset of chronic fungus infections, and on occasion may disappear abruptly with no therapy other than yeast suppression — this suggests a relationship between *Candida albicans* and the unknown changes in the immune system that allow or cause allergic reactions to occur.

Once therapy is initiated, the symptoms of approximately one in five patients will worsen. This is called a Herxheimer Reaction which will be described in the next chapter. Some doctors call this a "dieoff reaction" and others may even call it a "healing crisis." It occurs when a large number of Candida organisms are killed off during initial stages of treatment, resulting in a sudden release of toxic substances that results in an immune response and intensified symptoms. It normally lasts no longer than a week and is frequently confused as an allergic reaction toward the therapeutic agents.

The use of nutritional supplements and therapeutics, as opposed to drugs, tends to lessen the intensity, duration and frequency of these symptoms. However, when symptoms are severe, treatment should be backed off to tolerable levels and built up over time.

When the Herxheimer is too severe, I usually recommend that patients cut the dosage of their medication in half for a week and then go back to the original dosages.

If symptoms persist, alternative options for treatment may be given.

Patients should continue treatment for this condition for at least three to four months before stopping treatment. If treatment is discontinued before the patient gets the condition under control, all their symptoms will usually return.

After the fungus overgrowth has subsided and the yeast is killed down to a normal level (and this takes at least three to four months) the medications and supplements are gradually decreased over a period of six to eight weeks and the patients are allowed to gradually add previously forbidden foods to their diet.

Foods You Should Avoid In Your Diet When Treating Candida Fungus Overgrowth

The Candida fungus grows on sugar and starch and high carbohydrate foods and is fed by gluten containing grains. Gluten grains include wheat, oats, rye and barley. The fungus also grows and is fed by other yeast molds, and yeasty foods. It is known that yeast, molds and fungi cross-react.

When taken in food or even breathed in high concentrations, they trigger symptoms and diminish the body's resistance to Candida overgrowth.

Bathrooms and air vents should be kept clean and dry. Yeast molds and fungi should be minimized in foods. Therefore:

1. Do not eat any sweets or desserts of any type and this includes products made with honey or molasses as well as any form of sugar or products listed on labels that end in "ose," such as fructose, glucose, maltose, lactose, etc.

2. Do not eat wheat, oats, rye, barley, or corn. Starchy foods such as rice, potatoes, buckwheat, beans and corn, should also be excluded from the diet while treatment is being undertaken. Two rice cakes each day are allowed, however. A bowl of oatmeal is allowed each day, if desired.

3. Milk (even raw) encourages Candida fungus growth. Try to avoid milk, and milk products, except butter and plain unsweetened yogurt and especially avoid any yogurt that has fruit or sugar in it. Patients on this program are allowed one glass of either sweet milk or buttermilk each day.

4. Yeast is used in food preparation and flavoring in all commercial breads, rolls, coffee cakes, pastries, cakes and this, of course, includes hot dog and hamburger buns, cookies, crackers, biscuits and pastries of any kind. You must be very careful with any flour products or even meats fried in cracker crumbs as well as all cereals. All beer, wine and all alcoholic beverages contain yeast and therefore must be avoided. You should also avoid commercial soups, potato and corn chips and dry-roasted nuts. Vinegar and vinegar containing foods such as pickled vegetables, sauerkraut, relishes, green olives and salad dressings all contain yeast and should not be used. Don't forget that soy sauce, cider and natural root beer also contain yeast. Also, all malted products contain yeast, as well as catsup, mayonnaise, pickles, condiments, and most salad dressings. The citrus fruit juices either frozen or canned usually contain yeast and only home-squeezed fruit juices are yeast

free. All dried fruits such as prunes, raisins and dates contain yeast, as well as all antibiotics.

5. Yeast is the basis for most vitamin and mineral preparations. Nearly all vitamin and mineral preparations purchased at a drug store or from a large pharmaceutical manufacturer is loaded with yeast and should not be taken. If the patient has any doubts about other supplements I ask them to please check with me or my Clinic before taking them. Some vitamins purchased in health food stores that claim to be yeast free are not really yeast free and one must be careful or they can really aggravate your fungus overgrowth.

6. Molds build up on foods while drying, smoking, curing and fermenting. You should therefore avoid pickled, smoked or dried meats, fish and poultry, including sausages, salami, hot dogs, pickled tongue, corn beef, pastrami, smoked sardine or other fish that have been dried or smoked. You should not eat any pork of any type as pork is usually loaded with molds and yeast. Dried fruits, such as prunes, raisins, dates, figs, citrus peels, candied cherries, currents, peaches, apples and apricots should be avoided. All cheeses (including cottage cheese), sour cream, and other milk products, such as mentioned above, should be avoided. Chocolate, honey, maple syrup and nuts accumulate mold and should be avoided.

7. Melons (especially cantaloupe and watermelon) and the skins of fleshy vegetables or fruits accumulate mold during growth.

8. Avoid canned or frozen citrus, grape and tomato juice. Avoid all canned or frozen foods which contain citric acid.

9. Mushrooms, truffles and many herbal products such as black tea, are loaded with yeast and should be avoided if at all possible. Don't forget that teas including herb teas and spices are dried foods and accumulate molds, so you should avoid these.

10. Eating fruit will boost blood sugar levels and will encourage yeast growth. But one fruit is allowed each day under this program, with the exception of melons and grapes. Bananas are probably the third highest sugar containing fruit and should be limited in amounts.

Be sure you read through this list of forbidden foods numerous times in order that you can familiarize yourself with what you can and cannot have to eat. Once you're familiar with these foods, it will enable you to select acceptable foods while dining in a restaurant or while visiting friends or neighbors at meal time. You should definitely learn those foods that you must stay away from if you want to get the best results in your treatment.

I'm sure you may be thinking "what else is there left to eat." We'll describe those, but meanwhile it is absolutely necessary that you carefully look at all labels on the canned and packaged foods and consult the above list constantly, or you will continue to suffer needlessly the consequences of the fungus overgrowth in your body.

You can eat out in a restaurant but order very carefully. Skip the cocktails. Have virgin olive oil and lemon juice on your salads. In fact, I routinely prescribe one tablespoon of virgin olive oil each day for patients being treated for Candida fungus overgrowth, because it not only has some good fatty acids in it, but the olive oil kills Candida.

When dining out, order fish, chicken, turkey or lean red meats (other than pork) or other animal proteins that are prepared without sauces which might contain sugar, mushrooms or wheat as a thickener, and other harmful ingredients. Broiled or plain items are obviously the safest choice. Steamed vegetables are perfect but you must skip bread, crackers and desserts of any kind.

Remember, you must totally and absolutely avoid:

1. All sweets and desserts and sugar foods in any shape, form or fashion.

2. All breads and flour products (including whole wheat) of any kind.

3. All cheeses while on this program.

4. Any kind of alcohol beverages which are strictly forbidden since they contain sugar and yeast.

Candida Diet Allowables: What you Can Eat on This Program

Vegetables

Artichokes Asparagus Bamboo Shoots Beet Greens
Broccoli Brussels Sprouts Cabbage Caraway
Carrots Catnip Cauliflower Chicory Collards
Dandelion Dulse Egg Plant Endive Fennel
Green Beans (Fresh) Green Peas (Fresh) Kelp Mustard Greens Okra
Peppers Rhubarb Squash String Beans Swiss Chard
Turnip Green Water Cress

To wash vegetables, use one tablespoon of bleach or Clorox in one gallon of cool water (Or see prior chapter on H_2O_2.)

Salad Vegetables

Alfalfa Sprouts Bamboo Shoots Broccoli Cabbage

Caraway Catnip Cauliflower Celery
Chard Chives Cress Dandelion Dulse
Endive Fennel Kale Kelp Leeks Peppers
Rhubarb Spinach Squash Swiss Chard

Water Cress Fresh tomatoes and onions are also allowed, along with summer squash and zucchini — all types of squash.

Meats and Proteins (All Lean Cuts)

Beef Chicken Clams Crab Eggs
Ham Lobster Salmon Shrimp Tuna
Turkey Veal

Also all game birds and animals such as squirrel, rabbit, quail, duck, goose and venison are allowed. Nuts and Seeds

In limited amounts (one ounce) — Walnuts, Sunflower Seeds and Pumpkin Seeds.

Oils Use only cold pressed or expeller pressed or non-hydrogenated oils. Also, you should take one tablespoon of virgin olive oil each day on your salads or vegetables. You can add lemon juice to this if you so desire. The best salad dressing is virgin olive oil in lemon juice.

Other Items

You may have two rice cakes daily.

Eat real butter and totally avoid all margarine.

You may have plain unsweetened yogurt but no yogurt with fruit or sugar in it. You may have one cup of oatmeal (the old fashioned kind) per day.

One small to medium fruit per day is permitted, but no melons or grapes.

You may have any unsweetened, decaffeinated drink. Any coffee you drink should be decaffeinated and your tea should be weak. If you must drink diet drinks they should be caffeine free and sugar free and you may have no more than two each day, maximum. You may have either two packages of Nutri-Sweet® or Equal® or Aspartame® as sweeteners, but no more each day, whether they are in packages or in your diet. You may, however, have Sweet and Low® or saccharine in any amounts you desired. [Stephan Cooter, Ph.D. says that "It might be of interest to know that Aspartame or Nutri-Sweet, when metabolized, is half transformed into aldehydes responsible for the diet drink `hangover': H.J. Roberts, *Sweet'ner Dearest*, Sunshine Sentinel Press, ISBN 0-9633360-1-5. *Citizens for Health Newsletter*, for instance, reported that the FDA had over 5,500 complaints against Aspartame in 1992, uncomfortably and closely related to worsening of Multiple Sclerosis and arthritic symptoms, tied to aldehyde toxicity"[92] We encourage you to use Stevia or xylitol instead of Nutri-Sweet® or Equal® or Aspartame® as sweeteners: Ed.]

You may use salt, pepper, garlic or onions if you desire.

For those patients who tend to lose weight easily, and especially those who should not lose any weight, I recommend that these patients eat three or four large tablespoons of homemade mayonnaise each day.

You must not use store bought mayonnaise as it contains hydrogenated oils. The mayonnaise recipe listed below contains 120 calories per tablespoon which will help prevent any excess weight loss by eating this each day.

Of course, if you are overweight you should avoid this mayonnaise.

The recipe for mayonnaise is as follows: Take two fresh eggs, preferably at room temperature (take out of the refrigerator for a couple of hours before using) and add two tablespoons of freshly squeezed lemon juice (no bottled lemon juice) and add one teaspoon of salt (preferably sea salt [Hint: All labeled "Sea Salt" is not necessarily recommended. Try Grain and Salt Society, Inc.; Ed]). Mix this in your blender and add slowly one and one-fourth cup of cold pressed or expeller pressed or non-hydrogenated safflower oil. [The editor has used Virgin Olive Oil, as well as other safe oils. Not all safflower oil is recommended.]

This is an excellently tasting mayonnaise and when refrigerated will last two to three weeks. Don't forget that the diet in this treatment is absolutely vital and failure to comply with this diet will result in failure of treatment of your fungus overgrowth condition.

[Stephan Cooter, Ph.D. would also remind arthritics that an additional screening of the Candidiasis diet may be necessary to avoid the Nightshade family tobacco, potatoes, tomatoes, green peppers, and eggplant[92].]

Medicines Used

Dr. Prosch uses a variety of substances to kill *Candida albicans* overgrowth, among which are: Micocydin®, Paramicrocidin®, Par-Qing®, Borage Oil, SAM EPA®, *Lactobacillus acidophilus*, and various forms of Caprylic Acids and Olive Oil.

Most organic fatty acids are fungicidal. S.M. Peck and H. Rosenfeld demonstrated that Undecylenic Acid is about six times more effective as an antifungal agent than caprylic acid[93].

Candida Purge

William (Bill) G. Neely, D.C.[94] of Johnson City, TN successfully uses a Candida Purge that contains a mixture of items to be used in a certain way, which will kill overgrowth while also helping to scrape fungal Candida from the intestinal tract. The mixture contains Caprol (Caprylic + Oleic Acids), Psyllium, Bentonite and *Lactobacillus acidophilus*.

The Caprylic Acid is fungicidal for *Candida albicans*. It is harmless to friendly intestinal flora, and effective against the invasive mycelial form as well as the yeast form, because it is absorbed by the intestinal mucosal cells. Caprylic Acid is metabolized by the liver and does not get into the general circulation. It must exert its fungicidal effect in the intestinal tract or not at all. According to studies, just ten minutes after oral intake of straight caprylic acid, more than 90% can be traced in the portal vein on its way to the liver. Consequently, Caprol should be taken with Psyllium Powder which will form a gel in the intestinal tract and release the caprylic acid trapped within over a period of time.

Oleic Acid (major component of Virgin Olive Oil: 56-83%) hinders conversion of *Candida albicans*

yeast to the more harmful mycelial fungal form.

Psyllium gradually scrapes away *Candida albicans'* breeding ground (fecal encrustations) from the colon wall, absorbs toxins within the colon and carries them out, reduces toxic overload ("die-off reaction") from poisons released by dying Candida during treatment start-up and forms the gel which binds Caprol into a timed-release formulation. This powdered product gives slippery adhesive bulk to help loosen and dig out old, congested, solidified fecal matter that often coats the colon walls, thereby providing a breeding ground for *Candida albicans*, and other undesirable microorganisms. Because psyllium is not absorbed itself, toxic wastes are carried out in the feces.

Lactobacillus acidophilus arrests intestinal *Candida albicans* overgrowth, and is also effective against many pathogenic bacteria, thereby strengthening the immune system by lessening its workload.

Bentonite directly adsorbs *Candida albicans* and flushes them out, adsorbs toxins within the colon and flushes them out, and reduces toxic overload ("die-off reaction") from poisons released by dying Candida during treatment start-up.

According to Frederic Damrau, M.D.[95] "Bentonite is a native, colloidal, hydrated aluminum silicate.

. . . It has been established in vitro and in vivo that hydrated aluminum silicate adsorbs toxins, bacteria and viruses. This property helps explain its therapeutic usefulness in acute diarrhea of diverse etiology. By virtue of its physical action bentonite serves as an adsorbent aid in detoxification of the intestinal canal."

Because bentonite is not itself absorbed, whatever it adsorbs is removed in the feces. This includes miscellaneous intestinal poisons, toxins generated by Candida (especially during treatment start-up), and the Candida itself!

Patients with severe Candidiasis (up to 50% of the cases) may experience certain uncomfortable effects within the first week after initiation of the Candida Purge program at the intensive level of therapy, such symptoms as flu symptoms (stuffiness, headache, general aches, diarrhea) skin rashes, and vaginal irritation/discharge may result from the release of toxins from a rapidly dying *Candida albicans* population. The exact symptom picture will depend upon the individual case and is often dramatic — anything from "lead feet" to mental aberrations. The exact symptoms are neither important nor do they lend themselves to explanation, and they'll all disappear in a few days, as also happens when the Herxheimer effect is incurred in the successful treatment of other diseases.

Search for Goodbye Candida on the web. Whoever is handling it will probably have all of the Candida

Purge ingredients.

Garlic, Aloe Vera, Pau D'Arco Tea

In the foregoing, Gus J. Prosch, Jr., M.D. mentioned that there are other substances that can be used also, such as garlic, aloe vera, Pau d'Arco tea and other items.

Garlic[96] is certainly an important supplement that will speed your recovery by killing off *Candida*

albicans and preventing formation of lipids in the membrane of Candida, thus obstructing their intake of oxygen.

The use of an odor-modified garlic extract (Kyolic®) seems to shift lipids into the bloodstream, causing initially higher serum lipid levels, but the lipids are then broken down and finally excreted from the body, according to Benjamin H.S. Lau, M.D., Ph.D.[20].

The use of this odor-modified garlic is dose dependent, and over six months of daily usage, the good lipids, HDL, increase and the bad guys, LDL/VDL, decrease.

Garlic has long been known as a natural antibiotic, without damage to the "good guys" microflora, but now Dr. Lau and many other scientists and physicians have shown that *Candida albicans* drastically reduces in the blood stream throughout six months of continuous usage. More than that, however, is evidence that shows increased protection from radioactivity damage, environmental pollution, cancer protection, damage from stress, and it is generally an immune booster, a nutritional supplement, antioxidant, detoxifier, anti-clotting agent and anti-microbial.

The studies by Dr. Lau were performed chiefly with cold-aged garlic preparations from Wakunaga

Pharmaceutical Co., Osaka, Japan, but can also be purchased in the United States[96].

Molybdenum Approach to the

Handling of *Candida albicans* Aldehydes

Dr. Stephan Cooter[98] writes of a novel and new way to utilize the damaging byproduct of *Candida albicans*, that is, ethanol, and its descendant, aldehyde.

Dr. Cooter says that ethanol is not bad in itself, but when we receive too much of it, it converts to aldehydes. "If you have adequate amounts of glutamine, selenium, niacin, folic acid, B6, B12, iron and molybdenum, aldehydes continue to be metabolized into acetic acid, which can be excreted, or converted further into acetyl coenzyme A. If these nutrients are in poor supply, aldehydes begin collecting in

the body's tissues.

So when Candida is fully nourished (or we are), Candida furnishes the body with a necessary part of the Krebs energy cycle necessary for the health and maintenance of all cells. When our digestion is unbalanced, we incompletely convert sugars into poisons and they remain poisons in our human systems. When our digestion is balanced, or we give it what it needs in terms of supplements, a potential poison is transformed into a source of energy: i.e., aldehyde poison becomes acetyl coenzyme A[98]."

The metabolic pathway described by Dr. Cooter is that ethanol converts to aldehyde to acetic acid to acetyl coenzyme A.

Cooter writes that, "Within days of taking 100 mcg of molbydenum three times a day, I could feel the poisons from

Candida garbage transforming themselves into heat and energy. Where I had

experienced pain in my neck and shoulders, I felt warmth. A stiff back that felt like a wall of steel was transformed into copious sweat. My muscles relaxed and were pain free. At the same time, the person I was who found it difficult to get out of bed, became someone who needed only 4 to 8 hours of sleep rather than 10 or 12. Where I had been confined within a prison of fatigue, the fatigue was translated into an open expanse of energy and possibility. An intellectual fog that had filled my head for years scattered itself the first day I took molybdenum. I had lived with an aldehyde hangover for so long, I had no idea what it was like to experience mental clarity[98]."

Dr. Cooter stated that 100 mcg tablets of molybdenum amino chelate were chewed or sucked three times a day for 30 days in volunteer studies performed by himself and Walter Schmitt, Jr., D.C, with gratifying success for about two-thirds of the people who did try the supplement[98]. Their studies included changes in chronic fatigue, chronic weakness, joint pain, muscle pain, headache frequencies, mental concentration, depression, memory, and insomnia.

As Drs. Schmitt and Cooter have addressed the one problem that few other doctors have been able to find a solution for, i.e., the aldehyde poisoning caused by *Candida albicans*, they are to be commended. A Candida treatment was also formulated called "Exspore." Dr. Schmitt's clinical findings were published in 1991, *Digest of Chiropractic Economics*, 31:4:56-63, and it was his insalivations protocol Dr. Cooter followed for both himself and the 31 people in Dr. Cooter's study. Dr. Cooter says, "Of special interest to me, was that Dr. Schmitt's discussion of aldehyde oxidase, the primary enzyme that metabolizes aldehyde into acetic acid and then acetyl coenzyme A, requires molybdenum for the conversion. Also Drs. Henzi, Ponzi, and Schwyzer in Switzerland and Germany have found, for instance, that B12 and folic acid, provided a different metabolic pathway for the metabolism of formaldehyde in multiple sclerosis patients (*Let's Live*, January, 1993: 66-68.)[92]"

We believe that the findings of Stephan Cooter/Walter Schmitt are well worth investigating for yourself.

Dr. Prosch's Patient's Preliminary Diagnostics: Yeast Overgrowth Index

Directions: Check each line item that applies to you. Make your choice to the best of your ability and memory.

First Set How many mercury amalgam dental fillings? Have you been vaccinated within past 5 years?

All other questions refer to the past year, only.

Have persistent Prostatitis or Vaginitis. Have taken Cortisone type drugs.

Have taken birth control pills. React badly to cigarette smoke. React badly to chemical fumes. Symptoms worse on damp or muggy days. Have had athlete's foot and/or Jockey itch. Have cramps

with my periods.

Crave alcohol (beer, wine, whisky). Feel helpless at times. Seem to have lost interest.

Lost or decreased sexual desire. Shaky or irritable when hungry. Cannot seem to concentrate. Stomach gets sore all over. Ears itch at times.

Had bladder infections.

Had urinary frequency or urgency. Vaginal discharge

Feel weak all over.

More nervous than usual.

Often am dizzy or light-headed. Heart pounds or beats fast. Had constipation and/or diarrhea. Mouth ulcers

Total Number of Check Marks for Set One.

Second Set

Took antibiotics 3 times in past few years? Took antibiotics 3 times in past year? Have Premenstrual

Syndrome (PMS).

Have Mitral Valve Prolapse. Have allergic symptoms often. Strong perfumes make me sick. Have had a skin or nail fungus.

Crave sugar, desserts or chocolate. Crave breads, and/or pastries.

Have trouble thinking clearly. Noticed numbness or tingling. Pains in my stomach. Hypoglycemia (low blood sugar). Chronic rashes or itching skin. Had nausea and a "sick" stomach. Joints ache at times.

Feel tired most of the time. Feel "drained" and exhausted. Stomach bloats frequently. Have a poor memory.

Feel "spacey" and unreal. Muscles ache more often. Have depression fairly often. Have headaches frequently. Headaches are getting worse.

Total Number of Check Marks for Set Two.

Patient's Name

You've now shown me that you really want to get well! I sincerely appreciate the time you've spent filling out this questionnaire. Don't forget to bring it with you for your first office visit. With the above answers, I can start your program to get you well and in the best of health. **Thanks for your efforts!**

Please don't write below this line.

For Physician's use only:

First Set:

Total number check (V) marks X 1

Last Set

Total number check (V) marks X 2

Total Score

1. Below 6 — No yeast overgrowth.

2. 7 to 12 — Minimal yeast overgrowth.
3. 13 to 20 — Moderate yeast overgrowth.
4. 21 and higher — Severe yeast overgrowth.

Scoring

The Herxheimer Effect Dr. Paul Pybus, a surgeon, acupuncturist and Englishman, resided in South Africa. He was our friend and former Chief Medical Advisor for The Arthritis Trust of America.

In the 1960s he worked with Roger Wyburn-Mason, M.D. the man who brought us our first consistently successful treatment for otherwise crippling arthritis.

From early teachings by his mentor, Wyburn-Mason, Paul Pybus developed our technique of intraneural injections that is so successful for the pain of both Osteoarthritis and Rheumatoid Arthritis, and which may explain one of the causative factors of Osteoarthritis. (See Amazon.com at Kindle or Nook at Barnes & Noble) That story is elsewhere[99].

An article prepared by Dr. Paul Pybus at the same time as the above mentioned *Intraneural Injections*

. . . booklet was titled "The Herxheimer Reaction History." Paul prepared this material because of the extreme importance of noting and accounting for the Herxheimer effect when treating arthritics and many other infective diseases such as Candidiasis. It is a pity that many modern-day physicians have not been taught the Herxheimer, or, if they have, do not understand its importance when treating a number of diseases.

It's a phenomenon that results when there is an intensification of the disease symptoms and often an expansion of similar symptoms to other parts of the body, all of a temporary nature, after which the patient is improved or well. Often it appears to some as if they have the flu, and so is described as "the patient having flu-like symptoms." "Flu-like symptoms" is an over-simplification of what happens in varying cases and with varying patients.

When treating Leishmaniasis, Syphilis or Tuberculosis, the phenomena is called Herxheimer, when treating Leprosy it's called Lucio's Phenomena. Other rare tropical diseases also call it the Herxheimer. When treating Candidiasis, patients and doctors call it the "die-off effect."

When experiencing the Herxheimer there is the appearance of a war or tussle going on inside the body akin to the antigen/antibody warfare, where the body produces fever, sweat, aching and swollen joints, diarrhea, nausea, and so on, in varying proportions with varying degrees depending upon state of metabolism, genetics, source of disturbance and so on.

It is our belief that some prescription drugs wrongly are described to be toxic because, on observing a Herxheimer reaction in the patient trying the new drug, the drug researchers (and others' observations during subsequent follow-on research and use of the drug) do not fully understand the Herxheimer and believe the cause is the drug's "toxicity." Even with a full understanding of the Herxheimer effect a pharmaceutical company must follow the "rule of over-caution" to satisfy FDA requirements for the "health and safety" of us more ignorant citizens. Thus, even with knowledge of the Herxheimer effect, a physician researcher is not necessarily in a position whereby he can, or wants to, discriminate between drug toxicity and the Herxheimer effect.

It is necessary for the successful treatment of many diseases, therefore, that the physician fully comprehend the distinctions between specific drug toxicities and the Herxheimer effect. This distinction probably can come only through the experiences of applied clinical practices.

Drugs do have toxicities of their own, but the essential importance is to be able to discriminate between the two: the Herxheimer effect and drug toxicity.

This is unfortunate, as it clouds otherwise desirable treatment modes, not just those recommended in our treatment protocols. From another viewpoint, those who fully understand the distinction between the Herxheimer effect and drug toxicities find themselves with a guiding clinical tool that permits the physician early in the treatment regimen to determine the probability of success for a given patient.

Through our Physicians, we have learned that, generally speaking, the more severe the induced Herxheimer, the more probability of wellness — which is not to say that one who has a very light Herxheimer may not also get well.

Prior to Dr. Paul Pybus' work developing intraneural injections, it was felt that Osteoarthritis and Rheumatoid Arthritis had little in common, except that here and there folks with Rheumatoid Arthritis might also have some Osteoarthritis. Perhaps it is still true, that the causes are indeed distinguishable.

But one very interesting set of experiences has come forth from the application of the WyburnMason/Pybus/Prosch Intraneural Treatment on both Rheumatoid and Osteo victims: joint pain and joint damage in both diseases seem to stem from the same source, namely a disturbance in certain key trigger points along the peripheral nervous system. The peripheral nerves are usually those nerves close to the surface of the body, and have no insulative layers — similar to an electric wire passing current without insulation — called the C fibers, or "unmyelinated" fibers.

It might very well be that Osteoarthritis can be halted with Pybus' intraneurals, along with good diet, including proper supplements, hormones and changes in life style.

Those possibilities, along with Pybus' Intraneural injections are told elsewhere in our literature.

The Herxheimer Reaction History

by Dr. Paul K. Pybus, M.A., M.B., B. Chir (Cambridge), M.R.C.S., M.R.C.P. (London), D.R.C.G. (London), F.R.C.S. (England)

"This reaction was first described by an Austrian dermatologist Jarisch Adolf Herxheimer[100]

working in Vienna and Innsbruck in 1895 and shortly after this, confirmed by his brother Karl

Herxheimer[101, 102] also a dermatologist working in Frankfort.

"They were both mainly called upon to treat syphilitic lesions of skin by means of mercury and later arsenical and bismuth preparations. They both noticed that when treating these patients many of them developed signs of high fever, profuse perspiration, night sweats, nausea and vomiting. What was more they also observed that the skin lesions became larger and inflamed before settling down and healing. In addition they found that those cases that responded in this most violent manner healed the best and fastest. The patient was quite ill for 2-3 days after which the syphilitic lesions resolved.

"Jarisch Herxheimer accounted for this reaction as a toxic manifestation caused by the foreign proteins released from the dying spirocheates. Meanwhile his brother Karl[101, 102] described in detail the Herxheimer fever. There is first a febrile phase with pyrexia, malaise and often a sore throat. The lesions are then aggravated and the ash if present becomes more marked with tension in the regional lymph nodes being more pronounced. In addition the primary ulcer would become oedematous and painful (the primary chancre is characterized by its painlessness). [In a letter to *The Lancet*, p. 340, Feb. 12, 1977, it is suggested that two of the three identifying features of a Herxheimer were known since the end of the 15th century when arsenical ointment was first used to treat the great pox which had just arrived in Europe from the New World: Ed.]

"During this reaction many other signs appeared such as histologic changes such as transient acute inflammation in the lesion, a leucocytosis and lymphopaenia which was greatest as the pyrexia was at its zenith.

"It was suggested by another surgeon Heyman[103] that these histologic changes indicate that the reaction was hypersensitivity phenomenon of the delayed type similar to the tuberculi hypersensitivity type of reaction.

"Theories as to Cause

"1. *Herxheimer et al.* [101, 102, 103] The phenomenon is caused by the release of endotoxin of spirochaetal breakdown products following treatment. These products are reacting with sensitized syphilitic tissue to produce exacerbation of the lesion.

"2. *Milian.* [104] Suggested it was due to stimulation of the spirochaetes and inadequate medication.

(Bradford and Allen state that 'The purpose of endotoxin to the bacterium that produces it is to act as a semipermeable membrane, limiting and regulating the nature of substances that may enter and provide nutrient for that organism. for this reason endotoxins reside solely on or near the surface (cell wall) and are shed into the surrounding medium only upon the death of the organism. This fact may well be an explanation for what has become known as the Herxheimer reaction in which a patient becomes worse following the administration of anti-biotics or other form of treatment that kills the causative organism[105].')

"3. *Jadassohn.* [106] Suggested that the direct effect of the anti-syphilitic drug on the tissue was an entirely toxic reaction.

"4. *Fleishman.* [107]Suggested this reaction was of a vascular reflex mediated by the autonomic nervous system.

"In 1943 Mahoney et al[108] first described Jarisch Herxheimer Reaction in syphilitic patients treated with penicillin and since then it has been observed that other chemotherapeutic agents that are effective with syphilis also produce a Herxheimer reaction.

"Moore et al[109] regard the reaction as all or none phenomenon but it was found that if the dose was less than 10 international units per kilogram bodyweight the reaction did not occur. The increase of the dose, however, did not increase the degree of the reaction. It also occurred equally in the seropositive and seronegative patient.

"Joulia et al[110] reported that during the Jarisch Herxheimer reaction the eosinophils decreased showing it to be an antigen antibody reaction. However, Heyman found that using antihistamines had no effect on the reaction whatsoever.

"The Jarisch Herxheimer reaction occurs in other diseases treated with antibiotics. It has been noted in:

1. Yaws treated with penicillin.
2. Vincent's Angina treated with metronidazole.

3. Relapsing fever (also a spirochaetal disease) treated with tetracycline.

4. Rat bite fever (also due to a spirillum) treated with penicillin or tetracycline.

5. Leprosy where it is known as the Lucia phenomenon treated with Dapsone.

6. Brucellosis treated with chloramphenicol.

7. Glanders treated with erythromycin.

8. Anthrax treated with aureomycin.

9. Rheumatoid Disease treated with metronidazole [and other drugs: Ed.]

10. Psoriasis treated with metronidazole [and other drugs: Ed.]

11. [Systemic Lupus Erythematosus and Scleroderma treated with metronidazole and other drugs: Ed.]

"In 1972 Gudjonsson[111] investigated the Herxheimer reaction in adult seropositive and negative syphilitics and found a febrile reaction in 60%. It could be produced with doses above 10 International units per kilogram. However, in 30% of cases no reaction occurred until as much as 600,000 I.U. per kg, were given and so it would appear that the higher doses produced a stronger reaction than the lower ones and this was at variance with the observations of Moore.

"He also noted an increase in the neutrophils and a decrease in the lymphocyte count which occurs when the temperature is greatest. The Eosinophil decreased and may be due to the degranulation of their cells as they phagacytose the breakdown products of the treponemes. This is also an observation in my own series of treated rheumatoid arthritis cases with metronidazole as the eosinophils are completely removed from the blood in most cases with a positive Herxheimer reaction.

"**Effect of Prednisone on Herxheimer reaction**. Here the Prednisone clearly influences the febrile response at a daily dose of 40 mg. The leucocyte changes are not affected and so the Prednisone influences only the febrile component and not the other manifestations of the reaction. Gudjonsson concludes that the reaction is not of an allergic nature, but is caused by some leucocyte pyrogen released by phagocytosis of the treponemes.

"**Discussion**

"If we say that Gudjonsson is correct and that the reaction is due to the release by the leucocytes of a pyrogen when something is phagocytosed, then this further suggests that the Herxheimer reaction seen when treating rheumatoid arthritis [and other diseases] with certain drugs is due to the phagocytosis of an infective agent. Thus, although no one apart from Stamm and Wyburn-Mason[112] have found amoebae for certain [in arthritics], this is strong evidence for an infective cause of the disease. [See "Free Living Amoeba & The Effects of Anti-amoebic Drugs on Rheumatoid Disease," "The Free-living Amoebic Causation and Cure of Activity in Rheumatoid and Auto-Immune Diseases," http:// www.arthritistrust.org.] An Herxheimer reaction is the one constant finding in all our search and the strength of the reaction correlates very closely to clinical improvement as shown separately by Prosch, Bingham and Pybus[99] [and now others: Ed.].

"Furthermore in my own recent series the correlation is shown to be 100% correct.

"I have also shown what would occur should these cases that I have done be analyzed on a doubleblind study by someone who was not acquainted with the Herxheimer reaction.

"Herxheimer reaction is becoming the cornerstone of our present research and unless full account is taken of its occurrence any double-blind trial performed will tend to be misleading. The mere fact that it occurs will influence any such trial and would probably be more advantageous if the final assessor could be suitably blinded as to the previous occurrences of the Herxheimer reaction.

"I had sincerely hoped that this was being done at our double-blind studies. I have strongly advocated that it be done." [The Herxheimer reaction was not taken into account at our double-blind studies at Bowman Gray School of Medicine. This study was reported separately in the "Research" section on http://www.arthritistrust.org: Ed.]

"The symptoms of the Herxheimer can be most severe. They can discourage not only the patient, but also the doctor and anyone running a trial not knowing of these, will assume they are toxic symptoms and remove the patient from the trial [as occurred at our Bowman Gray School of Medicine study on use of Clotrimazole: Ed.]

"This also occurred in the original Guy's[113] trial when they came to the conclusion that

metronidazole had no effect on rheumatoid arthritis and this lack of recognition of the Herxheimer reaction did untold damage to our cause. Not only were the numbers in the trial inadequate, only 20, but other medications were not stopped [Nonsteroidal anti-inflammatories: Ed.] Follow-up was only for 6 weeks (they should have waited at least two months), strike dosage was usually inadequate either to produce a Herxheimer or clinical improvement (400 mg b.d.) and the one case that did produce a reaction [The Herxheimer effect: Ed.] was withdrawn because of these 'side effects.'"

"**Recent Progress**

"This year I have made an analysis of 24 cases of Rheumatoid Arthritis (RA) and this revealed many interesting facts.

"In a total of 288 metronidazole nights there were only 47 nights or 16.32% when nothing happened at all. All the rest (241 or 83.68%) showed some reaction and were divided up according to the following:

Heavy perspiration and night sweats	54
Flu-like symptoms	47
Rigors	32
Fever	2
Headaches	85
Malaise	43
Diarrhea	19
Nausea	49
Vomiting	8
Pain in other joints previously unaffected	79

Burning Micurition 21
Bone pain 39
Itching 33
Flushing of skin and red patches 39

"These figures are all the more remarkable when one considers that in the normal person without rheumatoid disease, this dose of metronidazole produces no symptoms whatsoever.

"Thus, in our campaign in the treatment of rheumatoid disease, two points stand out markedly: (1.) Metronidazole and our other recommended medicines work in the treatment of Rheumatoid Diseases; (2) That a Herxheimer reaction occurs in at least 83% of metronidazole nights.

"These two points seem to prove that an infection must be at least at the root of the rheumatoid disease problem."

[I find it most interesting — and consistent — that Dr. Pybus found 83% suffer a Herxheimer reaction, and subsequently show improvement or alleviation of this disease, and that Gus Prosch, Jr.,

M.D.[114] has shown a cure/remission rate of about 80% since 1982, using these oral medications combined with intraneurals and proper diet. Other physicians report about 50% remission rate: Ed.] [It is stated and referenced in Roger Wyburn-Mason's[112] various works that The Herxheimer response only occurs when an organism more complex than a bacillus is being killed by an antibiotic and due to the Herxheimer, this fact "proves" that the infective agent must be of a complicated structure. Ed.]

"In South Africa, our research has been based on the effect of metronidazole on moving cells found in joint fluid. It has been shown that the macrophage-like cells found in the rheumatoid fluid, when challenged with metronidazole, first respond with an increased movement of a writhing character. These movements after 15 minutes largely subside to be replaced by the slower movement and eventually after 309 minutes they are mostly crenated and absorbed. Thus, the metronidazole would appear to kill the macrophage [*in vitro*: Ed.].

"Wyburn-Mason stressed that the *Amoeba chromatosa* was often confused with macrophages, and that they had the power of independent existence for a long time, which fact some of us have corroborated. [He may have viewed clusters of cell-wall deficient bacteria: Ed.]

"Kwang Jeon[115] [University of Tennessee, U.S.A.] cultured these cells in joint fluid that were up to one week old and showed that they would develop into fibroblasts. However, the fluid that had been treated with metronidazole grew nothing.

"Davies[116] has noted these macrophages in penassy fluid left at room temperature were still fresh (active) for as long as 24 days.

"Wyburn-Mason[117] described the macrophage in great detail and gave it great prominence in his book on the reticulo-endothelial system. He concluded it was not mesodermal in origin as is so often claimed and said, but not proved, to develop from the monocyte, but rather was it neuroectodermal in origin and was developed from the trophic nerve ending.

"Later, when working with Stamm[112], he was convinced that these were in all probability amoebae. Furthermore, they both claimed that they had cultured them, but attempts by all of us have failed to repeat this.

"However, these macrophages have been grown at the University of Tennessee by Kwang Jeon and this, I feel, is a great step forward."

For those who are interested in pursuing the easing of the Herxheimer, the following suggestions have been *made, in addition to various traditional allopathic remedies.*

As the "die-off effect" is the same as the well-known Herxheimer effect, one might also ease the pain of temporarily increasing toxins by use of a steam (dry or hot) sauna or sign-up for a complete detoxification as practiced by members of the Church of Scientology. Any Church outlet can steer you to the closest detox center. This detoxification is rather severe, requiring a physician's approval, and also the daily replacement of specific vitamins, minerals and fatty acids, as it is the lipids (fats) in the cells that hold toxins and therefore must release them. [See the chapter on "Allergies and Biodetoxification]

Russ McMillan, D.D.S., D.P.H., Dr. P.H. suggests "something that helps with the rather debilitating symptoms that accompany the Herxheimer effect after medication. I take a saltz bath which consists of adding 1 cup salt, 1 cup soda, 1 cup Epsom salts, 1 cup aloe vera, to a hot bath which I remain in and keep hot for about 1-1/2 hours all the while consuming about 2 quarts of warm water. Evidently the

perspiration and osmotic pressure removes the causative toxins. I find it quite helpful[118]."

One short note to the unwary. Our civilization throws aspirin or Non-steroidal Drugs (NSAIDS) at children or adults at the least showing of fever. While some very high temperature fever can be damaging and should be brought down by a professional, most fevers are the body's method of fighting off and killing an invasive organism. By shutting down the fever one is encouraging the invasive organism by eliminating the body's weapon against it. When treating many diseases based on an invasive organism the Herxheimer can become so intense that one welcomes symptomatic relief. Usually no harm is done by relieving some of the Herxheimer symptoms. Keep in mind, though, that the body is doing what it needs to do for the moment to achieve wellness.

Hydrochloric Acid for Untreatable Bacterial Infection

The idea of injecting hydrochloric acid (HCl) into your plumbing might scare you a bit, but consider these facts: (1) everything you eat is saturated with HCl in your stomach so that food's chemistry can be torn apart and reassembled into nutrients that each cell requires; (2) your immune system, in part, already utilizes HCl to kill invasive microorganisms.

The amount of HCl we're reporting on here is far, far too dilute to harm you. From personal experience it is about the same as injecting pure water, such is the dilution.

There is much in the news media of late concerning the great danger of antibiotic-resistant bacterial infections. We have a few bacteria now for which there is only one expensive antibiotic that will contain them. There has been dire warnings that the time may not be far off when there will be deadly bacteria resistant to all antibiotics. For treatment of some antibiotic resistant strains of tuberculosis the time is already here. No antibiotic will kill these super-evolved germs and, as usual, the allopathic intransigent attitude is to find an antibiotic that will work, never mind the folks now suffering and dying. Don't step out of the pattern that bullying pharmaceutical companies have laid down, develop another antibiotic no matter the cost in money or lives!

We talked to a doctor who was the Chief Medical Officer for a city/county government. His function was to oversee public health concerns, such as sexually related diseases and tuberculosis. When discussing the problem cases of incurable tuberculosis we asked, "Why don't you use HCl therapy on those who don't respond to antibiotics? It's been around since before WWI, and will absolutely kill any bacterial infection by stimulating the body's natural immune system."

His answer: "I don't dare use anything that's not in the public health manual!"

This is real — but really unreal! This is the state of our allopathic medical system dictated to by special interests — medical application via written down recipes. What was all the medical training for? To read and follow an inapplicable recipe though death is certain?

During the past twenty four years the Arthritis Trust of America was been fortunate to have Wayne Martin as one of our most esteemed advisors. Wayne was not just a knowledgeable advisor, but also a fine friend, one who unstintingly gave of his medical knowledge to whoever inquired.

Wayne Martin graduated from Purdue University with a BS in Chemical Engineering in 1933 with major emphasis on biochemistry and bacteriology. Depression years of the twenties and thirties prevented him from obtaining a medical degree, his first love, but did not stop him from a lifetime of interesting synthesis of the world's medical literature, often resulting in discoveries of interesting treatments used today by many complementary/alternative medical practitioners.

His professional work in Chemical Engineering also resulted in remarkable findings results of which are still used by people everywhere. Ninety percent of the beryllium copper alloys used worldwide contain 1.80% of beryllium instead of the more expensive form of 2.2 to 2.5% beryllium set by Germans at the Siemans and Haliske Company. Working at the Beryllium Corporation, Wayne Martin in

1935 discovered that the 1.80% beryllium to copper alloy (Berylco 180) was superior in many ways and less expensive. For more than fifty years automobiles — and you — have used Wayne Martin's beryllium alloy.

Early in World War II, at the Sperry Gyroscope Company, and also as a "dollar-a-year" consultant with the Federal War Production Board (WPB), Wayne Martin developed two National Emergency (N.E.) aluminum casting alloys (319, 380). Ninety-five percent of today's aluminum castings are made of these two alloys. Sixty million pounds monthly of this aluminum alloy is currently used to produce the modern automobile.

At end of World War II, the Beryllium Corporation was stuck with a plant owned by the Atomic Energy Commission for which they wanted a peace-time use. Wayne suggested that it be used to make potassium titanium fluoride. The entire aluminum industry uses it to grain-refine aluminum. After its return to the Atomic Energy Commission, Henry Kawecki, Wayne's friend, formed the Kawecki Chemical Company to manufacture potassium fluoride, becoming a multimillion dollar firm, all on Wayne's

ideas.

In 1950 Wayne Martin helped to place aluminum/magnesium alloy (AL MG 35) for which there was a large market. In 1960 he developed another aluminum alloy (Precedent 71) which, over a period of 20 years made his employer, U.S. Reduction Company, a great deal of money. (Think of airplanes, among other uses.)

Wayne retired in 1979, becoming a salesman with The Southern Aluminum Casting Company of Bay Minette, Alabama. Thereafter each retirement has led to further consulting jobs, so he never truly retired until his death in May 13, 2006.

So why was a Chemical Engineer who invented important metal alloys featured as a consultant in medicine?

Although the great American depression had steered him elsewhere for survival's sake, he never lost touch with medicine. His enquiring mind synthesized many medical articles and research papers to bring to light remarkable treatments in heart, cancer, and for possible solution in other medical problems.

In one example from years' gone by, in 1963 Wayne organized the Nutrition Research Products Company dedicated to doing something about the 600,000 deaths each year from heart attacks. His idea was carried to The Royal College of Surgeons and The National Heart Hospital in London, England, where Nutrition Research Products Company spent $200,000, and proved that his ideas were effective in preventing heart disease.

Wayne periodically gave himself weak hydrochloric acid shots because he'd learned — long before the advent of antibiotics — that administration of these weakened solutions stimulated macrophage and leucocyte activity, thus killing and/or warding off invasive infections.[119] His story about the

Harvard medical school graduate who became wealthy by specializing in this treatment for prostitutes in Las Vegas, NV was very educational as well as hilarious. After this physician's license was threatened in Massachusetts — apparently for curing folks the wrong way — the physician moved to Nevada where he specialized in treating prostitutes with the use of dilute HCl injections. He became very rich and at last retired in San Francisco as the owner of some very lucrative property. In the allopathic approach it seems to be not sufficient to cure someone unless it's done in the politically corrected and approved cookbook manner.

Wayne had a lifetime love affair with study of problems related to the heart and circulation and also with various types of cancers.

Many years before the expenditure of billions of dollars to "find the cure for cancer," Coley's toxin was bringing about remarkable "permanent remissions" in cancer. This so aggravated the medical monetary and power structure that the simple mixture was forbidden by the FDA. Having seen at first hand cures brought about by this mixture in his early adulthood, Wayne could never cease telling about it. Several years before his death he invested a goodly sum of his own money to have the product made in Brazil, thus making it available to any patient who wished to use it.

Again, alas! The long arm of "forbidden medicine" reached into Brazil, and the US supply was again halted.

Nonetheless, Wayne found another way to help cancer patients by publishing the formula for Coley's toxin so that any patient or doctor can make up their own supply, if desired.[120] (See http://www.arthritistrust.org for "Here is how to make Coley's Toxins.")

But even prior to his publication of Coley's toxin, certain (unnamable) doctor friends began manufacturing their own Coley's toxin and are having great success in bringing about "permanent remissions," among some of their patients!

In his youth, Martin's motorcycle accident resulted in loss of a leg. Phantom pain haunted him for years until he discovered that it could easily and safely be diminished thru the use of ginger tea.[121]

Martin was a remarkable human being, one who cared greatly for his fellow man, who gave without concern for rewards, who loved life, and who made each hour, each minute count toward bettering his fellow man.

We are so glad that he passed away peacefully — not in pain or suffering from degenerative disease — just a few months before his 95th birthday! But, we are not at all happy that he passed so early in his life — and we shall sorely miss this intelligent, generous, kind scientific advisor!

Wayne Martin's tips about the use of HCl follows. He writes:

"Here is a suggestion that we go back and have a good look at intravenous infusions of 10 cc of hydrochloric acid, from one part per 500 to one part per 3,000.

"This work originated with Burr Ferguson, MD of Birmingham, Alabama. During World War I he had been a battle surgeon in France where he was seeing the ravaging effect of bacterial infections in wounds. Dr. Ferguson picked up the concept of treating bacterial infections with intravenous hydrochloric acid from another surgeon, Dr. Granville Hains in 1927. Dr. Heins had been using intravenous hydrochloric acid one part per 3,000 in treating pruritus ani with success.

"Dr. Ferguson then began treating many kinds of bacterial infections successfully with intravenous infusion of 10 cc of 1 in 1000 hydrochloric acid. When he tried to publish his results he found that no leading medical journal would accept his reports.

"There was a medical news magazine then that reported on topics that today may be called alternative medical treatments. It was called *The Medical World.* In 1932 as a student at Purdue University, I subscribed to it, I think for $5.00 a year. Dr. Ferguson wrote extensively for this publication and many not-too-orthodox doctors read what he wrote and treated bacterial infections with hydrochloric acid infusions. Some of them reported success in so doing in *The Medical World.* (See *Three Years of Hydrochloric Acid Therapy* at http://www.arthritistrust.org)

"Dr. Ferguson reported that very soon after an infusion of hydrochloric acid, there would be a marked increase in white cell count and in phagocytes; also that red cells had an increase in oxygen content. He suggested that one infusion of hydrochloric acid would increase oxygen in red cells in excess over what would result from maintaining the patient in an oxygen tent. Dr. Ferguson reported that in treating gonorrhea with bladder irrigations of 1 in 1000 hydrochloric acid, he was able to get negative smears in two days with even more rapid relief from the symptom of burning and pain.

"I am going to give one case here of the use of hydrochloric acid in treating a bacterial infection, a case to show its remarkable fast antibacterial effect. The case was reported in *The Medical World.* The doctor was William Howell, MD of the small town of Lexington, Tennessee.

"He had gotten a supply of sterile 1-1500 hydrochloric acid but had feared using it. His story is as follows: 'On August

18, 1931, I found the case to use hydrochloric acid. Five days before I had delivered a girl of 15 after a prolonged and difficult labor using all possible aseptic precautions possible in a log cabin in the woods. The large baby lived only two hours. In spite of the small size of the mother (she weighed only 90 Lbs), lacerations were small in size. Three days later a message was sent to me that she had had a chill and a very high fever. It was a long trip to the river bottom where she lived so I suspected malaria and I sent quinine.

"'On the fifth day another message came telling of the grave condition of the patient and that my immediate presence was necessary. On going into the room, I sew that there had been no mistake in this urgent message. The little girl was delirious; temperature 106, pulse 140, respiration was 40; discharge from the vagina that was fetid in odor. Every other case, in the condition in which I found her had died of this infection.

"'With much trepidation I gave her an injection of 10 cc of 1-1500 hydrochloric acid. The following minutes were anxious ones for me, as I hardly knew what to expect as this was the first time that I

had even heard of acid being used in puerperal sepsis. The reports that I had seen of Dr. Ferguson's cases were of pyrogenic infections in gunshot or lacerated wounds. As I sat by that bed holding the radial pulse in that lonely log cabin, a flood of memories of teachings concerning the fatal consequences of injections of acid into the veins came over me. While in this frame of mind I noticed sweat on the neck and forehead of the patient and along with it a slowing of the pulse and in a few minutes more she was bathed in a profuse perspiration. With it there was a cessation of the chatter of her delirium

"'Thirty minutes following the injection of the acid I asked her how she felt. She said that she felt much better and she would like to go to sleep. Within one hour the temperature had dropped to 103, the pulse to 100 and the respiration to 22.

"'During the following four days, I injected the acid every day and on the fifth day temperature was 99, pulse was 72 and respiration was 22. Two days thereafter, I was called again and was told that the fever had returned. Found her with a temperature of 101 F, with a free discharge from the vagina. I gave her another injection as before. Save for weakness, all evidence of infection had disappeared the next day. She went on to an uneventful recovery with a complete disappearance of the mass in the left iliac region.'

"So here was a case where the patient was marked for death soon and within moments of one intravenous infusion of 1 to 1500 hydrochloric acid, the patient showed dramatic improvement. Was there ever a case where an antibiotic drug was so quickly effective?

"It is suggested that if bacterial infections are again treated with infusions of hydrochloric acid, it will be found that there is no such thing as a bacterium resistant to hydrochloric acid.

"In 1932 there was very little that could be done for the pain and suffering of a patient with a gonorrhea infection of the testicles. Dr. Howell reported that by then Dr. Ferguson had told him that treatment with intravenous infusions of hydrochloric acid was effective in treating any and all bacterial infections. In that year he was referred to such a patient. Dr. Howell said that after all of his training it seemed foolish to do an injection in the arm for a swollen and painful testicle. After the first injection of hydrochloric acid the patient had pain relief. This patient had a complete recovery from the infection following eight daily injections. He added that in time he had seen a few other cases of epididymitis like this one and they all responded to injections of hydrochloric acid just as had this one.

"If Possible Replace Antibiotics with Dilute Hydrochloric Acid when fighting bacterial infections!

"With the escalating cost of medical treatment, how nice it would be to replace expensive antibiotics with dilute hydrochloric acid, the cost of which is nil.

"Many antibiotics are greatly immunosuppressive and anything that is immunosuppressive will tend to cause cancer. How much better it would be to replace immunosuppressive antibiotics with immunostimulating infusions of hydrochloric acid in treating bacterial infections."

[Wayne Martin's letter was sent in to the TLfDP [*Townsend Letters for Doctors & Patients*] on 09-11-1999.]

On 10-04, *60 Minutes* on CBS devoted one-third of the program to tuberculosis. It was said that tuberculosis is a major disaster in the making. It was said that while tuberculosis is a minor problem in the USA today, it is a major problem now in Russia, especially in prisons for men. It was said that the tubercle bacterium in Russia for the most part is resistant to all drugs that in the past have been used to treat tuberculosis.

It was suggested that a single commercial aircraft flight returning to the USA had several passengers infected with the Russian type tuberculosis. It was also said that there are no new drugs in the pipeline to treat tuberculosis because there is almost no need for them in the USA and there is no money to be made on developing a drug to treat tuberculosis in Russian prisons. It was said that if this new strain of drug-resistant tuberculosis should get a foothold in the USA, it would cause thousands of deaths and cost billions of dollars.[Resistant tuberculin strains have been in the USA for some time.] There is notation in the *Medical World* of 1932 that Dr. Burr Ferguson had indicated that tuberculosis could be treated with intravenous infusions of hydrochloric acid. Dr. William Howell, referred to above in treating puerperal sepis and gonorrheal infections, has a report in 1932 of treating with success two cases of pulmonary tuberculosis with infusions of hydrochloric acid. Both patients before treatment had suffered severe hemorrhaging of the lungs. In these cases the infusions were of 1-1500 hydrochloric acid done three times a week for several weeks. In both cases the patient became free from evening fever and began to gain weight and live a normal life. In both cases there was a notation that infusions of hydrochloric acid would continue.

If the threat of pandemic drug-resistant tuberculosis is so great, it is hoped that some not-so-orthodox doctor in the world will try treating tuberculosis with intravenous hydrochloric acid, 1-1500 every second day. There were a few cases of treating cancer with success with injections of hydrochloric acid. One such case follows: The date was May 25, 1933. The doctor was O.P. Sweatt, MD of Waxahachie, Texas. The patient had epithelioma of the lower lip extending to within a quarter-inch of the chin. The cancerous area was the size of a silver dollar. There was much swelling and pain and an offensive odor with discharge. The patient had but little appetite.

Treatment was intravenous infusions of 5cc of 1-1000 hydrochloric acid every second day. After three such injections, they were changed to intramuscular injections due to the patient having poor veins. On the sixth injection the acid was changed to 1-500 and this caused a severe reaction. After only six injections the patient had shown improvement. There was less pain, the discharge was less and the odor of it was less offensive. The patient had a better appetite and the swelling had decreased.

In the reaction there was fever, rigor and painful aching which subsided in six hours. The next day the dose was reduced to 2.5 cc and then increased on a gradual basis back to 5 cc. Over the next 100 days, there were 50 such im [intramuscular] injections. There was steady improvement such that after injection number 18, this 77 year-old man was able to go out and chop thirty rows of cotton.

Then the injections were changed back to intravenous infusions for 20 more treatments. The statement was made that at this point the patient was not cured but that the tumor was reduced to the size of a five-cent piece. Another observation was made. It was said that a black scaly substance would form over the tumor and then fall away and that each time this happened the tumor would be reduced in size a bit. Also it was noted that during this treatment, the patient had no need for pain medication.

Here we see a case where intramuscular injections seemed to be effective. Also in this case there was notable regression after only six injections of hydrochloric acid. Here again, as in treating tuberculosis, over 50 injections were used over a period of many weeks.[122]

It's clear from the testimony above and as described in *Three Years of HCl Therapy* that the answer to invasive bacteria

— even extremely resistant bacteria — was known and used as far back as the 1930s. It's often more convenient to pop a pill consisting of the latest "breakthrough" than to use that which works — especially when collusion between the FDA and pharmaceutical companies wish otherwise.

Unfortunately injectable HCl requires a physician prescription in the United States. Otherwise each of us could follow Wayne Martin's suggestion of intramuscular injections.

There are some alternative/complementary physicians who provide their patients with this simple, inexpensive remedy against damaging bacterial infection. You just need to find them!

Universal Oral Vaccine: The Immune Milk Saga! Dream Cure!!

If our earlier chapters haven't made you angry, this chapter is guaranteed to make you furious! We'll discuss the dairy industry first, especially the non-value of milk and milk products.

From childhood onward we've been indoctrinated with a listing of "healthy" foods, among which is always milk. The food value of milk according to most alternative/complementary health professionals is vastly overrated. According to William Campbell Douglass, II, M.D. (and many others) milk adversely affects our health and, of course, uses up dietary dollars best used elsewhere.

Why?

First is the fact that it is pasteurized. We've all been fed a falsehood that pasteurization makes the milk safe to drink; we won't catch various diseases if the milk is pasteurized.

How do microorganisms enter the milk supply? Our environment contains an abundance of microorganisms that find their way to the hair, udder, and teats of dairy cows and can move up the teat canal. Some of these germs cause an inflammatory disease of the udder known as mastitis while others enter the milk without causing any disease symptoms in the animal. In addition, organisms can enter the milk supply during the milking process when equipment used in milking, transporting, and storing the raw milk is not properly cleaned and sanitized. All milk and milk products have the potential to transmit pathogenic (disease-causing) organisms to humans. The nutritional components that [supposedly] make milk and milk products an important part of the human diet also support the growth of the organisms. Drinking raw milk [presumably] causes food borne illness, and dairy producers selling or giving raw milk to friends and relatives are [presumably] putting them at risk.[123]

There are two main types of pasteurization used today: High Temperature/Short Time (HTST) and "Extended Shelf Life (ESL)" treatment. Ultra-high temperature (UHT or ultra-heat treated) is also used for milk treatment. In the HTST process, milk is forced between metal plates or through pipes heated on the outside by hot water, and is heated to 71.7 °C (161 °F) for 15–20 seconds. UHT processing holds the milk at a temperature of 135 °C (275 °F) for a minimum of one second. ESL milk has a microbial filtration step and lower temperatures than UHT. Milk simply labeled "pasteurized" is usually treated with the HTST method, whereas milk labeled "ultra-pasteurized" or simply "UHT" has been treated with the UHT method.[123]

Milk pasteurization has been subject to increasing scrutiny in recent years, due to the discovery of pathogens that are both widespread and heat resistant (able to survive pasteurization in significant numbers). One of these pathogens, *Mycobacterium avium* subsp. *paratuberculosis* (MAP), is linked to Crohn's Disease. Researchers have developed more sensitive diagnostics which have enabled testers to identify pathogens in pasteurized milk. [123]

Some of the diseases that pasteurization [is said to] prevent are diphtheria, salmonellosis, strep throat, scarlet fever, listeriosis, brucellosis and typhoid fever.[123]

Pasteurization is often an excuse to use unsanitary methods to milk, store, and transport the liquid because — after all — it will be pasteurized anyway. It's harder to keep milk clean than it is to just kill infected microorganisms in milk by heating it.

Second is the fact that pasteurized milk contains no utilizable calcium. OK!

We know you've been told for years that milk is a grand source for necessary calcium -to strengthen bones! The calcium is there, indeed, but after the milk is heated the calcium molecules are converted to a molecule that our bodies can no longer utilize for food according to William Campbell, II, M.D.![125]

Third is the fact of homogenization. Unprocessed milk consists of globules of milk fat suspended in a watery base containing dissolved proteins, sugars, vitamins, and minerals. If the globules are large enough, as with unprocessed milk from cows, the fat globules float upwards until they form a distinct cream layer at the top. Some animals, such as goats, produce smaller fat globules that remain mixed unless mechanically separated by centrifugation.[124]

You may like the idea of breaking up the fat globules in your cow's milk, but we do not. One reason we would drink milk is to intake the fat globules as they are.

Homogenization is a process that reduces the size of fat globules by forcing pressurized, hot milk through small holes, causing turbulence that breaks up the larger fat globules so that they remain suspended rather than separating in a cream layer at the top. The purpose of homogenization is to make milk more convenient to process, store and consume, eliminating the need to shake or stir the milk container to remix the separated cream layer and thereby increasing the shelf-life of the product.[124]

Notice that all but one of the reasons relate to the convenience of the milk producer and distributer, not to the consumer, especially that of increasing the milk's shelf-life!

Those opposed to homogenization argue that decreasing the size of fat globules may have unhealthy effects including allowing steroid and protein hormones to bypass normal digestion and increase their levels in the body. Concerns that uptake of the protein xanthine oxidase is increased by homogenization, leading to hardening of the arteries (atherosclerosis), coronary heart disease, milk allergy and milk intolerance, Type I and II diabetes were raised in the 1970s.[124, 125] While subsequent research "failed to substantiate, and in many cases has refuted a plausible effect of xanthine oxidase from homogenized milk on cardiovascular disease," many alternative/complementary doctors claim that the so-called refutations are questionable.[124, 25]

Fourth, the stupid [or grossly mis-stated] idea that eating or drinking fat causes folks to increase their own fat has brought about "slim" milk, 2% milk, and other names designed to attract the uneducated. These milks are simply less milk for a big price because water has been added to the container. The whole idea of drinking milk is to get nourished via the nutrients milk has to offer including fat globules.

One can get water cheaper at home. Increased fat is brought about by lack of appropriate exercise and especially from eating sugar and easily-converted-to-sugar products like flour, rice, potatoes and so on. Increased fat is not brought about by eating fat! Eating fat simply doesn't create excess fat! Fifth, once the milk has been brought to its high pasteurization temperature most of its valuable enzymes and anti-microbial features are destroyed. Some wise guy years ago said that cow's milk is great for calves and human female milk is great for human babies! Now we're going to explain why that is. The dairy industry and the gathering of milk have a long, honorable history. As the industrialization of a nation progresses so does the production, distribution and sale of cow's milk. There's already a huge industry worldwide to produce and distribute milk. So what follows would be a snap to implement worldwide were it not for the cozy relationship between the FDA, the US Agriculture industry and pharmacological big business.

In the dairy industry an oral vaccine could exist that is:

• 100% safe for 100% of those who use it;

• can be taken orally without any distaste;

• can be manufactured in virtually every country in the world with the technology available to each country;

• is so cheap that virtually everyone in the world can afford it;

• boosts the immune system, accelerates healing of injuries, helps repair nervous system damage, burns fat & builds lean muscle, increases vitality and stamina, and elevates mood.

• is ubiquitous, in that it will protect against any organism (including virus, rickettsia, parasite, protozoan, bacteria, mycoplasm, yeast/fungus, amoeba) or any allergen (including exogenous and endogenous sources), and might — just might — dry up to blow away a number of cancers?

• will not cause damage caused by vaccines, over-use of vaccines or by the preservatives placed in vaccines.

• does not require any needles and hypodermics to administer.

Over 4,000 clinical studies worldwide describe and/or support the use of this oral vaccine for hun*dreds of different diseases.*

Would you like to have this vaccine instead of Big Pharma's annual useless often dangerous shots?

Consider the Calf — or Any Other Newborn Mammal!

Bessie, our former pet milk cow, lived in a small pasture of not more than three acres. She munched on uncooked grasses during the summer and uncooked dry hay during the winter, licked mineral block, and drank from a rain-filled, surface-drained pond whose waters were loaded with a wide variety of microorganisms. The pond also held frogs, snakes, bugs, worms, snails, and so on. She often drank and urinated at the same time, recycling fluids from the pond even as she drank.

When she was ready to drop her calf, we led her to an old barn that had held forty head of cattle. One's nose almost stifled from sediments of dust, mold, fungi, and dried manure layered fifty years deep.

When Bessie's calf, Nina (pronounced "Neenya"), was born, the calf lacked effective defensive mechanisms against the blizzard of microorganisms that assailed her in every cubic inch of the air she breathed, the ground she stood on, or on the inexperienced tongue she extended to various surfaces. Almost by magic, thousands of potentially deadly microorganisms invaded her immature body.

Nina, as with all calves, was also born with a leaky gut!

Now pay attention here, because I know that many readers have a leaky gut, a condition where the stomach lining is so thin that whole, undigested protein molecules pass directly from the stomach into the blood stream. Once inside the blood stream these protein molecules are identified as foreign invaders, and we create antibodies to counteract them. This situation brings about food allergies.

Patients and their doctors both work very, very hard to get rid of the patient's leaky gut. Their leaky gut is considered the source of many degenerative diseases — or at least a major component of them. But Bessie and Nina had found a way to make the leaky gut a beneficial survival mechanism!

[A main difference between Bovid Mammary Gland and Human Cow's have a large cistern.]

When Nina wobbled to her feet and gently nudged at Bessie's milk sac, the very first milk to come was colostrum. As Nina prodded the milk sac with her nose and sucked as saliva dripped, she also injected her blizzard of rapidly multiplying microorganisms into Bessie's teat, and up into Bessie's milk sac into a portion called the "cistern."

Inside Bessie's cistern specialized cells that had been lying dormant came alive, and they started manufacturing — guess what? — "disease-specific antibodies," and "complement," and also flooding her cistern with "immunoglobulins" and "growth factors!"

"Antibodies" are molecules designed to attach to antigens (invaders and their toxins), making them amendable to later decomposition.

"Complement," plasma proteins, are molecules which assist (or complement) antibodies to overwhelm and to destroy foreign invaders, and they consist of twenty immunologically and chemically distinct forms capable of interacting with one another, with antibodies, and with cell membranes.

"Immunoglobulins" are a system of closely related proteins that can act as antibodies, and are identified as five major classes (with subclasses within), IgG, IgA, IgM, IgD, and IgE, each with different molecular weights.

According to research data, there are as many as 83 known substances (components) in colostrum, including growth factors, lipids, lactoferrin (iron-binding protein with antimicrobial qualities), cytokines [released from T cells, they inhibit replication of viruses and chemicals (cytotoxins) that kill the infected cell], etc.

The immunoglobulins (Ig's) are only one type of substance, and may not be the most important component.

All of these goodies are destroyed with high heat, that is, through pasteurization!

"Immune milk" is a "natural medicine" field that has been subjected to more than 80 years of research and yet there is much research to be mapped.

Very shortly after Nina introduced her stream of potentially dangerous microorganisms into Bessie's teat — then into Bessie's cistern — her mammary biochemical factory stimulated specialized cells that became active and began to create disease-specific antibodies and activated complement that mingled with Nina's first fluids, the colostrum, which Nina sucked back into her leaky gut from Bessie's teats.

The immunoglobulins, growth factors and these disease-specific antibodies and their helpers, the complement, passed directly into Nina's stomach and there they attached themselves to whatever corresponding organisms were present inside Nina's gut, killing many.

Now also the survival advantage of Nina's leaky gut came into play.

Because of Bessie's chemical factory many of these specially prepared biochemicals also passed directly into Nina's blood stream, and within her blood plasma they attached themselves to whatever microorganisms they'd been designed to destroy, thence a cascade of complement resulted [like rapid cloning], overwhelming the microorganisms one by one, so that never once was Nina placed in danger from the surrounding hostile environment whose every biological niche was filled with a wide variety of deadly microorganisms.

Growth factors in Bessie's colostrum also helped to heal Nina's leaky gut, and also strengthened

Nina in other ways.

Throughout 4.5 billion years our cellular and multi-cellular ancestors struggled to survive, creatively developing and utilizing a marvelously complex immune system. Throughout these aeons it has been eat or be eaten.

Our bodies utilize an extremely diverse army of cells and other molecules designed especially to protect us from the strategies of all of those would-be eaters. These finely tuned protective cells also work well as a team.

Researchers continue to uncover new and amazingly complex ways whereby protection from "outsiders" has developed. What is already known may sound complex, but please have patience. There's a point of great understanding in what follows.

There's an "innate" immune protective system. We're born with the ability to recognize certain microbes on sight, so to speak, and we can then destroy them.

There is an "adaptive" immune protective system. The "receptors" (as a lock is to a key) activated in the adaptive immune response are formed by piecing together gene segments, like piecing together a jigsaw puzzle. The available pieces are used by each cell in a different way to make a unique receptor, enabling cells to collectively recognize infectious organisms confronted during our lifetimes.

The end-point target of all immune processes is to destroy or otherwise protect from an "antigen," usually a foreign molecule from a microorganism.

The end-object of vaccinations is to confront the immune system with an antigen forcing the immune system to adapt to the foreign invader; that is, the immune system must learn to identify the foreign invader now and in the future.

One major end-result of such vaccinations is to develop a signal to specialized blood components, called "complement" (an enzyme substance) which is used to overwhelm and to destroy foreign invaders.

Specialized "antigen-presenting" cells, such as macrophages, roam throughout our bodies literally ingesting the antigens (invaders) and fragmenting them. These fragments are called "antigenic peptides."

Pieces of these peptides are layered on the surface of the cell called "major histocompatibility complex" (MHC). This joining produces a peptide-MHC combination.

Other specialized white cells called "T lymphocytes" have receptor cells that "recognize" different peptide-MHC. (The designation "T" means cells from the thymus gland.)

The T cells that are activated by that "recognition" begin to divide, and they also secrete a substance called "lymphokines." Lymphokines are chemical signals that mobilize other components of the immune system.

One set of those cells that responds to the lymphokine signals are the "B-lymphocytes" each of which also has receptor molecules of a single specificity on their surface. (The designation "B" means cells from bone marrow.)

However, unlike the receptors of T cells, those of B cells can recognize parts of antigens that are free in solution without the MHC molecules attached.

When the B-lymphocytes are activated, they divide and differentiate into plasma cells that secrete "antibody" proteins, water soluble forms of their receptors.

These antibodies bind to whatever antigens they find, neutralizing them or precipitating their destruction by enzymes derived from the molecule called "complement." Complement is a blood protein which can destroy pathogens on first encounter.

Complement activity — the end point of adaptive immunization, to develop a "complement" to antibodies — can be triggered in three ways.

(1) One type of complement called C3 can bind to any protein. Once bound to the microbe the C3 molecule causes other complement molecules to bind to the bacterium. This is called the "complement cascade." Their joint action overwhelms the bacterium. Our body's cells are protected from C3 by proteins that inactivate this molecule.

(2) Antibodies produced as a result of infection can also activate complement. After detecting an infection, a

macrophage secretes a substance called "interleukin-6." As it's carried through the blood stream, interleukin-6 reaches the liver causing the secretion of a "mannose-binding protein." (Mannose is a sugar formed by the oxidation of manitol.) Mannose-binding protein binds to the capsule of a bacterium, and this protein then triggers the complement cascade, thus overwhelming the bacterium.

(3) Antibodies produced as a result of infection also activate complement. B cells are activated if they bind to the bacterium and are stimulated by a so-called helper T cell. The binding stimulates the B cell to proliferate and to secrete antibodies. The antibodies bind to the bacterium and activate complement protein called C1Q, which activates other complement molecules — the "complement cascade" -thus overwhelming and killing the bacterium.

To make a rather long, complex story short, the many major immune defensive mechanisms we've inherited usually results in producing a complement cascade, which, working together with antibodies, overwhelms an invading organism.

The whole of the vaccination industry, which our biology ignorant Congressmen have excused from legal culpability, aims at stimulating the complement cascade against foreign microorganisms.

Billions upon billions of dollars are provided by us tax-payers to pharmaceutical companies to produce vaccines which will — allegedly — stimulate this long biological process so that our bodies can produce complement to surround and kill foreign microorganisms!

If your head aches by now, simply remember this — we inject foreign antigens in a process called vaccination. Our bodies go through some very complex reactions producing complement. Complement has the ability to attach to its counterpart, the antigen, also cloning itself and killing the invaders.

There's a cheaper, safer and easier way, as first discovered by University of Minnesota scientists!!! They called it "Immune Milk!"

According to Herbert Struss, Ph.D., former Senior Chemist, Food Chemistry Laboratory, Minnesota Department of Agriculture Laboratory Services Division — and also a scientist who was involved in much of the early clinical work testing this wondrously universal vaccine — those interested in "immune milk" (as it is called) during the '60s, made their astounding oral vaccine discoveries when they were trying to answer the question: "What's the survival advantage to being a mammal? After all, beetles have developed a wide variety of survival mechanisms that take up the major share of environmental niches allotted to insects; birds developed wings to escape ground predators, and, of course, microorganisms have adapted and thrive in virtually every imaginable niche, from deep rock, inside the hottest springs, beneath arctic cold, throughout fleecy white clouds above us, in us, and on us, and so on.

But why did mammals survive? What's the advantage to being a mammal?

Clearly, Nina's suckling at Bessie's teat, drawing a blood-like liquid called "colostrum" from Bessie's cistern was a possible answer to their question. The survival advantage was simply that an "acquired" or "adaptive" immunity could be transferred from mother to offspring, and that this adaptive immunity would extend for some period of time, thus providing the offspring with a distinct survival advantage!

In man, human milk may not be necessary for survival, as it is with multilayered placentas such as horse, goats, and cattle. But some immunity does pass from the mother to the human child. It's since become clear that a breast-fed human baby usually has an advantage over bottle fed, as the human mammary gland provides the same kind of acquired immunity to the child as that supplied by the cow to its calf. During the fifties and sixties pediatricians recommended against breast feeding. Those nurtured by bottle, rather than breast, did not receive a necessary boost to immune and digestive systems, or growth factors required after puberty. Vulnerability to disease and allergies was clearly greater!

So now that Nina is safe, and the survival of mammals seems assured in this eon, a second question was posed in the 1950's and 60's: Could Bessie's protective immunoglobulins and disease-specific antibodies and complement also be used by other species, such as man?

The answer to the question of Bessie's disease-specific antibodies and complement being transferable to other species, especially man, turned out to be an unequivocal **YES!**

Why?

Because: (1) the end products desired from all vaccinations against microorganisms are the same disease-specific antibodies and complement that can surround, attach to, and overwhelm it's counterpart invader one by one; and, (2) this disease-specific antibody and complement is the same regardless of whether or not it comes from a mouse, guinea pig, horse, cow, human, goat, lion, or any mammal on earth, so far as is known.

The Interactive Farm Ecology

Lee Beck, Ph.D., president Stolle Milk Biologics International, Blue Ash, Ohio, a company that holds about 300 patents related to the extraction, standardization, packaging and use of protective immune milk factors, provided a useful analogy:

Not more than a few generations ago (certainly during our lifetime) humankind was predominately centered around a farm community. Large families were the rule, each person having responsible chores for the good of the whole.

Farmer Brown's cattle grazed on open pasture, sharing and resharing microorganisms with all the other cows, calves and bulls.

Farmer Brown, or his wife and children, fed their cattle personally. Each of them transmitted many of their own microorganisms to the cattle. As they ate the meat and drank the milk produced by the cow, they received many of these same microorganisms back into their bodies.

Some of the cow's milk was fed back to the pigs and some milk was simply thrown away, or lapped up by their pet dog and cat.

Brown's pigs rooted in the cow manure. What the pigs didn't eat, the chickens and ducks scrambled for, inadvertently picking up a massive amount of shared microorganisms.

Farmer Brown killed cleaned and ate some of the chickens and ducks, collected and ate their eggs, and again unknowingly and, through handling and other contact means, he inadvertently received an infusion of their jointly shared microorganisms.

At least once a year, Farmer Brown and his family hitched up Dobbie to a wagon, and their work horse hauled their creaking wagon to the cow barn where Farmer Brown and his sturdy sons heaved cow manure into the wagon bed. Dobbie, of course, added his little bit now and then, but never mind; this was scooped up and added to the load.

The wagon moved out at last, and Farmer Brown and sons generously spread manure all over their garden-to-be.

Microorganisms worked their way into the soil which was tilled, planted and later, through the grace of God and the weather, brought forth abundant crops many of which were eaten by the Brown's family as well as their many animals.

Some of the microorganisms dried and blew back into the air breathed by farmer Brown and his family as well as his close-knit cluster of farm animals.

In short, this generous ecological sharing and re-sharing of both foods and microorganisms formed an almost closed ecological system so that vaccination and revaccination of Brown's family and his farm animals became a continuing on-going event.

Stories abound of isolated farm families who sustained great health until after a visit by a traveling stranger who was normally welcomed with open arms. Of course, an isolated Farmer Brown and family would not have had time to acquire immunity to the strange microorganisms brought into their ecological fold by this stranger and sometimes these tiny microbes devastated whole families, indeed, even whole communities, and sometimes tribes or nations. Think smallpox, for example, which decimated American Indian tribes by the tens of thousands.

Today we have predominately an urban environment. Rapid means of transportation, congested populations and a sparsity of loving, sharing farm animals that could process and reprocess our diseasecausing microorganisms daily have all conspired together to bring about a different world-wide ecology. This ecology consists of a multiplicity of microorganisms, humans, and animals, interacting, sharing one with the other, modifying, and sharing again.

A disease — Hong Kong flu, for example — appearing at one part of the globe can sweep toward any other part as fast as it takes airplanes to fly, and, it mutates just as rapidly.

We're all of us on one huge ecological farm, called "Earth" without specific community-center help from Bessie, Dobbie, or any other common farm animals, except in isolated farm communities. Our primary reliance seems to be on a deceptive, over-protective FDA and the unlikely veracity and assumed grace of giant pharmaceutical companies.

Suppression of A Vaccine With Broad Scope

Back in the 1950s and '60s — stemming from University of Minnesota research — a general solution to all infections and allergies was discovered, implemented, and suppressed.

Suppressed by whom? — by the FDA and the U.S. Department of Agriculture, of course!

While succeeding admirably during these early days with FDA approved clinical studies on rheumatic disease, rheumatoid arthritis, multiple sclerosis, and allergies, the initial approval granted by the FDA was suddenly revoked without a rational excuse.

But the FDA was not alone this time. When charged with repeating a study to substantiate a key patent claim related to "immune milk," members of the U.S. Department of Agriculture deliberately falsified experimental results, according to court records.[126]

Impro Products' Mary Collins (deceased) of Waukon, Iowa fought the U.S. Department of Agriculture. She demonstrated to the court's satisfaction that the U.S. Department of Agriculture had falsified experimental data, apparently to prevent Collins' patent on immune milk. Her patent became only the second in U.S. history to obtain an extension of time by act of Congress, due to governmental interference.

To emphasize further — this general solution encompassed the specific solution to all known antigens, bacterial, viral, yeast/fungal, amoebic, mycoplasmal, pollen, and simple protein.

In other words if you have a health condition that is based on any microorganism or allergen, and some chemical sensitivities, there is already known a simple, inexpensive process to solve the problem.

Scope of Protection From Immune Milk

As already stated, appropriate scientific studies carried out in the early 1960s found promising success. They included rheumatoid arthritis, multiple sclerosis, rheumatic fever, and pollen allergies. Subsequent research has expanded this list considerably, including drying up some cancerous tumors.

According to Herbert Edwin Struss, Ph.D., one unpublished report showed "spectacular" survival rates for small children from a poverty area in Mexico who were treated against colon bacteria with this method by cooperating Mexican physicians.

Immune milk pioneer, contemporaries and co-workers were original innovators Drs. Berry Campbell W.E. Peterson, and Herbert Edwin Struss, Ph.D. Dr. Struss was former Senior Chemist, Food Chemistry Laboratory, Minnesota Department of Agriculture, Laboratory Services Division, St. Paul, Minnesota and one of the key men to initiate FDA approved human clinical studies with specially prepared colostrum. Dr. Struss was also Director of Research for the W.E. Petersen Research Institute and editor of the *Journal of Immune Milk* published in the early '60s by the International Association on Immunity.

As a general principle, this method of preparing disease-specific colostrum will transfer adaptive immunity safely against any allergen or antigen — any substance which, when introduced into the body, creates antibodies (such as allergenic pollens, house dust, animal hairs, or microorganism proteins). For allergy prevention, one can use a mixture of hair (cats, dogs, cattle), making a bovine cisterninjectable vaccine. Other allergens, like pollens, can also be introduced into the cow's cistern resulting in colostrum that has the beneficial effects of developing resistance to the antigens that produce the allergies.

Experimental studies in the patents listed in the references attached include: "bacteria, viruses, proteins, animal tissue, plant tissue, spermatozoa, rickettsia, metazoan parasites, mycotic molds, fungi, pollens, dust and similar substances . . . exemplary antigens include: bacterial — S*almonella pullorum, Salmonella typhi, Salmonella parathypi, Staphylococcus, aureus, a Streptoccous agalactiae, g Streptococcus agalactiae, Staphyloccus albus, Staphylococcus pyogenes, E. Coli,* pneumococci, streptococci, and the like; viral — influenza type A, fowl pox, turkey pox, herpes simplex and the like; protein — egg albumin and the like; tissue — blood and sperm."

In an experiment using immune milk conducted at Notre Dame University's Lobund Institute, Impro Products, Inc. substances reduced tooth decay in laboratory animals as much as 87 percent. (Although bacteria are usually blamed, the work of dentist Dr. Trevor Lyons clearly demonstrates a synergism between protozoans and bacteria, and the devastating effects of certain protozoans.[127])

Trial mammals protected according to various immune milk patents were mice, cows, goats, chickens and pigs.

The immune milk method is also good for chickenpox, cold sores, genital herpes, Cryptocides sporidium, and for anti-inflammatory conditions, as it is heavy with complement (C3B) and anti-complement, substances that assist in the destruction of invasive organisms.

Other Sources than Immune Milk

Although not as economical or as easy to obtain as bovine or goat colostrum, the same diseasespecific antibody and complement can also be obtained from other sources than colostrum. For example: (1) donors with high (cell-mediated) immunity to known antigens (cloning); (2) from human placentas, and (3) the spleen from immunized eggs, pigs or ducks, or even from humans who have good (cell-mediated) immunity to the relevant antigens.

Because these substances — called "transfer factors" — are so cheap, widespread, and easy to use, various countries outside of the United States use it, including China, Czechoslovakia, Germany, Poland, and Hungry. In Japan, the only high-wage country where it is used, forty Red Cross Centers provide transfer factor produced from pooled leukocytes (white blood cells) of normal healthy donors to 400 hospitals for use in a wide variety of conditions.

(Use of transfer factor does not cause hepatitis, but is effective against hepatitis, does not cause AIDS, and may be helpful in some of the diseases associated with AIDS.)

There are many particles that can transfer immunity. Subsequently confirmed by other scientists -in reporting on membrane filtered (dialyzable) white blood cells (leukocytes) to obtain "transferfactors" — they found that transfer of immunity had taken place in the following conditions:[128, 129, 130]

1. Familial T-lymphocyte dysfunction with severe recurrent infection (white cell dysfunction)

2. Herpes infection (viral)

3. Cytomegalovirus infection (viral)

4. Candidiasis (yeast/fungus)

5. Parasitic infection (e.g., pneumocystis carinae, cryptosporidiosis, etc.)

6. Mycobacterium tuberculosis infection refractory to antibiotics

7. Behcet's syndrome (skin condition/arthritis)

8. Lupus erythematosus

9. Pemphigus vegetans (skin disease)

10. Wiskott-Aldrich Syndrome (immune deficiency disease with decreased blood platelets and skin rash)

11. Florence Nightingale Disease (aka Chronic Fatigue Immune Dysfunction Syndrome)

12. Bone metastases after surgical removal of breast cancer

13. Bone metastases after surgical removal of kidney cancer

14. Guillian Barre' (disturbance of two or more nerves, after viral or mycoplasma infection)

15. Amyotrophic lateral sclerosis (Lou Gehrig's disease; one subset)

16. Retinitis Pigmentosa (inflamed retina: one subset, 50%; Dialyzable Leucocyte Extract-Transfer Factor — filtered through a membrane — does not reverse the disease but prevents additional visual loss)

Also reported by Fudenberg and Pizza,[128, 129, 130] but not yet confirmed by others were:

1. Mycobacterium fortuitum infection (mycoplasma)
2. Mycobacterium avian infection (mycoplasma)
3. Alopecia totalis (hair loss over entire body)
4. Alzheimer's disease (one subset)
5. Autism (one subset, 70%)
6. Osteosarcoma (prevented metastases to lungs)
7. Epidermal dysplasia (multiple skin malignancies)
8. Certain food and chemical hypersensitivities

9 Burkitt's lymphoma, etc. (B-cell malignancy)

Reported by other than Fudenberg and Pizza[128, 129, 130] were:

1. Lepromatous leprosy
2. Leishmaniasis (parasite affecting skin, nasal cavity and pharnyx)
3. Rat diabetes (Type I-immunologic) (trials in humans not yet reported, 1993)
4. Myasthenia gravis (great muscular weakness)
5. Subacute sclerosing panencephalitis (slow virus disease, affecting thinking and movement)
6. Atopic dermatitis (skin)
7. Bronchial asthma (lungs)
8. Recurrent otitis media (ears)
9. Varicella (virus)
10. Hepatitis B — acute and chronic (virus)
11. Brucella (bacteria affecting man and other mammals)
12. Asthma
13. Nasopharyngeal carcinoma (cancer)
14. Stomach carcinoma (cancer)
15. Colon carcinoma (cancer)
16. Non-small cell lung carcinoma (cancer)

17. Spontaneous abortions

According to H. Hugh Fudenberg and Pizza,[128] "The potential for bovine colostrum-transfer factor treatment of human diseases is fantastic since one can obtain so much more [transfer factor] extract at little cost." It is found free and in high concentration in colostrum; but can also be obtained from donors with high cell-mediated immunity to known antigens (cloning); or from human placentas, and also spleen from immunized pigs, chickens, eggs, or ducks, or even humans who have a good cell-mediated immunity to the relevant antigens." The definition of a transfer factor is "a substance that is produced and secreted by a lymphocyte functioning in cell-mediated immunity, and that upon incorporation into a lymphocyte which has not been sensitized, confers on it the same immunological specificity as the sensitized cell." This means that transfer factors stimulate and modulate the immune system against infectious disease. Some companies have chosen to sell isolated transfer factors instead of whole colostrum.

Patents obtained by Stolle Milk Biologics International, as well as their present commercial partnership with the New Zealand Dairy Board also demonstrate that bovine intramuscular inoculations can result in a whey product containing the desired antibodies and complement.

Some commercial laboratories in the United States have followed up on Dr. Fudenberg's research, reportedly producing excellent antigen specific antibodies and complement.

So, clearly, there are many sources and paths to obtain the desired immunity factors that can be used sublingually or orally, rather than expensive, sometimes damaging vaccinations.

Early Clinical Trials

In the late sixties, Herbert Struss, Ph.D., working with the Borden Company of New York City, held a FDA IND (Investigate New Drug authority) for studying the use of bovine derived "Specific Serum

Protein Capsules." Using 10 strains of Streptococcus, 2 strains of Staphylococcus and 1 strain of Diplococcus in properly prepared cows, these lyophilized (freeze dried) serum proteins derived from colostrum were prepared in 250 mg capsules, and contained the gamma globulin fraction (protein in blood which helps resist disease) of the antibodies and immunity which enabled seventy percent of the Rheumatoid Arthritis victims to overcome the disease or receive marked benefit, once again demonstrating a close relationship between an infectious microorganism and some Rheumatoid Arthritis.

Cyril M. Smith, M.D. conducted a sample survey of 199 persons who used antibodies produced by cows in the treatment of arthritis symptoms. Smith reported that antibodies were successful in 56.8% of cases reported. This improvement occurred within 3 months. (The greatest improvement was noted between the second and fourth weeks. However, in some cases it required more than 6 weeks before a marked improvement was noticed.)

Twenty-three percent who found relief from symptoms while taking antibodies experienced an increase in pain prior to their improvement. This "increase in pain" was most likely the Herxheimer

Effect described earlier and as summarized by Dr. Paul K. Pybus.[19] The great majority of the persons who experienced pain made marked improvement.

It's extremely remarkable that such a high percentage of cure rates would occur using only a fraction (Staphylococcus, Streptococcus, Diplococcus) of the suspected multitudes of microorganisms related to arthritis! Based on presumption of totally different organisms than those used to develop arthritis-specific antibodies and complement, both Roger Wyburn-Mason, M.D., Ph.D. (protozoan) and Thomas McPherson Brown, M.D. (mycoplasma) -and their practitioner followers -have achieved higher rates of cures, especially when proper diet and consideration for candidiasis and food allergies are also included in the treatment protocols.[131]

An extremely brief summary of uses for transfer factors follow:

In Animals Uses

There's another route for protection called "transfer factors."

• Bovine . . . extract-transfer factor made against the parasite coccidioides protects not only cows but also mice from an LD 90 dose (the dose necessary to kill 90% of a population). Bovine dialyzable (filtered) leucocyte (white cell) extract devoid of transfer factor has no protective effect;

• Bovine antigen-specific transfer factor is effective in treatment of human herpes infections;

• Bovine created for nematodes, *Haemonchus contortus*, *Trichostrongylus axei* infections is effective in sheep;

• Bovine . . . extract, from both lymph nodes and colostrum, against virus and parasitic diseases, have been used in dogs (canine parvovirus), pigs (swine transmissible pharynogeolaryngeotracheitis), chickens (bursal disease, Newcastle's Disease, and other viral diseases);

• Coccidioides destroys $250 million per year of prize cattle in Texas. Lymph Node Leukocyte (white cell) Extract (with Transfer Factor) can protect cattle against this infection, and also prevents mastitis in cows, and death from infection in newborn calves;

• Horse dialyzable (filtered) leucocyte (white cell) extract is effective against rheumatism in horses.

In Human Uses

• Bovine dialyzable (filtered) leucocyte (white cell) extract (with transfer factor) has been given repeatedly to humans without adverse reaction;

• Eradicated cryptosporidiosis in humans with diarrhea;

• Coccidioides derived transfer factor, eradicated diarrhea and eliminated ova and parasites from stools;

• Being used on 6,000,000 people in China to prevent acute and chronic infectious hepatitis;

• Many other conditions, as previously mentioned.

Colostrum Pitfalls

In most health food stores you'll find a product called "colostrum" often touted for its ability to "strengthen the immune system."

It's quite possible that a particular batch or manufacturer has produced colostrum that has beneficial effects in the strengthening of your immune system. It contains, after all, a multiplicity of important immune "transfer factors" common to all mammals.

And — it's even possible that a particular batch of colostrum will favorably affect the course of an allergic reaction to an allergen (pollen-based) or disease from an antigen (microorganism-based).

But — unless the manufacturer has injected into the cow's cistern dead microorganisms specific to your disease (or allergens), the expectation of the cow's naturally derived antibodies and complement matching those that you must have to counteract a particular dysfunction, based on a microorganism, is considerably less than the probability of one Powerball ticket winning a $100,000,000 jackpot. Keep in mind that the cow will only have immunity factors related to the antigens to which it has been exposed — and most modern dairies isolate their cows from most humans, thus preventing the nice, comfy farm ecological relationship once known to man, Bessie, the cow, and her family of farm animal friends.

During your life time you're likely to encounter at least 600,000 types of germs. If only one percent of these are capable of causing disease, that's still 6,000 germ types. A commercial colostrum manufacturer is very unlikely to utilize 6,000 germs to create their immune milk. Then, too, we haven't even factored in the possibility that the commercial colostrum found in your health food store has been properly stored. Then, too, the odds increase more the farther away one is from fresh, unpasteurized, whole colostrum! — except for a handful of "immune milk" companies who have applied modern technology in preserving most of the active ingredients in a dry powder or liquid form for use by all farm animals.

The hundred or so rheumatoid diseases, including rheumatoid arthritis, for example, are caused by many factors among which are nutritional, genetic predisposition, hormonal, and microorganism-based antigen/antibody immuno-complexes which are not easily swept out by a clogged up lymph system. Most standard colostrum preparations for rheumatoid arthritis are based on injections of Staphyloccus and streptococcus antigens. We know that many organisms, such as mycoplasms, corneybacteria, klebsiella, candidia and others can be the antigenic stimulation in the human that results in the symptoms of rheumatoid arthritis.

On a hit or miss basis, then, if you happen to be a person suffering from a tissue sensitivity to staphylococcus and streptococcus, and you are suffering from an overwhelming invasion of staphylococcus and/or streptococcus, and you happen to buy colostrum containing antibodies and complement resulting from the effects of these two organisms as developed in the cow's cistern, and the material you've purchased is still strong and active, then you might very well respond favorably to this particular colostrum.

But if your arthritis stems from a mycoplasm, corneybacteria, candidia or klebsiella (among many other possible microorganisms), you're just out of luck. "It didn't work!" you'd report to your friends, and the overall idea of using colostrum would be invalidated for you and your friends.

You're better off placing your money on the Powerball jackpot!

But "Yes!" Many of these desirable immune factors can be purchased for protection of farm animals, but not for man! Even so, the likelihood of getting the right product for you at the health food store, prepared and preserved in the right way, is so remote as to be inconsequential.

There are exceptions which we'll mention shortly.

So, as you learn about the miracle of colostrum, don't run out to the health food store and buy colostrum with the expectation of solving your health problems!

Colostrum must be collected and preserved correctly, and administered properly, before this universal vaccine will work for you.

By the way, colostrum prepared and used properly has little to do with whether cow or goat milk is good or bad for you. Indeed, one of the allergies that the right colostrum can solve is that of allergic reactions to milk!

How to Obtain Properly Prepared Colostrum
The Simplest Procedure?

Ordinarily the simplest way to obtain the proper antibodies and complement required for your particular medical condition would be to purchase products manufactured by a company that has many years of experience preparing these products. Such products are available for animals from several companies, but — unfortunately — by law their specially prepared disease-specific products cannot be sold for human use, only to farmers who wish to protect their animals from disease cheaply and simply. As a matter of fact, the company with the most experience is so terrified of legal involvement and possible bankruptcy from the FDA and U.S. Department of Agriculture that they refuse to permit their name to be used in connection with this or any other article. For purposes of this article they shall be called Farm Products, Inc.

This is very much reminiscent of governmental restrictions on the use of DMSO (dimethylsulfoxide), an inexpensive by-product of paper production that is a very strong antioxidant and can be used to rapidly relieve pain. Any veterinarian supply house has it for sale to farmers for animals, but humans are not supposed to use it except under strict physician supervision.

Some marketers sell colostrum as a nutritional substance guaranteed "to contain a minimum of 30% immunoglobulin content." Their colostrum is often obtained from New Zealand Dairies and advertised to be from "healthy, pasture-fed, dairy cows that are pesticide, antibiotic and hormone free." That last, by itself, as compared to milk products produced in the United States, is something of a miracle! I have no knowledge of whether or not these products are more than a good protein product, or if, in fact, it contains valuable antibody/complement nutritional factors.

In an article by Morton Walker, D.P.M. in connection with Symbiotics,[132] (quoting a number of investigators), therapeutic components found within colostrum include a wide-range of substances such as immunoglobulins, lactoferrin, proline-rich polypeptides, leukocytes, lysozymes, enzymes, cytokines, glycoproteins and trypsin inhibitors, lymphokines, oligo polysaccharides and glycoconjugate saccharides, and many other substances. This multiplicity of factors helps to neutralize toxins and counters microbial attacks, reduces incidence of cancer and chronic fatigue, regulates the thymus gland while stimulating and regulating immunities and also interferon production to slow viral activities, boosts immune system and T-cell activity, and so on.

According to some investigators, one of whom will be mentioned shortly, not all is yet known about the beneficial actions of colostrum!

Lucky Nina!

Whether or not standard colostrum products sold in farm supply stores — such as for *E. coli* — is effective even for animals probably depends upon many factors far beyond the control of the average consumer, such as production method, length of shelf life, specificity, bacterial strains used, and so on.

Standard products for a dairy herd include colostrum preparations against salmonella, staphylococcus, streptococccus, *E. coli*, pseudomonas, cornyebacteria, klebsiella-pasteurella, *Candida albicans*, clostridium, aerobacter aerogenes, proteus, and chlamydia.

Former Iowa Congressman Berkley Bedell suffered from Lyme Arthritis disease caused by *Borrelia burgdorferi* a spirochete bacterium from a tick usually found on deer.

Lida Mattman, Ph.D., Professor Emeritus, Department of Biology, Wayne State University, Detroit, says that it is bad for a state's tourist trade to admit they have any Lyme disease and therapy against the disease is expensive. Its better to let the patient disintegrate into a wheel chair or a mental institution. Actually, this spirochete disease, like the syphilis spirochete disease of the 13th century, has invaded every block of every city in the civilized world. However, unlike syphilis, this [disease] is spread by mosquito, tick, mite, probably household contact, as well as trans-placentally. Like syphilis this disease is the great imitator, attacking joints, heart, brain, etc. We looked at spinal fluid, blood, and synovial fluid of over 500 cases who had symptoms of Lyme [arthritis disease], and found the spirochete of the same genus, in most patients."[134]

About 10% of Lyme Arthritis victims do not get well by traditional medical treatments, and former Iowa Congressman Bedell was one of those. Bedell[135] says, "I left Congress because I came down with Lyme Disease which I contracted while fishing at Quantico Marine Base, and which conventional treatment failed to relieve. After three series of heavy antibiotics infused into my veins over a period of two years, I finally turned to unconventional treatment. My symptoms disappeared and today I am clearly free of Lyme Disease.

"Let me tell you about that treatment. There is a company in our own state of Iowa, Mr. Chairman that produces a product for livestock by injecting killed germs into the udder of a cow prior to the time the cow has a calf. When the cow has the calf they then take the first milk that the cow gives, which is called colostrum, and process it into whey so that it will keep.

"The theory is that the cow will communicate the disease to the unborn calf, and will develop the antibodies, or whatever, in the colostrum to protect the newly-born calf from that disease.

"After I took a teaspoon of this whey every 1-1/2 hours for a few weeks, my symptoms of Lyme [Arthritis Disease] disappeared, and I no longer suffer from that disease. Because of the publicity of my case, I get frequent phone calls from desperate people who have been unable to get relief from Lyme [Arthritis Disease] with conventional treatment. It breaks my heart that I cannot tell them about my treatment, because no one has been willing to spend the millions and millions of dollars necessary to get FDA approval to market this special whey. I can tell you it cured what appeared to be arthritis in my knee in 15 minutes."

"I have talked to a doctor in Wisconsin who was using this material. He claims 80-90% success in treating patients like me for whom conventional treatments have not been effective. He has now been advised by the Iowa producer that the material will no longer be available because the producer is afraid of the FDA."

Because of Congressman Bedell's success with colostrum treatment against Lyme Arthritis disease, and from other non-standard medical treatments, he and Iowa Senator Tom Harkin convinced the U.S. Congress to establish an Office of Alternative Medicine under the National Institute of Health. This Office has now been upgraded to a Center by Senators Tom Harkin and Arlen Specter, and Representative Peter DeFazio, but its functions have strayed far afield from the intent of its originators.

It has been mentioned that the U.S. Department of Agriculture can also act as a strong determent, preventing healing when using colostrum.

We hope and pray for a much more mature Department of Agriculture and FDA who will grant permission to renew studies on the use of this already well-developed technology. These products especially prepared for maintaining the health of farm mammals should be easily available for us, too. After all, we're also mammals and deserve equal consideration! The US Army purchased antigen specific complement prepared from chicken eggs from one supplier. This substance was then mixed in K rations. Apparently some branches of the government know what is what!

A Second Possibility is to Bootleg the Treatment

Herb Saunders, the dairy farmer who cured Congressman Bedell when no licensed physician had been able to do so, was prosecuted on the report of the FDA in St. James, Minnesota by the state prosecuting attorney for practicing medicine without a license.

Saunders had been treating — and curing — humans of a wide variety of diseases for many years, including cancer. For the most part, he used standard products prepared for treatment of cattle, and, when necessary, he used (dead) microorganisms (such as *Borrelia burgdorfi* bacteria) passed through the cow's cistern prior to collecting the colostrum.

When all else failed, he'd pass human blood from the sick person through the cow's cistern. Each person's blood contains a wide variety of microorganisms — especially when sick — that is unknown, or unacknowledged by most physicians, but are recognized and acknowledged by the cow.

The colostrum thus obtained for the next 10 days was fed back to the sick person just as would be the standardized products made for the use and health of cattle.

According to immune milk pioneer, Herb Struss, Ph.D., colostrum obtained by injecting whole human blood into the cow's cistern does not produce auto-immune reactions to one's own blood. "It's one of the first things we checked," Struss says.

Herb Saunders was selling bovine colostrum ("first milk") as a potential cure for cancer. "Saunders would sell each patient a cow for $2,500 but keep the cow on his farm. He would inject a sample of each patient's blood into the cow's udder [cistern], and then sell the colostrum to the cow's owner for $35 a bottle. Saunders told an undercover state agent who posed as a cancer patient that he would 'cough out' his cancer within months if he would take colostrum, [and to] refrain from chemotherapy. Dairy farmer Herb Saunders, Odin, Minnesota, was prosecuted for practicing medicine without a license twice but was freed by a grand jury twice. Saunders had treated and cured by means of immune milk a large number of diseases, including most of the major ones named in this article.

"After two weeks of [court] trial — the longest this small community had ever seen — the result was a hung jury. The 6-person jury voted 5-1 to convict, but the last holdout, a part-time social studies teacher, apparently couldn't decide whether Saunders was practicing medicine without a license or offering an alternative type of care that is not medical practice."[136]

Attorney Calvin Johnson, Mankato, Minnesota, without charge, defended Herbert Saunders before a grand jury twice against the charge of practicing medicine without a license, and won! Calvin is a staunch supporter of the use of immune milk. Former Congressman Berkley Bedell provided $21,000 for Saunders' expenses.

Reported by attorney Calvin Johnson, Herb Saunders' second trial once again resulted in a hung jury, reportedly more hung than the first one, with 3 jurors resisting indictment.

The district attorney dismissed the case on May 30, 1996, and will not retry Saunders!

Sanders approach seems to be well substantiated by the work of many scientists over a period of more than 40 years.

It's up to you to find dairymen and to convince them to risk prosecution as they secretly treat you. If blood is to be drawn from you, it should be injected into the cow's cistern immediately on being drawn from your arm at least once a week for four weeks before the calf is born.

Buy Your Own Cow or Goat

In answer to the technical questions of how immune milk is obtained, Herbert Struss, Ph.D. suggests that a "springing heifer" be used to prepare the right colostrum for you. A "springing heifer" is a cow that has not given birth to prior calves.

He reports that immune milk is obtained by inoculating into the cistern with the use of a 20 ml syringe — about 5 milliliters of the antigenic or allergenic material is passed through each of the four teats with a cannula (specially designed reed or tube) at weekly intervals one month before the calf's birth.

He also reports that those who must inject human blood (for cancer, for example) as their antigenic material take about 10 milliliters from the human which is then distributed at 2-1/2 milliliters to each teat, or bovine gland, immediately.

Ten days of milking, at most, is usable, although the first 24-48 hours of pre-milk produced from the cow's mammary gland after birth is usually defined as "colostrum."

According to Philip Derse (deceased) of Derse & Schroeder Associates, Madison, Wisconsin, who studied colostrum and transfer factors for thirty years, says that modern technology permits extracting many of the active transfer factors from whole milk long after the colostrum phase. One no longer needs to inject the cow's cistrum and capture at the correct time the colostrum. Proper antigen specific colostrum can be rendered from whole milk through the use of the proper dairy technology.

But we're speaking here of do-it-yourself methods!

After reading this foundation's first report on the good effects of immune milk, one retired dairy farmer purchased a milk cow and injected his daughter's blood into the cistern, eventually collecting the colostrum. His daughter suffered miserably from Epstein Barr Virus. Within 3 months of sipping on the colostrum his daughter was at last well.

One lady reported that, after being treated by Herb Saunders for Multiple Sclerosis, she's had no attack for more than 2 years! She also told us of a Multiple Sclerosis support group in North Dakota that chooses not to be identified as they have their own dairy herd and have been treating themselves.

Early virological and immunological studies have suggested that Multiple Sclerosis is an autoimmune disease triggered by a German Measles viral infection, also used to prepare the colostrum.

In a 1984 study reported in Medical Microbiology and Immunology.[137]

IgA-rich cow colostrum containing anti-measles lactoglobulin resistant proteases was orally administered to patients with multiple sclerosis. Measles-positive antibody colostrum was orally administered every morning to 15 patients with multiple sclerosis at a daily dosage of 100 ml for 30 days. Similarly, measles-negative antibody control colostrum (< 8) was orally administered to 5 patients. Of 7 anti-measles colostrum recipients, 5 patients improved and 2 remained unchanged. Of 5 negative (< 8) recipients, 2 patients remained unchanged and 3 worsened. These findings suggested the efficacy of orally administered anti-measles colostrum in improving the condition of multiple sclerosis patients ($P < 0.05$).

The Christmas of 1998 one of us spent watching the application of specifically prepared antigen/complement materials from bovine colostrum, the cow's first milk on calving.

What was personally observed was a kind of Christmas miracle. Nowhere had any of us previously read or heard of Psoriasis being related to staphylococcus. Here's what was observed:

A patient had gross, raised blotches of skin Psoriasis that would not heal no matter what standard treatments were tried.

A liquid preparation of colostrum staphylococcus antibody/complement was taken orally, 1 teaspoon each hour, and a cotton ball was also used to wipe the mixture on the Psoriasis blotches. The wiping on of the liquid was done every time itching occurred, and also occasionally throughout the next days. Also the oral treatment of the liquid was continued each hour.

Within minutes (literally) of the first wiping the blotches began to disappear. Within a day, all blotches were reduced in size. Within two days, only the longest standing and grossest blotches remained, though greatly diminished.

Finally, all marks were gone!

What a great Christmas present for the patient!

One doctor called The Arthritis Trust of America and asked what was available for treating Lyme

Arthritis disease.

Of course, Berkley Bedell's experience was quoted, and the doctor was advised that first s/he'd need a milk cow. Surprisingly, s/he answered that she had room for a milk cow at her farm.

Then s/he was told s/he'd need some dead *Borrelia burgdorfi* bacteria. Surprisingly again, s/he said she had this microorganism in her/his laboratory.

So here's another way: With others, or alone, buy a cow or nanny goat, get it pregnant, and do your own treatment!

The Proper Way

Doctors who treat tuberculosis patients are very aware of antibiotic-resistant tubercular mycoplasms on the swift rise. They could well consider for this and other diseases or allergies requesting the FDA's permission to run a double-blind study using specially prepared colostrum.

"Double-blind" means that neither the patient nor the doctor will know which one is receiving the presumably active ingredient, and which one is receiving the placebo, the inactive ingredient, until the study is completely run and ready for analysis.

Here's what's involved:

1. The doctor must prepare a research plan of action, a study proposal.

2. The study proposal, with all attached research references, must be submitted to an Institutional Review Board for review and approval. Usually, but not always, the Institutional Review Board is attached to a medical school.

3. If the study raises objections, it must be modified. When approved, it is then submitted to the FDA, spelling out exactly what's to be done, how the research is to be evaluated, and how the product is to be tested and how the placebo product will be prepared, labeled and used.

4. If approved by the FDA, the study is given an IND number, which means "Investigate New Drug number."

5. The study is then carried out, and final reports written for FDA review as well as for publication, if possible.

This sounds like a simple, straight forward procedure, but, considering the danger that is posed to the pharmaceutical industry, where specially prepared cow's colostrum is effectively producing cures while much touted and damaging pharmaceuticals are not, there will be many pitfalls placed between the honest doctor and final permission.

It is also a very expensive process, but probably would be nowhere near the expense of bringing in a new and unknown drug — providing the FDA plays square with you.

When University of Minnesota Herbert Struss, Ph.D. obtained permission from the FDA to use these products on rheumatic fever, rheumatoid arthritis, multiple sclerosis and allergies in the early

1960s, progress in patient wellness was quite obvious at different medical centers.

Dr. Struss was visited by FDA officials who, without adequate explanation, ordered him to cease and desist. He refused, explaining that their agency had granted him an IND — permission to conduct clinical studies.

His next FDA visitors were from higher up administrators who warned him that if he didn't stop his studies they'd put him in jail.

Having children and a wife to support Dr. Struss bowed to governmental suppression and did no further work on this amazing healing product throughout the remainder of his life.[59]

Perhaps the intervening 40 or so years has mellowed the FDA! Growing influence of the new Center for Complementary and Alternative Medicine under the National Institute of Health will provide an umbrella for submission of studies of immune milk on humans. Also, many prestigious medical schools are rapidly installing alternative/complementary medical courses and/or departments, and these are beginning to have influence on the politics of what should or should not be scientifically studied.

The Structural Research Center, Mobile, Alabama, headed by Walter Wilburn, Ph.D., had successfully accomplished the production of Lyme Arthritis antigen-specific immune milk from one of his certified scrappies-free goats. Using the methods of Stolle Milk Biologics International he developed patents for inoculating specific antigens in chickens. Eggs have also been produced which are sold

under contract to the U.S. Army for incorporation in Army K-Rations.[59]

Using Dr. Fudenberg's research on transfer factors, Chisholm Biological Laboratory, http://www.forresthealth.com/chisolm-biological-laboratories/, developed a number of antigen specific immune factors, for physician use, including, but not limited to: HIV, *Pneumocystic carinii*, Human tuberculosis, *Borrelia burgdorferi* (Lyme Arthritis), Bovine Tuberculosis, Babesia, Ehrlichia, Epstein-Barr Virus (EBV), *Chlamydia pneumoniae,* Cytomegalovirus (CMV), Staphylococci, *E. Coli*, Herpes 1, Herpes 2, Human herpes virus 6 (HHV6), *Candida albicans*, Cryptosporosis, varicella zoster, and *Mycobacterium avian*. (See *Lyme Disease and Rife Machines: When Antibiotics Fail* by Bryan Rosner for latest information. Rosner provides additional information for Lyme disease patients — Fortunately, though, a new Lyme-specific transfer factor product has become available: LymPlus, made by Researched Nutritionals at https://

www.researchednutritionals.com/store/products.cfm?category=Transfer%20Factor&catid=17

These sources may have excellent products. We don't know. The only product that the authors have had experience with is that of Impro Products, Inc. colostrum from Waukon, Iowa. When used on humans it is decidedly effective. However, they can sell only to dairy men and veterinarians.

A Homeopathic Approach

Exempted from FDA over-surveillance are standardized homeopathic remedies.

The preparation of these homeopathic remedies is begun by using the colostrum from specially prepared allergens or antigens as a "mother."

A "mother" is the initial brew or dissolved substance that is the "active ingredient" used to make homeopathic remedies. A 1X (read as "one time) homeopathic remedy is 1 volume of mother to 9 parts of distilled water; 2X is 1 volume of the 1X solution to 9 parts of water (or 1 of the mother to 99 of water), 3X is 1 volume of 2X solution to 9 parts of water (or 1 of mother to 999 parts of water) and so on, until the mother has been diluted 1 part mother to 999,999 parts of water to achieve a 6X dilution.

Homeopathic remedies are prepared by and can be purchased from Beaumont Bio-Med, 23 1st Avenue Ne,Waukon, IA 52172 -

Ingredients for "rheumatism" for example, include Rhus tox (poison ivy) 12X, Causticum (potassium hydrate) 12X, Lac vaccinum (cow's milk) 30X, in a base of lactose, 20% alcohol and distilled water. A 2 fluid ounce bottle lasts about 2 months. Properly prepared colostrum, of course, is the basis for the "cow's milk" ingredient. The milk products used are defined in the Homeopathic Pharmacopoeia of the United States.

Additional homeopathic remedies prepared in the same manner include preparations made from specific microorganisms for cold and flu, sore throat, fever and inflammation, stomach ache, skin, acne and muscle and joint pain.

Among those patents filed and dated from 1945 to 1992 are found some exemplary studies related to animals using homeopathic remedies.

Groups of four mouse test subjects, using deadly *Pseudomonas aurogenosa* challenges were conducted using test categories of water, colostrum and milk as the raw materials. A first mother was prepared from the first cow's colostrum and also used to produce a second mother by passing the first mother's colostrum into the cistern of a second cow, after which homeopathic remedies were prepared from the second mother derived from the second cow at 3X and 6X potencies.

In the first table described in the patent, mouse survival was higher for 6X than for 3X for both colostrum and milk mother sources, but surprisingly, even higher results were obtained when both the

3X or 6X potency quantities administered were cut by one half or one quarter in both colostrum and milk, resulting in nearly 100% mouse survival rate in most cases! This surprises us, but would not have surprised Hahneman, founder of homeopathy who stated two principles: (1) the more dilute, the stronger the homeopathic effects; (2) the less quantity used, the stronger the effects.

A second study (replicated) gave similar results.

One hundred and thirty cows having udder congestion and/or abnormal milk contributed milk samples. Staphylococcus aureus, a *Streptococcus agalactiae*, g-*Streptococcus agalactiae*, and *E. Coli* were collected and used to make a first homeopathic mother from a healthy cow.

Homeopathic material was prepared to the 6X potency, whence these were bottled under 50 ml sterile conditions, of which ten 50 cc bottles were sent to the veterinarian.

"Each month the cows in a herd having high cell counts (disease indicator) are listed on the owners required report (DH1A) for treatment. The high [bacteria] cell count cows in the herd were treated with

2-4 cc (ml) doses of the homeopathic product orally in their feed at twelve-hour intervals with the results shown in the third table in the patent."[142]

In the third table, results showed that in most cases, a High Somatic Cell Count (SCC) of greater than 1,000,000 reduced to less than 200,000 within two weeks of treatment.

A similar study was performed, with similar results, using the cow's colostrum instead of milk.

The Vaccination Process

Zoltan Rona, M.D., in *Nature's Impact*,[140] says, "At one time, conventional medical doctors were enthusiastic about using colostrum as an antibiotic. This occurred prior to the introduction of sulfa drugs and penicillin. In the 1950s, before the wide-scale use of corticosteroids as anti-inflammatory agents, colostrum was used to treat rheumatoid arthritis. Dr. Albert Sabin, developer of the polio vaccine, discovered that colostrum contained anti-bodies against polio; he recommended it for children

susceptible to catching the disease. For thousands of years, Ayurvedic physicians have used bovine colostrum for medicinal purposes."

When vaccination against microorganisms or pollens takes place, antigens or allergens are introduced into the human body. The object is to induce the body to produce vast quantities of antibodies which, presumably, result in (memory cell) protection against antigens or allergens.

According to Harold Buttram, M.D. and Richard Piccola, MHA, (*Our Toxic World: Who is Looking After Our Kids?*), vaccinations over-challenge small infants, depress the immune system, transfer into our bodies undesirable viruses including additional damaging contamination, disturb brain and nervous tissue, interfere with natural immunity-developing processes, bring about death or disability in some, and are probably responsible for chronic fatigue immune dysfunction syndrome as well as some other degenerative diseases.

If the end object of vaccination with the use of antigens and allergens is to bring about production of antibodies and cooperating complement — and/or protective transfer-of-immunity factors (called "transfer factors") — when under attack by the microorganism or allergen, then why not introduce the antibodies and complement and other transfer factors directly, thus saving money, time, energy, and health, especially to that of immature immune systems, such as babies?

This grand concept makes sense only if (1) there is a cheap source for antigen-specific antibodies and complement, and (2) the developed antigen-specific antibodies and complement are identical to that of humans.

The antibodies, complement and other transfer factors produced via other mammals, such as cows or goats, are low in cost and indeed identical to that of humans as has been repeatedly demonstrated over more than 70 years of research.

While it is considered optimum to use raw colostrum properly prepared — the farther from raw colostrum during handling and treatment, the more opportunity to damage or weaken the diseasespecific components, according to Herbert Struss, Ph.D. — the active transfer factors can be very carefully pasteurized and freeze-dried (lyophilized). During Philip Derse's past thirty years or so of research (Derse & Schroeder Associates), he learned that the active components can also be obtained from milk produced by specifically [antigen] challenged cows, when the milk is properly processed. This discovery increases by vast amounts the available active ingredients from specifically [antigen] challenged cows, and therefore lowers cost further.

Finally, the active products can be made to go farther and lower costs even further if the active ingredients are rendered into homeopathic remedies having specificity for given microorganisms — or

allergen-based diseases.

According to Fudenberg and Pizza, the FDA "approved" bovine Transfer Factor for human use again in 1985 and bovine colostrum in 1980.

Also according to Fudenberg and Pizza, two federal courts (one a Medicare court in a suburb of Washington and the other a health and human services court in San Francisco) ruled in 1987 that in diseases where no prescription medicine exists

Transfer Factor preparations are not experimental and furthermore ruled that insurance companies must reimburse the patients for the cost of Transfer Factor

preparation.[138] [We wish you lots of luck if you try this!]

Stolle Milk Biologics International

Beck and Zimmerman,[139] divide the history of immune milk discoveries into two general eras: (1) The Peterson Era (1950-1958) where Drs. "Pete" Peterson, Barry Campbell, and colleagues at

the University of Minnesota used killed bacterial antigens injected into the teat of a cow, and collected the first ten days' colostrum, as after the tenth day milk antibodies were almost entirely absent for immunization purposes.

"Peterson's interest in human diseases was concentrated on rheumatoid arthritis and allergies. . . ."[139]

Peterson's work, and its acceptance by the scientific community, was greatly limited by the state of knowledge of immunology of the times, according to Dr. Beck.

Impro Products of Waukon, Iowa received licenses from Peterson and went on to file some of the early patents, also supplying to this day a variety of products for use as a veterinary product. As a layman you're forbidden to purchase these wonderful products. However, any dairyman or veterinarian can do so. Impro produced an opaque 3.2 ounce bottle containing a wide variety of colostrum prepared by specific antigens. For example, gram negative, gram positive, *Borelia burghdorfia, Streptococcus, Staphylococcus, Salmonella, Escherichia coli,* and so on. In fact, Impro has long demonstrated the technical ability to provide an antigen specific colostrum against virtually any antigen.

A whole tray of antigen specific colostrum can be purchased by either the veterinarian or the dairy farmer. They also produce homeopathic remedies based on these products which can easily be purchased by the lay person. Apparently neither the FDA or US Food and Agriculture departments fear competition against pharmaceutical companies from homeopathic remedies.

(2) The Stolle Era (1958 to present) began with Ralph Stolle, businessman and owner-operator of the SanMarGale Farm in Lebanon, Ohio.

Ralph Stolle was a businessman with far-reaching vision who built his financial empire upon innovation, and who was drawn to the concept of immune milk by the work being performed by Dr. Peterson and colleagues.

Stolle early concluded that the Peterson method of introducing antigens through the bovine's teats had commercial drawbacks and he set out to develop new methods that would permit system-wide standardization of the vaccination of antigens, separation of antibodies and other transfer factors, their safe storage and later use by humans.

That Stolle Biologics International and their team of scientists — Lee R. Beck, Ph.D., President, Daniel A. Gingerich, D.V.M., M.S., Peter Fuhrer, Ph.D., Director of Biochemistry, Robert Stohrer, Ph.D., Associate Director Biotechnology Division, and others — were successful is certain.

At the time of our interview [1998] Lee R. Beck, Ph.D. had 26 years of research and business experience in the field of milk biologics. His earliest work was as Director of Reproductive Research at the University of Alabama, Birmingham Medical School, directing a staff of 15 scientists, and where he was a pioneer in the field of controlled drug delivery. Dr. Beck worked as a consultant to the Stolle Research & Development Corporation from 1972 to 1985, also working with Mr. Ralph Stolle to manage and build Stolle's research laboratory becoming Executive Vice President and Director of Research for Stolle R & D in 1985. He became President of Stolle Milk Biologics International in 1995 when Stolle R & D and the New Zealand Dairy Board formed the Stolle Milk Biologics International venture, located in Blue Ash, Ohio.[59]

Stolle Biological obtained more than 300 patents that cover methods of production and composition of immune milk, isolation of anti-inflammatory factors, methods for treating vascular and pulmonary systems, prevention and treatment of arthritis, treating protozoal gastrointestinal disorders, production of immune suppressive product, passive immunization of mammals using avian and/or bovine antibodies, antibodies derived from bovid milk and avian egg, general mammalian immunization, dental caries inhibiting products, deodorants containing antibacterial antibodies, longevity factors, prevention of suppression of t-lymphocyte functions, protein antibodies derived from bovid serum, and use of honey as a vaccine.

These patents were filed and granted in the United States as well as in many foreign countries and, indeed, Stolle also formed a limited partnership with the New Zealand Dairy Board, where uncontaminated milk reigns supreme.

Using Stolle technology,[59] the New Zealand Dairy Board inoculates cows with a wide range of

standardized bacterial antigens, and, without interruption of the flow of milk and milk products pro-

duces a dried, standardized, pasteurized whey substance that is then packaged and sold in Taiwan, Japan, Korea, New Zealand, and Hong Kong, with plans to broadened nutrient supplement sales in other countries, as well as to increase the range of protective substances and their means of delivery.

Method Used by Stolle Milk Biologics and New Zealand Dairy Board to Produce Nutrient

Substances Containing Large Quantities of Antibodies and Anti-Inflammatory Factors for Human Use[59]

Cows are inoculated using standardized vaccines containing known antibodies. The cream is drawn from the milk from which ice cream and butter are made. Skim milk is then processed further by addition of rennet to produce casein, cheese and whey.

Whey is further separated by ultra filtration into “Whey Protein Concentrate” (containing high molecular weight proteins and IgG antibodies) and “permeate” (containing low molecular weight proteins and anti-inflammatory factors).

The permeate is run through an ion exchange column washed with 0.15 Moles NaCl, then freeze dried.

Permeate and antibodies are combined together after removing the lactose from the permeate, producing “Whey

Protein Isolate," a product that is spray dried and sold as a commercial product.

Numerous research studies clearly show that the Stolle products have desirable impact on strengthening the immune system, but, of course, none are aimed at solving a specific disease condition, such as Lyme arthritis disease, surely the next great commercial step in the immune history saga.

Dr. Struss reported that a method other than rennet was used by original researchers. This was glacial acetic acid. They found that the agglutinating titers were higher than when using rennet, which is a proteolytic enzyme. This resulted in a larger quantity of specific antibodies and complement. When using only rennet, the casein had to be washed out or dissolved to obtain its entrapped antibodies/ complements.

In a trip to New Zealand (1999), Herbert Struss, Ph.D. reported that two kinds of colostrum are produced, disease specific and non-specific colostrum.

When you go to a health food store and purchase colostrum, you're buying the non-specific colostrum, which means that a variety of antigens were used for its production but the probability of the antigens matching those that you need for the moment is virtually zero. Colostrum sellers will argue that their product will strengthen your immune system. Perhaps it will. Good Luck!

There you have it. For more than three quarters of a century members of the FDA and Department of Agriculture have suppressed a natural, low cost, absolutely safe means to conquer nearly every kind of disease or allergen. Since this would also reduce political income and power from the large pharmaceutical companies our senators and representatives have provided tons of our tax money to those who produce vaccines under the guise of necessity, advertising loud and long that our children will suffer if we don't let them get inoculated with too many and too dangerous of vaccines. Even their legal liability for possible damage has been removed from them, permitting the vaccine companies to go "hog wild!"

Beneath this long-standing deception is immune milk! Safe, cheap, wide-spread, with all of its critical variables already worked out!!! Are you yet wildly angry?

Is this or is this not the definition of evil?

Bee Pollen: The Perfect Food

In the search for health one's attention is constantly drawn to the evolutionary aspects of man's nutritional needs, the so-called cave-man diet. Everyone knows that man did not have processed sugar

during his stone age — and probably the only direct source for fructose, sucrose and glucose was fruit and vegetables — with the exception of nectar from flowers and its concentrate, honey from wild bees.

What I knew of bees and their importance to our health was virtually zero until a reading of Royden

Brown's book, *How To Live The Millennium: The Bee Pollen Bible*, available through C.C. Pollen Company[150]. It was clear that Royden Brown loved the products of the beehive as a hobby, a profession and, like some of us, was a health nut! It's furthermore clear that Royden Brown had studied bees and their products personally, and also he'd had translated virtually all of the important scientific papers from every country in the world. We highly recommend that you purchase a copy of the above mentioned book for a more thorough reading. This chapter, therefore, will be limited to a generalized summary of Royden Brown's book — of what we didn't know about bees and their products and how those products can influence our health. The content herein and all quotes are used by permission of Royden Brown before his untimely, accidental death.

Background on Bees and Their Products

"Renowned healers of antiquity employed [honey, bee pollen, propolis, and royal jelly] . . . . It was when the laboratories of the world community of nations confirmed that bee pollen contains all nutrients necessary in human nutrition that an efficient way to harvest bee pollen for the use of man became a necessity.

"In the course of her work, a pollen forager [the bee] will visit as many as 1,500 blossoms. A single granule of bee pollen contains from five hundred thousand to five million live pollen spores.

"Pollen is the male seed of flowers. It is required to fertilize the plant. The tiny particles consist of

50/1000ths of millimeter corpuscles, which are formed at the free end of the stamen. Every variety flower in the universe puts forth a dusting of *pollen*.

"Once a honeybee arrives at a flower, she settles on the stamen and nimbly scrapes off the powdery loose pollen with her jaws and front legs. She then moistens it with a dab of the honey she brought with her from the hive.

"When her baskets are fully loaded, the microscopic golden dust has been tamped down into a single golden granule.

". . . pollen . . . cannot be duplicated in a laboratory.

". . . raw honey in the comb is rich with pollen particles and bears little resemblance to the honey you find in the supermarket.

". . . , what was needed was a device of some kind which would dislodge a measure of the pollen as the bees enter the hive, while permitting the bees to retain a sufficient portion of the life-giving golden dust for the maintenance of the colony."

Royden Brown invented such a trap. "It is equipped with a series of scientifically-designed wire grids through which the bees must pass to gain entrance to the colony. As they make their way through the grids, approximately sixty percent of the pollen is gently brushed out of their pollen baskets. It falls through a screen into the pollen drawer situated beneath the trap.

"[The pollen trap] allows sufficient pollen to pass through the grids into the colony for the care and feeding of the hive population, and insures the harvesting of the driest, cleanest pollen possible. Moistureladen wet pollen from low-lying humid areas ferments quickly, or develops mold. This type of pollen must be heat-treated immediately to preserve it for use. But high heat processing kills the enzymes and reduces the nutrient value considerably, transforming the pollen into a dead food.

"When bee pollen is improperly stored and handled, it will lose up to 76 percent of its nutritive value within twelve months.

The only satisfactory method of preserving fresh, live bee pollen is flash-freezing at zero degrees to maintain hive-freshness indefinitely and to preserve all vitamins, minerals, and other nutrients intact. Allowing pollen to remain in the trap for as little as ten day's results in nutrient loss or worse. Beekeepers who harvest for the C.C. Pollen Company are required to gather bee pollen two times

per week. Each maintains a large chest-type freezer right alongside their honey extractors in the bee house. The C.C. Pollen Company mandates that all freshly gathered pollen be immediately flash-frozen in small batches.

"Honeybees have a flight range of twelve square miles and are masters at seeking out sources of pollen and nectar.

"The population of your hive will consist of one queen, approximately 20 to 100 thousand workers, and a few hundred drones.

"There are many bee farms in the U.S. which are maintained only for their honey production. Much of this honey ends up in the supermarkets as a refined liquid sweet with all the bits of pollen and propolis strained out. Unfortunately, only a true unrefined raw honey can be classified as a nutritive food. This type of honey is getting harder and harder to find. A few unrefined honeys still find their way into supermarkets, but health food stores are the place to be certain of finding this unrefined liquid gold, cloudy and rich with suspended bee pollen.

"The C.C. Pollen Company offers multiblended bee pollen harvested in environmentally-clean areas where man has not intruded with harmful chemicals, or polluted the surrounding countryside with the by-products of civilization, such as car exhaust and worse.

"Because it would be a disaster of huge proportions if the population of their hives were exposed to some of the dangerous agribusiness chemicals, migrating beekeepers are extremely careful to place their hives with farmers who use only harmless chemicals which pose no danger to the bees. The experts say the difference in yields in fields pollinated by the bees can amount to hundreds of millions of dollars per year across the U.S.

"This bit of amber [in the American Museum of Natural History] has been dated at 80 million years, but the bee preserved inside it may be much older than that. Chemical analysis indicates that the resin components which produced this amber actually came from a family of early conifers which proliferated in the Cretaceous period, from 135 million to 65 million years ago. The grand sequoia of today is a relative of those early pines."

Bee pollen will survive in a hard encasement that surrounds it for millions of years, and is often used to date archeological sites. This husk must be cracked for human usage. The C.C. Pollen Company developed a means for doing this without use of heat, chemicals, radiation or alcohol.

"Propolis is often called 'bee-glue.' Bees, then as now, collect propolis, take it back to the hive, mix it with flakes they secrete, and use it to chink up stray holes. Because propolis is the strongest natural antibiotic and disinfectant known, the bees also use it to insure that the interior of the hive remains hospital-clean. If a foreign object too large for the housekeeping bees to move contaminates the hive, it is coated with propolis and sealed off. This little bee [in the American Museum of Natural History] was undoubtedly on a propolis-gathering mission when she was caught and held fast in the sticky resinous sap of some ancient leaf bud.

". . . experts have long theorized that bees came into being at least 125 million years ago when flowering plants began blossoming in profusion. Bees and flowers are so dependent on one another for their very existence that the experts say they must have 'invented' one another. . . . Bees must have the carbohydrates they glean from the nectar present in the hearts of blossoms, as well as the proteins they require from the pollen they collect. Fossilized remains of pollen, leaves, and even flowers have been dated back to when dinosaurs ruled the land, more than 125 million years ago.

". . . bees have changed very little in the past 80 million years.

". . . we do know that primitive man not only fought the bees for their honey, but also feasted royally on the bee pollen stored in the comb and even ate the eggs and larvae. Aboriginal tribes still feast on bee grubs and still regard bee pollen and honey as well worth the price of a few stings.

". . . every age has regarded the bee as benefactor of mankind and accords this little creature almost

holy status.

"The Bible, the Talmud, the Torah, the Koran (the Code of Islam), along with the scrolls of the Orient, the writings of the ancient Greece and Rome, the legends of the Russian and Slavic people, even the relatively recent Book of Mormon (1830), all praise the industrious honeybee and her highly nutritious and healing products of the beehive.

"Hebrew scholars of the Torah, the Old Testament of the Christian Bible, say that early translators mistakenly used `honey' in many scriptures in place of the more accurate phrase `products of the beehive'." Royden Brown replaces the proper word in various biblical sentences, clearly making the meanings different when the words "pollen," "honeycomb," and so on are used, rather than the generalized

inaccurate term, "honey."

The ecologists of today reckon that over 100,000 species of plants would die out and become extinct without the pollinating work of the bee. Without these plants, life as we know it, perhaps all life would become impossible.

Health Benefits of Products of the Hive

"Writings over 2000 years old reveal that Egyptian physicians called honey the `universal healer'. In ancient China, honey was used to treat the victims of smallpox. The sticky stuff was smoothed over the entire body of the infected person. According to old records, this very contagious and disfiguring disease was stopped in its tracks and no pitting or scarring ensured.

"In light of present day scientific studies by the U.S. Bureau of Entomology showing that typhoid germs are destroyed in 48 hours and dysentery bacteria killed in less than 10 hours, when these bacteria strains are placed in a lab dish with a bit of raw honey, those old-time healers were onto something big. Raw honey is rich with the bee pollen particles we now know are the true source of honey's remarkable healing powers. . . . British researchers at England's Norfolk & Norwich Hospital tried raw honey to treat infected wounds with notable success. In days of old, raw honey was often the treatment of choice for dressing battle wounds." [Raw honey also contains hydrogen peroxide which explains some of its antimicroorganism status, and may also contribute to some of the health effects, according to Walter O. Grotz. See the chapter on Hydrogen Peroxide Therapy: Ed.]

Bee Pollen

Contents of Fresh Bee Pollen

(Percentage follows the ingredient in parenthesis.)

Amino Acids by dry weight: Arginine (4.4-5.7), Histidine (2.0-3.5), Isoleucine (4.5-5.8), Leucine (6.7-7.5), Lysine (5.9-7.0), Methionine (1.7-2.4), Phenylalanine (3.7-4.4), Threonine (2.3-4.0), Tryptophan (1.2-1.6), Valine (5.5-6.0).

Minerals by percentage of ash: Potassium (20-45), Magnesium (1-12), Calcium (1-15), Copper (0.05-0.08), Iron (0.01-.0.3), Silicon (2-10), Phosphorus (1-20), Sulfur (1), Chlorine (0.8), Manganese (1.4).

Vitamins and Hormones in micrograms/gram: Thiamine (5.75-10.8), Riboflavin (16.3-19.2), Nicotinic acid (98-210), Pyridoxine (0-9), Pantothenic acid (3-51), Biotin (0.1-0.25), Folic acid (3.4-

6.8), Lactoflavine (0.2-1.7), Alpha/Beta Carotene (A) (avg. 1.53), B_2 (16.3-19.2), C (152-640), D (0.2-0.6), E (0.1-0.32), Inositol (30-40), B_{12} (avg. .0002).

Pigments: Flavoxanthine, Xanthophyll epoxide, Carotene, epiphasic Carotenoids, Flavonols, Eth-

ylic Ether, Quercitin, Zeaxanthine, Lycopene, Crocetin, others.

Other Components: Water (3-4%), Reducing sugars (7.5-40%), Non-reducing sugars (0.1-19%), Starches and other carbohydrates (0-22%), Etheric extract (volatile fatty acids falsify the quantitative analysis of humidity beyond 70^0C.) (0.9-14%), Proteins (7-35%), Free amino-acids (10%), Human

Growth Hormone Factor (not measured), Hormones (gonadatropic estrogenic) (not measured), Rutin (not measured), Ash (1-7%).

Bee Pollen Miracles — Testimonials

1. A young man had acne — pimples and pustules — for over five years. Tried everything without success until at last observed his brother who used 3000 mg per day. In just three days, brother's redness was almost gone. Tried it himself, and quit worrying about his complexion thereafter.

2. Middle aged man cleared up long-standing (7 years) San Joaquin Valley fever. Had tried everything. After three months of bee pollen condition cleared up at least 50 percent.

3. Forty year old woman suffered for years with serious depression. She could hardly function. After a week or so of fresh bee pollen granules, slept less. After two months, found depression gone and took long walks and did housework cheerfully. After one year on the granules, lost twenty-five pounds.

4. Twenty-eight year old, overweight by 67 pounds, easily tired, took granules for four months and started losing two to three pounds per week. No longer too tired to exercise, noticed personality changes becoming more outgoing and having more self-confidence; increased mental alertness, too.

5. Young woman of twenty-four suffered from hypoglycemia. Switched to an all-vegetarian diet and eliminated all types of sugars, including honey. Began taking bee pollen with breakfast. After two weeks noticed drastic improvement in symptoms. Another woman of thirty-eight, 20 pounds overweight, also with hypoglycemia changed from constant fear and depression to calm cheerfulness with energy.

6. Forty-seven year old at 257 pounds was diabetic. After taking insulin for five years, has not taken any now for five months. Also has not taken ulcer or arthritis medicine for one year.

7. Health-food store owner and her husband took two capsules of *Pollenenergy* per day at breakfast for two months. Stopped both of their snoring.

8. One person's colon infection cleared up on taking six caps per day for four weeks. Six months of doctoring could not kill the colon's bacterial strain.

9. One doctor says, "I give this honeybee pollen to all my patients. It is an excellent product. I certainly recommend it to my fellow physicians as the best of its kind."

10. Fifty-two year old man with atherosclerosis and blockage of heart chamber deemed inoperable, suffered stroke. Condition improved greatly after taking bee pollen.

11. Woman, late twenties, suffered numerous health problems: had stopped menstruating, lost hair, frequent headaches and backaches, fatigued, and sensitivity to cosmetics. On taking bee pollen had more relaxed feeling in her body, and in just days was sleeping better. After eight months on pollen began having regular menstrual periods for the first time in seven years. Had increased strength, sounder sleep, more cheerful disposition, thicker and healthier hair, no more problems with chills. Another woman, after giving birth to last child, was depressed and hormones messed up, with irregular periods. Within three months of taking bee pollen, started having normal periods and moods leveled off. Nails started growing strong and long, and no longer split and chipped off.

12. Woman, aged seventy-two, suffered great pain from arthritis in knees, feet, hands, back and right hip complicated by osteomyelitis which had left one leg shorter than the other. Took teaspoonful of bee pollen granules before meals for thirty days, whence had more energy than for a long time. . . . At age seventy-five, and still on bee pollen, a recent physical exam found her in "text-book perfect" health with perfect blood pressure and an excellent blood analysis.

13. Male of fifty-five had had psoriasis for fourteen years. Two heaping teaspoons of granules for two months noted a reduction in areas of psoriasis, with more energy and strength.

14. Eighty-one year old former scoutmaster could not walk alone and not far even with help. After two months on bee pollen he can now walk a mile, and does not lean on wife's arm to walk any longer.

15. Elderly lady with senility vastly improved by fresh granules daily.

16. Senior citizen feels wonderful with bee pollen. no longer drinks beer or other alcoholic beverages.

17. Fighting radiation sickness, feels better with bee pollen.

18. Two skin lesions about face and head had refused to heal for over six months, have now vanished. More endurance and stamina and requires less sleep.

19. Allergies much improved; no problem with irregularity.

20. Gray hair is turning back to black! Another says that thin hair is really thickened, lustrous and jet black as it used to be.

21. No longer have to get up every two hours to relieve kidneys and no longer chronic constipation or fatigue.

22. Don't take antacids anymore.

23. After taking bee pollen for ten months, arthritis of spine no longer wears me out and constant dizziness is gone; have good complexion.

24. For a year and a half suffered with eczema. Fingers cracked open and bleeding. Now healed.

25. Four pound poodle with arthritis could hardly drag himself. One teaspoon in food and he no longer suffers from arthritis. Preacher says he had arthritis in painful state in left foot and limped. Now it's completely gone.

26. Leg pains gone, have lost fifty pounds and works every day of five day week.

27. Have had no cold, flu, or digestive troubles.

28. Suffers from emphysema, but now breathes more easily and is eating better.

29. Took pollen for forty-one days which took away bloatedness and is helping arthritis.

30. Seventy year old Noel Johnson, based on exercise, diet and bee pollen, was able to reverse longstanding heart condition, going from bed-ridden to champion long-distance runner, boxer and, as he describes it, stud at 80. Also lost arthritis, gout and bursitis.

Scientifically Established Miracles of Bee Pollen

A doctor wrote about a five year old child: "This is a severely developmentally delayed floppy child whose differential includes a structural abnormality in the brain or a genetic abnormality, some of which may be diagnosed by chromosome analysis or genetic screen." Parent's tried every possible approach with no improvement. The Easter Seals Rehab Center listed the child as "(1) Severe receptive and expressive speech/language delay; (2) Immature neuromotor functioning; (3) Delay in development of play/cognitive skills; (4) Questionable hearing acuit/perception; (5) Severe delays in all areas of development; (6) Severe hypotonia."

Her mother began to give Bee-Young tablets, and slow progress began: lost rag-doll floppiness, clung to mother when held. Later noted that her eyes fixed on colorful objects with interest; able to scoot body forward while sitting on couch; rolled over for the first time; reached with operational arm for articles; skin color better; able to drink from cup.

Improvement continued onward: Colleen is alert and interested in things around her — this fact alone is "medically impossible" — she is beginning to speak — she smiles and laughs, loves hugs and kisses. "A British physician rediscovered this old treatment and now successfully treats hay fever patients with his own unfiltered pollen-laden honey. He reports that during the first year of treatment, attacks are

reduced. During the second year of treatment, his patients are entirely free of hay fever symptoms. "Leo Conway, M.D. . . . treats his patients directly with pollen itself by oral ingestion, explaining, 'All

patients who had taken the antigen (pollen) for three years remained free from all allergy symptoms, no matter where they lived and regardless of diet. Control has been achieved in 100 percent of the earlier cases and the field is expanding. . . . Ninety-four percent of all my patients were completely free from allergy symptoms. Of the other six-percent, not one followed directions, but even this small percentage were partially relieved nonetheless. **Relief of hay fever, pollen-induced asthma, with ever-increasing control of bronchitis,** ulcers of the digestive tract, colitis, migraine headaches and urinary disorders were all totally successful'."

In nutritional tests, "Hundreds of mice have demonstrated that pollen is a complete food and that it is possible to let several successive generations be born and live without the least sign of distress while nourishing them exclusively on pollen."

"Bee pollen stimulates the production of hemoglobin . . . we have noted counts rising to 4 to 4.5 million. The large proportions of free amino acids, especially methionine, a specific medicine for the liver, explains the favorable action of bee pollen on that organ.

"Bee pollen contains all the essential components of life; it corrects the failings due to deficient or unbalanced nutrition.

Lecture by Gunther Vorwhol at a recent German Apiarist Convention in Sontra,Germany: ". . . the vitamin balance can be improved by eating this complete food from the bee hive," but additionally, "rutin

. . . favorably influences the permeability of capillaries. . . ." and there are "important hormonal factors, substances which act like the estrogenic or gonadatropic hormones which so greatly aid the human reproductive functions, both male and female. . . ." and also, " bacteria-inhibiting effects of the pollen collected by bees. . . . medical experience teaches that the ingestion of bee pollen is recommended in the case of digestion difficulties, arteriosclerosis, and liver dysfunctions. It also improves the hemogram (blood production)."

Published in *La Revue de Pathologie Generale et de Physiologie Clinique* "The Physiological & Therapeutic Effects of Various Bee Pollen Extracts," Bee pollen contains "variable quantities of an antibiotic potent against *E. coli* and Proteus, as well as a substance which significantly accelerates healthy growth of mice receiving a complete and balanced diet from other sources. . . . the effect of bee pollen acts favorably on the intestines, on the hemoglobin level of the blood, and in the renewal of strength in convalescents and in the aged."

From the Institute of Apiculture, Taranov, U.S.S.R.: Bee pollen has a "very high content of the nucleics, RNA and DNA."

Alain Callias, Ph.D., Academy of Agriculture, Paris, France: "Bee pollen is richer in proteins than any animal source. It contains more amino acids than beef, eggs, or cheese of equal weight."

From *Techniqures du Directorat des services Veterinaires*: "There exists in bee pollen a principle which accelerates healthy growth. . . . Experiments have shown that bee pollen contains an antibiotic factor effective on Salmonella and some strains of Colibacillus."

From Romania, in a paper by G. Calcaianu and F. Cozma entitled, "Treatment with Bee Products of the Behavior Troubles in Young People in the Period of Puberty and Teenage," Given regularly, bee products (pollen, royal jelly, and honey) lead to favorable results. . . . we can prevent important behavioral troubles."

In "Administration of Biological Pollen Products to the Undernourished," translated from Spanish Children's Hospital of Cordoba: [Out of thirty children under two years of age with varying degrees of malnutrition] "red blood cells and hemoglobin increased in 14 cases; calcium increased in 12 cases; urinalysis improved in 10 cases; proteins increased in 19 children. There was an 83.33 percent improvement in appetite."

In a special reporting from *Naturheilpraxis*, "A Summary of Clinical Tests Concluded With Bee Pollen,". . . a reduction of cholesterol and triglycerides and also of S-lipo-proteins and albumins, while K and S globulins increase. A normalization of cholesterol count . . . in 40 patients who suffered from cerebral sclerosis. . . . A treatment with a combination of bee pollen, royal jelly, and honey has positive effects during the biological crises of puberty and adolescence, during behavioral disturbances, with problems of adjustment, learning disabilities, neurotic disturbances, and excessive neuromuscular sensitivity. . . . increase work performance and favor blood circulation in the brain.

Mice Following the Ingestion of Pollenized Food," by William Robinson, Bureau of Entomology, Agriculture Research Administration: Mice that were bred to produce tumors were supplied bee pollen, while a control group was not. Tumor incidence was 100% in the control group after 31.3 weeks, as expected. The bee pollen group delayed onset of tumors 41.1 weeks. Seven mice were tumor free at 56 and 62 weeks when the tests were terminated. Conclusion: . . . bee pollen contains an anticarcinogenic principle that can be added to food."

L.J. Hayes, M.D., Apiculteur Haut-Chinois, Guebwiller in Mittelwigen: "Bees sterilize pollen by means of a glandular secretion which is antagonistic to tumors."

Sigmund Schmidt, M.D., The Natural Health Clinic, Bad Bothenfelds: "Bee pollen contains all the essential elements for healthy tissue and may well prove to be the natural cancer preventive all the world is seeking."

Ernesto Contreras, M.D., cancer specialist: "To my knowledge, there is no better and more complete natural nutrient than honeybee pollen."

Dr. Peter Hernuss, University of Vienna "conducted a study of 25 women suffering from inoperable uterine cancer. . . . [Surgery being impossible, they were all given chemotherapy]. . . . The lucky women given bee pollen with their food quickly exhibited a higher concentration of cancer-fighting immune system cells, their antibody production increased, and the level of their infection-fighting and oxygencarrying red blood cells markedly improved. . . .The control group receiving a placebo did not experience relief."

In a Yugoslav paper, "Therapeutic Effects of Melbrosin in Irradiation of Diseases," [Melbrosin is a Swedish preparation of bee pollen, royal jelly, and honey.] ". . . 84 female patients were separated from a group of tumor-dose irradiated patients who suffered from gynecological carcinoma and who showed clear signs of X-ray disease: fatigue, lack of dynamism, anorexia, nausea, vomiting, diarrhea, headache, unconsciousness, insomnia, heat and perspiration strokes, tachycardia, increased temperature, etc. . . . After taking the preparation [Melbrosin], 30.5 percent . . . had no sign of fatigue; 66.7 percent felt light fatigue; only 2.8 percent still complained of severe fatigue; 38.9 percent no longer suffered from anorexia; 41.6 percent exhibited light anorexia; 8.3 percent moderate anorexia; 44.4 percent suffered no longer of nausea; in 50 percent, nausea was reduced to the mildest form; in only 5.6 percent did the intensity remain unchanged. Great improvement was also achieved in psycho and neurovegetative complaints. . . . it was possible to conclude that improvement was obtained in 88.8 percent of the cases. . . " From the Argonomic Institute, Faculty of Zootechnices, Rumonia, an animal study showed the "immune-strengthening effects of bee-pollen."

From Yuogslav, by Prof. Dr. Izet Osmanagic, University of Sarajevo, "Reduced Sexual Potency:" "Summary: . . . forty patients were examined. Eighty percent suffered from relative or absolute reproductive impotence and some from reduced capacity for intercourse. . . . 1. An improvement in the general state of health and subjective condition. 2. An increase in sexual activity. 3. Improved sperm production . . . obvious proof of the positive effects of the preparation in cases of reduced sexual and procreative potency."

A joint Swedish/German study of 212 male patients using twelve different urologists, showed improvement in a variety of sexual dysfunction and chronic prostatitis.

Using Cernilton, a Swedish pollen preparation, Dr. Gosta Leander of Stockholm reported in "A Memorandum Concerning a Statistical Evaluation of the Results of a Clinical Investigation of Cernilton," stating, ". . . it can be confirmed that a statistically highly significant effect of the compound could be demonstrated in prostatovesiculitis, estimated on the basis of a double-blind control study of 93 patients, 50 of whom received the compound, and 43 of whom received the placebo. A 92 percent ascertained improvement was confirmed in the group given the compound. The effects of the compound found during the course of this study have been established as statistically highly significant."

From Kyoto, Japan, "Use of Cernilton in Patients with Prostatic Hypertrophy . . ." ". . . Of the ten cases which showed improvement, three were in the first degree of hypertrophy, four cases in the second degree, and three cases in the third degree. In two cases, symptoms recurred within one month after withdrawal of the drug; these patients eventually underwent prostatectomy. All patients in the third degree of hypertrophy subsequently underwent prostatectomy."

A later Japanese study concluded, "Of a total of 15 cases in the Cernilton group, 10 cases were effective; 3 cases slightly effective. Results obtained in the placebo group were much less favorable; effective in 7 cases; ineffective in 9 cases." No side effects reported in the 38 cases.

Egyptian scientists, F.A. Soliman and A. Soliman, in "The Gonad Stimulating Potency of Date Palm Pollen Grains," from the French journal *Experientia*, "Several investigators have extracted estrogenic materials from palm kernels and date pollen grains. . . . a gonad-stimulating principle was extracted from pollens. . . . combined activity of the two hormones present in 1 gram of pollen is close to 10 I.U."

From Rumania, Gh. Salajan and Gh. Baltan, in "Influence of Maize Pollen on Ovulation: Results of Incubation & Biological Value of Hen Eggs," Pigs, chickens and calves, pollen protein reduced food consumption, stimulated growth, increased ovulation, and in eggs, improved quality of incubation and the biological value of eggs.

From Yugoslavia, L. Pokrajcic and I. Osmanagic, entitled, "The Treatment With Melbrosin of Dysmenorrhea in Adolescence." [Melbrosin is a bee pollen/royal jelly compound.] One hundred and twenty 15 to 20 year old girls were included in this study which showed good results on "patients with underdeveloped constitutions and irregular menstrual cycles."

From Yugoslavia, Endocrinological Department of the University Clinic for Women at the Medical Faculty in Sarajevo, in "A Clinical Testing of The Effect of the Preparation Melbrosin on Women Suffering from Climacteric Syndrome," ". . . it may be said that in addition to causes of menopausal disturbances in general, this treatment offers justifiable indications that the preparation should be used in the treatment of all patients subjected to irradiation."

"A two-year study conducted by former Russian Olympic coach, Remi Korchemny . . . this study confirms that bee pollen actually does improve the crucial recovery power of athletes after stressed performance."

"A study reported by *Aerospace Medicine & Life Sciences* proved that the average daily consumption of food falls by 15 to 20 percent when bee pollen is a regular item on the menu."

Dr. Lars-Erik Essen, M.D., . . . dermatologist of Halsinborg, Sweden, says, "Through transcutaneous nutrition, bee pollen exerts a profound biological effect. It seems to prevent premature aging of the cells and stimulates growth of new skin tissue. It offers effective protection against dehydration and injects new life into dry cells. It smoothes away wrinkles and stimulates a life-giving blood supply to all skin cells."

G. Liebold, a holistic physician and psychologist of Karlsruhe, Germany, in *Bee Pollen: Valuable Good Nutriment & Remedy*, "Bee pollen should be used as prophylaxis and therapeutical treatment against all the disease of modern civilization. . . . Bee pollen is an excellent prophylaxis and therapeutical treatment against all the precocious symptoms of old age. It should be considered a universal geriatric treatment in the form of a natural remedy."

Naum Petrovich Ioyrish, Chief of the former Soviet Academy of Vladivostok reported, "Long lives are attained by bee pollen users. It is one of the original treasure-houses of nutrition and medicine. Each grain contains every important substance necessary to life."

Propolis

"Propolis is the sticky resin which seeps from the buds of certain trees, the bees prefer poplar, and oozes from the bark of other trees, chiefly conifers."

Sometimes called "bee glue," propolis is blended with flakes "secreted from special glands on the underside of the bee's abdomen. It is used by the bee to (1) reduce the size of the hive entrance, (2) plaster up unwanted holes to the outside, (3) cover over and sterilize dead organic matter [insects] that are too huge for the bees to remove, (4) line the interior of brood cells, and (5) to keep the hive antiseptic.

Propolis offers "antiseptic, antibiotic, antibacterial, antifungal, and even antiviral properties." Propolis was hand mixed as varnish for Antonius Stradivarius (1644-1737), "for his incomparable musical instruments."

Part of the antimicrobial properties against various bacterial and fungal infections is due to galangin, caffeic acid, and ferulic acid.

Empirical evidence, testimonials, and scientific evidence for the benefits of propolis "are as many and varied as are those for bee pollen," but not widely known in the United States.

Royal Jelly

"Royal Jelly is the rich royal milk fed to the Queen bee for the whole of her life." By feeding larvae Royal Jelly, a Queen is produced, otherwise the outcome is not a Queen bee.

"Royal Jelly, a thick fluid of creamy consistency and milky-white in appearance, "is synthesized in nurse bees' bodies during the digestion of bee pollen, accounting for its remarkable quantities of hormonal substance and the strong proteins found in its highly nitrogenous composition."

Contents of Royal Jelly

"Royally jelly is chemically very complex." Moisture content is "66.05%; proteins 12.34%; lipids 5.46%; reducing substance 12.49%; minerals. 0.82%; with unidentifiable elements totally 2.84%. "It is . . . exceptionally rich in natural hormones, offers an abundance of B vitamins (including thiamine, riboflavin, pyridoxine, niacin, pantothenic acid, biotin, inositol, and folic acid) plus vitamins A, C, and E. With twenty amino acids, royal jelly is a highly concentrated source of rich proteins, including cystine, lysine, and arginine. It possesses important fatty acids, sugars, sterols, phosphorus compounds, as well as acetylcholine. . . . rich in nucleic acids . . . DNA (deoxyribonucleic acid) and RNA (ribonucleic acid) . . . Gelatin, one of the precursors of collagen . . . gamma globulin . . . immunostimulating factor . . . decanoic acid which exhibits strong antibiotic activity against many bacterial and fungal infestations."

Scientifically Established Benefits of Royal Jelly

From Dr. A. Saenz, Head of the Laboratory of the Anti-Rabies Institute of Montevideo, Uruguay, later joining the Pasteur Institute of Paris, in a paper, "Biology, Biochemistry & The Therapeutic Effects of Royal Jelly in Human Pathology," says:

"When those who are suffering from arteriosclerosis are subjected to royal jelly treatment, the readings correct themselves. This correction of the plasma protein dispersion thus reestablishes normal activities of the metabolic process where lipoproteins originate."

". . . . very significant improvements in thromboangeitis obliterans (Buerger's disease).

"Simple stress, physical or mental exhaustion, so frequent in modern life, is rapidly corrected by treatment with royal jell.

"In manifestations of sexual involution, as well as in endocrine asthenias, royal jelly in association with classic therapies accelerates the normal re-establishment of disturbed functions by means of its action on the adrenal cortex."

Effects on weight of nursing infants are clearly evident, and improved tonic effect on child. "Mimics [the action of] amphetamines without the harmful side effects.

"Cases of anxiety, depression, shock, and senility all benefit by royal jelly treatment . . . . insomnia

. . . . corrected."

In gastroduondenal ulcer, "Its specific action is due especially to the presence of pantothenic acid, known to be necessary in the protection of the mucosa and the healing of ulcerations.

Several cases have been published of arthritics being helped.

"A satisfactory remission of Parkinson's disease. . . .

"Several specialists have employed royal jelly treatment with success in eczema, in neurodermatitis, and in impetigo. Its use is indicated in skin ailments with a very alkaline pH. Royal jelly has an acid pH which re-establishes the acid mantle of the skin."

H.W. Schmidt, M.D., in a lecture before the German Medical Association, topic, "Royal Jelly in Diet, Prophylaxis, and Therapy," says "The action of the active substances and nutrients contained in royal jelly takes place throughout the entire body and acts to regulate all the functions of the body. . . . it is apparent this is a powerful agent composed of hormones, nutrients, enzymes and biocatalysts which starts up and revives the functions of cells, the secretions of glands, the metabolism, and blood circulation. . . . it is the interplay of all the complex factors present in royal jelly which works to preserve life and strength in the organism, which delays the aging process, and which retains for as long as possible the youthful physical freshness of the body, elasticity of the mind, and psychic buoyancy."

How to Shop For Bee Pollen

1. Do not run to the nearest store and buy bee products without first learning about how they must be harvested, shipped, packaged and stored!

2. Buy bee pollen that comes from a widely varying geographic distribution, where its bulk source is from many different plants, and where the pollen has been blended and standardized.

3. Do not buy flower pollen, as the bee adds to the pollen, making it nutritionally active for human use.

4. Buy only bee pollen that has been deep frozen at the site of collection, and kept dry, unpolluted and frozen until packaged. Heat-treated pollen is robbed of nutrition. Pollen collected in humid climates is often poor.

5. If you can, buy pollen collected from unpolluted sources: no pesticides, herbicides, as far away from industrial pollution as possible.

6. Your taste test should be "sweet, fresh, and delicious;" your see test should note pollens of varying shades of gold, ranging from pale straw through oranges, browns, purples, to almost black; your feel test between thumb and middle finger should be soft and springy. If it crunches in your mouth and refuses to dissolve on your tongue, it has been destroyed and has little nutrient value.

7. Insure that the husk which surrounds the pollen has been prepared for human digestion and assimilation by means other than heat, chemicals, radiation or alcohol.

8. Insure that the bee pollen purchased and used has available a listing of nutritional content, and that the content is not deficient in certain appropriate vitamins, minerals, etc.

9. Purchase from only a reputable, reliable dealer.

In the words of *Health Freedom News*, October 1990, "From the Forum," by James F. Scheer: "What other health product contains 185 of the known nutritional ingredients — 22 amino acids and higher amounts of the eight essential ones than most high protein foods, 27 mineral salts, the entire range of vitamins, hormones, carbohydrates and fats and more than 5,000 enzymes and coenzymes, necessary for digestion, healing and for the continuity of life itself?"

The Arthritis Trust of America expresses its appreciation and thanks to C.C. Pollen Company for permission to use the foregoing materials, and especially to Royden Brown who had diligently researched and applied his findings for the purpose of bringing to us the very best possible bee products.

Proper Nutrition For Everyone By now you're asking yourself why we never mention nutrition. Nutrition, you're ready to tell us, is the foundation of all health and the cure for all diseases. Just because bee pollen contains all the

essential components of life and corrects the failings due to deficient or unbalanced nutrition, one can't live on bee pollen alone.

You're absolutely correct!

A few principles that many nutritionists fail to comprehend are these. More than six billion humans on the planet earth are to some extent genetically the same, but they also have remarkable differences. As we featherless bipeds expanded across our globe we encountered external conditions that weeded out many and selected others who bred entire generations that subsist on foods from which their forefathers would have sickened. Eskimos (Esquimaux) have inhabited the polar regions from eastern Siberia across Alaska, Canada and Greenland. Their bodies can subsist on foods that yours and mine most likely cannot. Many Africans lack enzymes to digest milk which the federally recommended food pyramids always enclose as a "must" to the health degeneration of our own Afro-Americans. Some folks do just fine on an all-vegetable diet. Some survive well on a mostly meat diet.

So, therefore, one principle to understand is that there is no one magic diet that will serve all human beings.

Smoking tobacco, drinking hard liquor, eating lots of sugar is always recommended as nonos — but, there are folks who live beyond a hundred who smoke tobacco, drink hard liquor frequently and constantly consume sugar. The chances of yours or our genetic composition tolerating these "nonos" are slim — but the point is that some folks can do so!

Those who claim (as so many do) that their diet is the one for you are probably wrong, or at least mostly wrong!

When healing the body it is almost always true that you must have good acidic conditions in your stomach but the balance of your tissues should be somewhat alkaline, not acidic. The food that you eat can switch those other tissues back and forth from acidic to alkaline and back again to acidic.

Most germs thrive in an acidic environment and die off in an alkaline diet! Your tissues metabolize, grow and remain healthy in a somewhat alkaline diet!

Therefore, any diet that you settle on should strive to reduce acidity (except in the stomach) and increase alkalinity!

Before we present one of the founders of the Arthritis Trust of America, Gus J. Prosch, Jr., M.D. (deceased) recommends that he must warn that very little of the food that you buy or eat is suitable for human consumption. From childhood on upward through every form of communication you are inundated with food falsehoods. As one brilliant biochemist put it, there are two things people place in their mouths. One is called "food" and the other is called "nonfood." He said, "I'll define "nonfood" first. "Nonfood" is everything that has been canned, frozen, packaged or in any way treated to provide longer shelf-life for your grocer. "Food" is that which you gather from your garden.

We know that this truism is a very difficult statement to swallow because all of your life you've been able to run down to the store and pick up something that's easy to open, warm-up and serve. It fills the stomach, doesn't it?

To can food or to freeze it or to preserve food for future use requires heat that destroys necessary enzymes and to some extent natural, important molecules are changed. This change is most profound when exposed to microwave ovens. No knowledgeable health professional will approve any kind of food — even water — that has been heated by microwave.

"Gus J. Prosch, Jr., M.D. says: I've spent thousands of hours in research and many thousands of dollars to be able to write this article. It's been a primary goal of mine for the past twenty five years to develop the Perfect Plan in an effort to help my patients achieve a state as close to Perfect health as possible. Now, perfect health does not just mean the absence of disease. It involves many factors that not only *help keep you disease* free, but also factors that help to keep you feeling good, happy and content, sleeping peacefully, and energetically enjoying your work and existence.

"As a physician, I've been extremely concerned and even deeply worried, that the American people today are not getting the quality of medical care that they need, much less deserve. For generations, very wise men and women have reminded us that nothing — that's right — NOTHING — is as important to us as our health. Now, if you are like the many patients I treat every day, people from all walks of life, you're not getting very vital information and training that can help you avoid disease, have more energy, or even get rid of any medical problem you may have.

"You see, I sincerely care about your health. It's my job to care. In fact, my work is much more than just a job. It's a lifelong dedication and a passionate commitment to help you live a healthier life than you ever thought possible or even dreamed of. That is the purpose of this brochure: to make available to you the proven facts to attain Better Health, the information and condensed knowledge that once applied to your everyday lifestyle, will do absolute wonders for your health and existence.

I will provide this information to you in this paper, but it is up to you to act on it. I CANNOT DO THAT FOR YOU. If you act on this knowledge, whether young or old, rich or poor, no matter what race, sex or religious preference, you will live longer, healthier, and happier than you can even imagine. I've always tried to educate my patients about better health and one primary reason is because of the truth and wisdom I once read in an ancient proverb.

"If you give a man a fish, he will make a meal. If you teach him to fish. he will have a living. If you are thinking a year ahead, sow seed. If you are thinking ten years ahead, plant a tree.

If you are thinking one hundred years ahead, educate the people. By sowing seed once, you will harvest once.

By planting a tree, you will harvest tenfold.

By educating the people, you will harvest one hundred fold.

"I would like for this to be a manual of instruction for you to attain better health. Just like when you buy a new car, you get an owner's manual which explains how you can get the most efficient performance from your new car. This manual tells you what grade of oil to use, what type of gasoline is best, how to safely drive the car, and the proper way to lubricate and service the vehicle. If you do not follow these instructions, you could have disastrous results. You wouldn't put water in the gas tank or battery acid in your radiator and expect your new car to give top performance, or even run at all. This brochure is your owner's manual to attain better health with proper nutrition.

"The Healthless Generation

"Our generation may well be called the 'healthless generation.' With today's pollution or our air, water and food, good health or even normal health for the average person is an impossible dream. Degenerative diseases, which were almost unknown a century ago, are becoming epidemic today. Every physician who treats patients is seeing an increase in all the chronic degenerative diseases every year such as arteriosclerosis, arthritis, diabetes, cancer, heart disease,

Alzheimer's disease, obesity and hypertension — the list goes on and on.

"However, to me, even more significant than these major diseases that are increasing is the almost continual minor illnesses nearly everyone is developing nowadays, which are blindly accepted and endured by tens of millions of Americans. So-called 'minor illnesses,' like colds, flu, sore throats and ears, indigestion, joint and muscle pains, allergies, tooth and gum disease, fatigue, viral and fungus infections and a multitude of other conditions are robbing many people of good health. Unfortunately, these 'minor illnesses' are usually accepted today and simply taken for granted. I've seen many such 'sick and tired' people even brag about their health — right up to their dying day. Some people seem to believe that merely being alive means they have health. I cannot understand how these people settle for this when anyone deserves more.

"You can have better health, be a whole person and be free of disease. You can be whole physically, emotionally, mentally, socially, and spiritually as God intended you to be. You can be free from any health limitations whether major or minor if you simply follow the enclosed guidelines on how to eat, drink and live for life abundantly — not deficiently. BUT YOU MUST CARRY THE BALL YOURSELF AND PLACE YOUR HEALTH IN YOIJR OWN HANDS. NO ONE IS GOING TO DO THIS FOR YOU, BUT YOU YOURSELF, so it's really simply up to you and you alone. I'll teach you how, but you must apply the knowledge.

"Why The Increase In Diseases

"In the 1960s and 1970s, extensive studies were conducted by the Ford Foundation, as well as several U.S. Government agencies, concerning the health of America. The conclusions derived from these studies proved that the chronic degenerative diseases were increasing each year, behavioral and scholastic problems in all our schools were increasing nationwide, no matter how many millions of dollars were thrown at these problems and good health in general is deteriorating in America. No psychological or social factors studied could account for the above conclusions and much evidence pointed to a biological cause — perhaps a nutritional basis as a primary factor in reaching these conclusions.

"In 1982, the W.K. Kellogg Foundation commissioned Joseph D. Beasley, M.D. of the Institute of Health Policy and Practice at Bard College Center, to undertake a detailed study to determine why the conclusions of the Ford Foundation were happening in America. The conclusions of this study were just published in 1991 and the results are startling. The study concluded that no one factor determines our health or any disease. Health is a quality, the most important quality of life. It is a state of being — of countless interrelationships in what is called 'the web of life.' Neither the most brilliant scientists nor the world's most sophisticated medical centers understand the 'web of life' in enough detail to manage or control it. The fact that they also cannot prevent or cure the chronic conditions, suggests that these are not so much diseases as symptoms of the underlying state of our health, of something gone awry in the web of our lives.

"Great biological systems make up the web of life. Interacting in each of us continually, they yield our present state of health or illness. The existence of these systems has emerged into human awareness only in this century. Yet we know that if these systems are healthful — in good shape biologically — we humans will be healthy. We cannot manage health directly, for it is a quality. But we can protect and support the biological systems out of which life arose and on which our health depends, moment to moment. I came to these same conclusions twenty years ago and have tried to incorporate these principles in educating my patients each day.

"Of these biological systems, the above study concluded that there are 5 which are absolutely essential to achieve the best of health in today's society. THESE 5 SYSTEMS ARE:

"1. Our personal genetics, our genes inherited from our parents, the body's unique cellular code or blueprint that guides all its processes.

"2. External events, accidents, luck or agents that cross our path by chance that affect our health such as a car wreck or flu bug or being in the wrong place at the wrong time.

"3. Nutrition — the sustenance and fuel we provide our bodies and minds every day and especially the 50 essential nutrients.

"4. The Environment, the milieu of natural and manmade elements, pollution, indoors and out, that supports or undermines human life and health.

"5. Our behavior or lifestyle in that environment, stressful or relaxed, sedentary or active, with or without smoking, alcohol, drugs or exercise and so forth.

"Of course, some might argue that these first two systems are factors that you can do nothing about, but I disagree because we can practice better safety habits (seat belts, protect against exposure to cold, etc.) and can, by better nutrition, stimulate our genes to work at maximum efficiency. The last three systems and their improvement have been the basis of my medical practice for the past twenty years and are the main factors. Physicians in America today are not taught in medical school about nutrition and the proper diet, or about pollution and toxic substances in our environment, and they are taught very little about lifestyle changes that must be made to attain better health. I'm very appreciative and feel honored that God has led and directed me to study and learn all about these important systems so that I can give my patients the truth as to how to attain better health.

"What Causes Sickness and Disease

"There have been a multitude of basic theories as to what are the main causes of sickness and disease and I will briefly discuss three of these theories.

"1. Germ Theory. This theory in a nutshell simply means that if you 'catch' a certain germ in your system, you will develop a corresponding disease. Most all physicians today believe this and don't even question it. I only partially believe the above in the sense that it is true that certain diseases are severely aggravated and initiated by certain germs. I do not believe that simple statement that germs cause disease because in order for a germ to cause a disease, you've got to have a body that is willing to accept that germ. If you don't have a body that's willing to receive the germ — if your body is healthy and your resistance is high, and you haven't inherited a weakened organ system willing to receive the germ, you will not develop a disease from contacting that germ.

"As an example, I'm sure you remember the incident some years ago during the American Legion Convention in Philadelphia, where there were 15 deaths from Legionnaires Disease. Investigations proved that the disease was caused by a relatively unknown viral type germ that was transmitted through the ventilating system of the hotel where the Legionnaires stayed and were holding their meeting, yet even though all 16,000 people were exposed to the germ, only 15 had a fatal outcome from the exposure. The truth is that germs are everywhere at all times and we are all exposed to them thousands of times each day and you cannot avoid exposure to these germs but you can avoid diseases initiated by the germs if you have a healthy immune system and other efficiently functioning body systems.

"2. Nutritional Deficiency Theory. The mainstream of medical practitioners have never believed this theory but numerous physicians and especially those involved in the study of nutrition believe that deficiencies in certain vitamins, minerals and other nutrients cause sickness and disease. I personally am convinced that nutritional deficiencies play a role in the development of diseases, but they are not the actual cause of diseases normally. Exceptions to this would be Scurvy (Vitamin C deficiency), Beriberi (thiamine deficiency), and Rickets (Vitamin D deficiency), and a few others. Nutritional deficiencies can cause malfunctions of numerous metabolic processes which weaken the body's immune system or the body's resistance but these deficiencies usually do not cause disease and sickness.

"3. Auto-Toxemia Theory. Proponents of this theory believe that our bodies remain healthy by continually ridding themselves of toxins through various organs of elimination. These organs are primarily the liver, kidneys, lungs, skin and colon. Physicians who believe this theory state that the body gets sick and disease develops when the body has more toxins and poisons than the elimination organs can dispose of and as a result, disease develops. I personally believe there is much truth in this theory but it is not the sole cause of disease and sickness. The excess toxins from air, water and food pollution do play a major role in weakening the organs of elimination, as well as the entire Nervous, Endocrine and Circulatory System and diseases will develop in these weakened organ systems if the source of these toxins and poisons are not removed. There are many steps a person can take to remove these toxins and

I'll mention several.

"What is the Truth?

"I have always believed and teach my patients that the truth lies in a combination of all these theories. There's much truth in all three, but I have felt for years that the real truth lies in the previously mentioned conclusions of the Kellogg Foundation Report showing that the primary systems involved

are not only genetics and accidents or luck, but good nutrition, environmental pollution and lifestyle changes. The reason I believe that a combination of these theories holds the truth is that I see good health develop every day in those patients who follow my suggestions.

"Diet and Nutrition

"Essential nutrients are those substances necessary for growth, normal functioning and maintaining life. These nutrients must be supplied by foods because they cannot be made by the body. In my thinking and discussions with patients, I usually extend the element of essential nutrients to include other components that are necessary for human life. These include oxygen, water, fiber and so on. . . .

"With the above, I have concluded that there are several categories of essential nutrients that must be addressed to attain proper nutrition and better health. These include the following categories.

1. Proteins — primarily in the form of amino acids.
2. Carbohydrates — natural sugars and starches.
3. Fats — primarily in the form of essential fatty acids.
4. Vitamins — fat and water soluble.
5. Minerals — essential and trace minerals.
6. Water— the most important of all.

7. Others — oxygen, fiber, specific anti-oxidants, etc.

"Recommended Daily Allowances

"Recommended daily allowances (RDAs) are merely guidelines to the quantities of nutrients that the body needs each day. They are set by committees and are simply opinions based on scientific evidence at hand. These recommendations are made on inadequate information and even differ from one country to another. All too often however, and unfortunately, many doctors cite RDAs as though they are the Gospel. This is far from the case and highlights the fact that the mere existence of RDAs can lead to a misunderstanding of what is actually occurring with any individual. Many recent studies made in the past ten years, are showing that even though many patients eat a 'balanced diet,' more than 90 percent suffer from the lack of one or more essential nutrients. The idea behind setting RDAs was to give at least some idea to the likelihood of groups of individuals being deficient in a specific nutrient when considering their dietary intake. This has severe limitations because people not only have different and unique fingerprints, but also different and unique nutritional requirements. In my opinion, the RDAs are useful only as a guide as to what amounts of these nutrients will prevent specific nutritional diseases like Scurvy, Beriberi, Rickets. To use them as a guide to attain better health can be catastrophic.

"1. Quality of food

2. Quantity of food

"Factors Influencing Nutritional Status

3. Efficiency of digestion.

4. Efficiency of absorption.

5. Efficiency of utilization.

"1. The Quality of the Food. Food grown on nutrient poor soil can be deficient in certain nutrients

The trace minerals in soils are largely governed by farming policy. Overworked soil and soils that have added chemicals such as pesticides, insecticides and herbicides, can adversely influence the quality of the food. Hormones, antibiotics and other chemicals fed to commercially grown cattle, chickens or pigs, to make them grow faster, definitely influences the biochemistry in our bodies. Certain processes that foods undergo during manufacture and storage influence their nutrient content. Even food preparation procedures in our kitchens influence the nutrient content of our foods.

"**2. The Quantity of the Food.** In America, under nutrition is not a problem. However, malnutrition can occur anywhere as a result of wrong food choices and a dependence on large amounts of heavily refined foods. Processed foods (foods in boxes, cans and packages) have had many essential nutrients removed and can definitely influence nutrition. Whole grain and unprocessed (fresh) foods are always superior and in fact, the 'health food nuts' of the past who insisted on whole grains and fresh vegetables have been proven right by modern science.

"**3. The Efficiency of Digestion.** A person who has an inefficient digestive system will naturally be more likely to have a poorer nutritional status than a person with an efficient digestive system. The former is often seen by physicians when certain patients do not have enough hydrochloric acid in their stomach to allow the stomach enzyme pepsin to work properly. This leads to impairment of other digestive enzyme activity.

"**4. The Efficiency of Absorption.** Digested foods must be absorbed properly from the intestine into the blood stream to provide the body with these essential nutrients. One example I see very often where patients do not absorb vital nutrients, is when patients have an overgrowth of yeast called Candidiasis. The yeast grows little finger-like projections that tend to 'plug up' the absorption tissues called villi and nutritional deficiencies can rapidly result.

"**5. The Efficiency of Utilization.** A person may have proper digestion and absorption of their food and nutrients, but previous deficiencies of certain vitamins and coenzymes may prevent certain vital chemical reactions from taking place in the various metabolic processes that are going on continually in the body. Some people with genetic defects may excrete excessive amounts of nutrients in the urine which definitely influences one's nutrition.

"**Truths and Myths about Nutrition**

"The idea that our Western diet is excellent and healthy needs to be debunked. Below, I've listed some myths that are still widely believed by many doctors and nutritionists in America.

"Myths

1. Animal protein is necessary for optimal health. But, according to some recent studies, animal protein is indicated for people with type O blood.

2. Nutritional deficiencies cannot exist in people on a so called 'healthy balanced' diet.

3. Sugar is an essential nutrient for energy.

4. Milk is necessary to maintain adequate calcium balance.

5. Food preservatives, colorings and additives do not affect good nutrition.

6. Skipping meals will help you lose weight.

7. Breakfast can be skipped and it won't hurt you.

8. Vitamins give you energy and make you hungry.

"Truths

The American diet contains too:

1. much animal fat,.
2. much salt,
3. much sugar and refined foods,
4. little fiber,
5. many processed foods,
6. much coffee, tea, alcohol and soda pop,
7. little pure water, also,
8. The American diet contains potentially harmful chemicals such as insecticides, pesticides, and herbicides, as well as damaging food colorings, flavorings, preservatives and additives,
9. Skipping meals will not help you lose weight and you should always eat breakfast every day,
10. Only calories from carbohydrates, proteins and fats give you energy. Vitamins themselves do not give you energy nor do they make you hungry.

"A Lesson in Chemistry

"This next lesson could well be the most important of all in helping you to understand why you must change your dietary habits if you ever hope to achieve better health. If you presently are sick or have any major or minor illness and sincerely desire to get well, you must remember that in order to make your life anew, you've got to change your point of view. You must remember that no matter whom you are and no matter what state your health is presently in, YOU CAN CHANGE AND IMPROVE YOUR HEALTH. You can slow down the aging process and eliminate the degenerative changes taking place in your body because with the information in this brochure, you will now be armed with the true facts as to what you must do. With my help, we will identify the major causes of your body's malfunction, then you must live as wisely as you can with the hazards you cannot remove. You see, there presently exist effective medical knowledge that is sufficient to prevent and/or to reverse the many malfunctions of body processes that are continually happening in our body systems. Unfortunately, most physicians do not understand these processes and are unable to advise their patients accordingly.

"Proper Chemical Balance Keeps Your Body Healthy

"If you sincerely desire to attain the best of health and to stay healthy, you should try to understand some basics of the chemistry of dissolved solids in your body fluids and how they work to keep you healthy and disease free. I must warn you, however, that the explanation is quite technical and unfortunately many physicians do not understand these processes as they are not taught in any depth in our medical schools because the processes involve colloidal chemistry — the chemistry of dissolved solids in liquids. If this section is too technical for you to understand, you may want to skip to the section entitled 'A SIMPLIFIED EXPLANATION.' I would prefer that you read this entire section however.

"SOME BASIC DEFINITIONS

"To clearly understand this next section, you must comprehend some basic definitions of chemistry language, so try to understand the following definitions.

"Atom. An atom is the smallest part of an element that can exist or that can enter into a chemical combination. Atoms have a negative or positive electrical charge.

"**Electrolyte**. Any substance or compound or molecule that can separate into ions when dissolved in solution, and thus becomes capable of conducting electricity. All salts as table salt (NaCl), Epsom Salt (MgSO4) or baking soda (NaHCO3), etc. are electrolytes.

"**Element.** The fundamental or elementary substance that cannot be broken down by chemical

means to simpler substances. All matter in the universe is made up or composed of one or a combination of 108 presently known elements. Examples of elements are hydrogen and oxygen, which combine to form water. Elements may be liquids, gases or solids.

"**Compound.** A compound is a distinct substance containing 2 or more elements chemically combined in definite proportions by weight. Compounds can be broken down into the elements that make them.

"**Molecule.** A molecule is the smallest uncharged individual unit of a compound and is formed by the union of 2 or more atoms. Water is a typical molecular compound and a single molecule of water consists of 2 atoms of hydrogen and 1 atom of oxygen giving the chemical formula H20. A molecule of table salt contains two elements; one atom of sodium (NA+) and one atom of chloride (Cl-) and when combined, form a single molecule of salt with the chemical formula NaCl.

"**Ion.** An ion is a positively or negatively electrically charged atom or a group of atoms. An ionic compound is held together by attractive forces that exist between positively (+) charged and negatively (-) charged ions. A positively charged ion is called a CATION (pronounced cat-eye-on) and a negatively charged ion is called an ANION (an-eye-on).

"**Colloid**. Particular matter (compounds usually in solution) in the size range of 10 angstroms (a unit of small-size measure) to one micron (another unit of measurement of larger size) in diameter which fail to settle out when in a solution or in a liquid suspension. When colloids are dissolved in or dispersed in a liquid or solution, this system is called a colloid system. All body fluids are examples of colloid systems as blood, urine, saliva, etc. In fact, blood and urine are a mass of colloids which include all electrolytes, protein particles, sugars and other dissolved solids.

"**Homeostasis**. The state of equilibrium (balance) of the internal environment and relative constancy of all body fluids with their chemical and physical properties. Ideal homeostasis exists when all normal body fluid chemicals and dissolved solid substances are in perfect balance.

"To summarize these definitions, I can state that one atom of sodium (Na+, an element and a cation) can combine with one atom of chloride (Cl-, an element and anion) to form one molecule of the chemical compound NaCl (table salt). Now, after dissolving the NaCl in water and when hundreds or even thousands of these NaCl molecules are dispersed (spread throughout the water) we then have a colloid system composed of the colloid form of NaCl whose molecular particle size keeps the NaCl dissolved in the water and the NaCl doesn't settle out. If too much salt is added to the water, the solution will soon become overly saturated with NaCl and the excess NaCl molecules will clump together (aggregate or agglutinate) and settle out to the bottom.

"**Understanding Colloid Chemistry— Vital for Good Health**

I feel that a terrible mistake is made in all our medical schools today, by not teaching colloid chemistry to all medical students. They are taught inorganic chemistry which is the chemistry of all elements (dead things) other than carbon and their compounds and they are taught organic chemistry which is the chemistry of the compounds of carbon (live things), and biochemistry which is the study of the specific molecular basis of life, but very little is taught about colloid chemistry which is what the body fluids are all about — the behavior of the dissolved solids and colloids in all our body fluids. As I've already mentioned, most physicians are so ignorant concerning colloidal chemistry that they cannot even give you a clear definition of what a colloid is. This is tragic. Without an understanding as to how these colloids or dissolved solids behave in our body fluids, IT IS IMPOSSIBLE FOR ANY PHYSICAN TO FULLY UNDERSTAND THE

MECHANISMS OF MANY DISEASE STATES AS WELL AS HOW TO TREAT THEM. This is one of the main reasons that medical students today are taught to treat symptoms of diseases with drugs and chemicals instead of being taught to treat the cause of the disease.

"Our Blood — Constantly Out of Chemical Balance

"Now, to put the aforementioned definitions to use to help you understand what is really happening concerning poor health in America, let me simply explain about what is happening with the cations and anions in all our body fluids, but with emphasis on the blood. When one is in good health and homeostasis and usually when a person is born, each liter (1,000 cc or slightly more than a quart) of blood contains approximately 2/3 anions and 1/3 cations. However, due to the pollution of our water, the polluted air we breathe, the chemicals and preservatives in the food we eat and the excessive amounts of prescription and nonprescription drugs and medications most people ingest, this ratio has reversed in most people to the point that most of us have about 2/3 cations and 1/3 anions in our blood.

"Your Drinking Water— Critical

"Most all city water filtration systems do an excellent job in making our drinking water germ free, but they do a miserable job in removing excess cationic dissolved solids that are increasing each year due to the pollution of our environment. Unfortunately, most bottled waters (with the exception of "distilled" water) do not address this problem and the majority of home water filtering systems on today's market does not remove these excessive cations. I advise all my patients to bring a pint of their drinking water to our clinic so we can check by a very sensitive electronic machine, the actual dissolved solids in their drinking water. I also advise my patients that before buying a home water filtration system to get a pint sample of the filtered water and bring it to the clinic to be checked before buying any water filtration system. I've found very few filtration systems that actually do what they claim to do, and those that do a good job are all using a reverse osmosis (R.O.) filtering system. Most of the waters from wells that I've been checking for my patients have much fewer cationic dissolved solids than most city waters. Therefore, to help eliminate this hazard in your health, you should drink distilled water or reverse osmosis (R.O.) filtered water from a good home water filtration system. I CANNOT EMPHASIZE ENOUGH TO YOU, THE IMPORTANCE OF DRINKING AND COOKING WITH THE CORRECT TYPE OF PURE WATER THAT DOESN'T HAVE EXCESS CATIONS.

"However, I'm not at all happy about directing you to distilled water, which is often "dead" water. One physician advises filtering your home water system with ceramic filter, activated charcoal filter, reverse osmosis unit, ultra violet light, and a magnetic loop around the tubing to remove homeopathic influences. These are laid out in the order given, with water reaching the ceramic filter first. This water is truly excellent!

"The Air You Breathe—Critical

"Another danger that gives excess cations in our blood is the increasing pollution in the air we breathe. All the smog, tobacco smoke, diesel and gas fumes, pesticides, herbicides, insecticides, detergents, deodorants, formaldehyde, phenolic compounds and many other chemicals polluting our environment today are primarily cationic in nature and only serve to add to the burden of excessive cations in our blood. One should therefore make every effort to avoid exposure to these pollutants, and some patients have to purchase special filters for their heating and air conditioning systems, especially at home.

"Chemicals and Drugs You Take — Critical

"The pharmaceutical and drug companies are making billions of dollars annually in selling over the counter and prescription drugs and medications. Most all the pain medications, antihistamines, cough medicines, antacids, and indigestion drugs, diarrhea medications, laxatives, sleeping pills, not to mention tobacco, alcohol, and illegal drugs, are primarily cationic in nature and when ingested, also serve to increase the excessive burden of cations in our blood and body fluid systems. It seems we are in a Catch 22 situation because the more drugs and chemicals we take in the sicker we become, which to most people simply calls for more drugs and chemicals to treat the symptoms, and we then begin to develop even more serious illness requiring more drugs. One must not forget that drugs and chemicals of all kinds are foreign to our bodies and only add severe stress to our already stressed-out systems, but they cause an excessive burden on the organs of elimination, suppress the immune system and severely compromise the imbalance of cations and anions in our blood, which in turn prevents maximum efficiency of all body processes throughout. Our health then suffers. No wonder the chronic degenerative diseases are increasing every year and the drug companies and many health practitioners keep getting richer and richer while unsuspecting citizens get sicker and sicker.

"The Food You Eat — Critical

"Probably the worse source of polluting cations in our blood and body is from our polluted food chain. All the ingredients added to our foods to make them look good, taste good, easy and convenient to prepare and all preservatives added to give longer shelf life, are cationic in nature and critically compromise the overburden of cations in our blood. In fact, at last count, there are over 60,000 different colorings, flavorings, preservatives, taste enhancers, emulsifiers, texture balancers and a multitude of other types of food additives that serve to increase the cationic imbalance in our blood and body systems. The processing of these foods alone, in addition to poisoning with cationic additives, only serves to make these foods deficient in vital nutrients such as vitamins, minerals, amino acids, and fatty acids. Many people today are eating only processed foods, so no wonder America is sick. If you are following this same pattern, then you are going to get sicker unless you take your health into your own hands and do something about your health. Unfortunately, most people do not have anywhere to turn to for advice because most physicians know very little about nutrition. They know even less about cations, anions, and colloidal chemistry, and the health of America continues to suffer, degenerative diseases increase, the pharmaceutical and drug companies and most doctors get richer and the cost of health care keeps sky rocketing.

"What a dilemma!

"Why Excess Cations are Dangerous

"The question now arises as to why these excessive cations are so dangerous in causing disease and why the depleted anions are protective and prevent the development of many disease conditions. When one does an in-depth study of colloids and colloidal chemistry and the behavior of these dissolved solids in our blood, one quickly learns that there are known and proven laws of behavior that regulate and control the actions of these dissolved particles of cations and anions. There are proven laws concerning Zeta Potential, Vander-Waal-London forces, specific conductance, surface tension, steric hindrance, surfactants, electrophoresis, anion gap, homeostasis, intravascular coagulation and other processes that are vitally important in controlling the behavior of these dissolved solids in our blood. It would take a full length textbook to explain what actually happens and why it happens in our blood when we reach the point of having excessive cations dominate our fluid systems.

"Hopefully a very simplified explanation will suffice to help you get an idea of what is happening in your blood when overburdened with excess cations. Cations are sticky in nature and you can imagine sticky substances in your blood trying to flow through your arteries and capillaries. A good portion of these sticky substances are going to stick to the lining of your blood vessels and this can build up over a period of time. (Could this be the actual cause of arteriosclerosis or hardening of the arteries?) These sticky cations will stick to the formed elements (red blood cells, white blood cells, and platelets) and they in turn will have a tendency to not only stick together (agglomerate) but also to stick to the blood vessel walls or lining. All of these sticky processes will finally terminate in a condition of electrolyte imbalance and intravascular coagulation where your organs and tissues cannot receive the proper nutrients (even if your diet has made them available), nor can the cells and tissues properly rid themselves of the cell products of waste metabolism. This results in a severe deterioration of cellular function and degeneration sets in. I've made a list of 64 different disease states where the above processes are playing a vital role in causing or aggravating these disease conditions. It's also been shown scientifically that heavy metal cations such as lead, mercury, aluminum, arsenic, cadmium, nickel and beryllium, are the absolute worst cations to initiate this intravascular coagulation. Our foods that are sticky are the high cation foods. All sweets and desserts, all processed foods (with additives of cations) like white flour foods, macaroni, spaghetti, pizza, chips and dips, most cereals, canned fruits, and all fatty red meats, but especially pork should be avoided as they are highly cationic. There are unprocessed foods like oatmeal and fresh fruits that are sticky and they have high cations but they also have high amounts of anions to balance them.

"The anionic foods are all the green foods, yellow foods, and slicky foods. If any vegetable is green, yellow, or slicky, it is high in the good anions. You can cut a cucumber and on rubbing it, the slickness is felt. The same holds true for squash, okra, broccoli, spinach, greens, cauliflower, cabbage, Brussels sprouts, as well as all the fresh green leafy vegetables. Yellow vegetables like squash, lemons, sweet potatoes, bananas or pumpkins, etc. are also highly anionic. The anions in the blood are slicky and all the formed elements (red blood cells, white blood cells and platelets) have a built in preference to have the anions coat their surfaces instead of cations, as well as the endothelial cells (lining) of our blood vessels. With adequate anions in the blood, you will find no intravascular coagulation (clumping or agglutination) and the circulation is greatly enhanced as those slicky cells slide quickly and easily through all our blood vessels and capillaries without clumping, and nutrients are efficiently delivered to the cells and tissues, and waste products from cellular metabolism are quickly removed from their source and carried to the excretory organs for proper elimination very efficiently. A person who has the proper amounts of the slicky anions will seldom be seen suffering from any of the 64 diseases listed.

"MOST PHYSICIANS DON'T UNDERSTAND THIS

"I want you to understand that the above subject and discussion is totally unknown, much less understood by 99% of the practicing physicians and health practitioners today. They haven't been taught colloidal chemistry and most doctors do not even understand the language of colloidal chemistry, much less comprehend the laws or principles involved in the forces that regulate the behavior of these dissolved solids (colloids) that our body fluids are composed of. So they will not even understand what I'm talking about and in all likelihood will ridicule, criticize, or scoff at the previous discussion because, human nature being what it is, I've learned that a law of human nature that usually applies is 'if they are not up on it, they are down on it.' (No one likes to admit their ignorance). Any honest and sincere physician reading this book will be compelled to call me to try to learn more about this vital subject in order to better treat their patients. The doubters and those that criticize this information are simply uninformed and ignorant (and maybe stupid), concerning these principles because there are basic laws concerning dissolved solids in the body fluids that work in certain ways under various conditions that I did not invent or make up or even discover, but these laws operate every day in our body fluids that control the behavior of these colloids. When we violate the laws we must suffer the consequences and our health deteriorates.

"My goal in life is to find the TRUTH concerning my personal, professional and religious life, and I've tried to pass on these truths to my patients in order to ensure that they attain better health. The previous discussion on colloids and dissolved solids in our body fluids are not my invention or conclusions. I'm not intelligent enough to figure out or to tie together all the processes involved because I am not a chemist, even though I have made an in-depth study on colloid chemistry principles. Numerous other physicians, chemists and scientists have made the discoveries and I have simply tired to help organize and tie these vital principles and laws together so that my patients can get well faster. I want no credit and deserve none for any discoveries or information produced in this brochure, but I have been able to help organize the ideas and principles into a format that will benefit my patients and help anyone who applies these principles and ideas to maintain superior health. I've never claimed to know everything and never will, but when I see the health of my patients improve by applying the ideas and principles recommended in this book, I feel obligated to share this information with anyone, physician or patient, who desires to achieve better health. These principles work and will enable you, if applied, to achieve the best of health for yourself and your family.

"TWELVE VITAL NUTRITIONAL AND HEALTH TOPICS

"There are twelve 'good health' practices and topics that needs further discussion and/or clarification to give you a crystal clear understanding of why you should incorporate them in your overall lifestyle. There is considerable confusion and false information that has been given out by various individuals and self interest groups concerning these subjects. Most of the confusion and incorrect fallacies have been spewed out to the general public in order for their perpetrators to make a profit on some 'health product' they are selling to an unsuspecting public. My desire and goal here is to bring you the truth, the facts, the proven knowledge to help you have the opportunity to use this truth to achieve better health — and I'm not trying to sell you any product or service. I just want you and your family to be healthy and avoid sickness. You may not be able to apply all of these principles to your lifestyles, but you will have the truth at your fingertips to use if you so desire. Again, IT'S UP TO YOU! I sincerely hope you put this information to good use.

"1. REFINED AND PROCESSED FOODS

"The food processing companies today are all in business to make money. You must never forget this fact. This is the American way, and I'm not being critical of them when I state this truth. There is tremendous competition among these companies and they are all striving to get you — the consumer -to buy their product instead of their competitors'. They do not want to harm you in processing their foods, but they simply want to make a profit from your purchases.

"These companies know that in today's society, in order for the average family to maintain the same standards of living that we are used to and the same standards our parents maintained as we grew up, it has become necessary for most husbands and wives to both work or be employed. The average wife (or husband) simply does not have the time or energy to prepare the wholesome and nutritious meals they feel they should feed their family. They must take short cuts and look for ways to save time, energy and money to give the family the necessary meals required. The easiest way to do this is to purchase processed, refined and prepackaged foods. Knowing this and trying to get your dollar, all food processing companies know that to be successful, they must make their packaged foods look good, taste good, and maintain a long shelf life. In order to accomplish this, they must remove many vitamins, minerals, fatty acids, much fiber and other vital nutrients from the foods and they have to add color and taste enhancers, emulsifying agents, preservatives and many other additives to keep the foods looking good and preserving them. All these added chemicals are cations and dangerous to your health. With some foods (like white breads) the U.S. Government requires that they add back 7 of the 23 nutrients removed. Most of the companies try to capitalize even on this by advertising that their product is "enriched" with the 7 nutrients they added back, but they never mention the other 16 vital nutrients removed from the flour. This is fraud and deception in my opinion as they are trying to make us believe they are 'enriching' the product by adding back some of the previously removed nutrients.

"Processed or refined foods are all packaged in boxes, bottles, cans or cellophane packages and include all sweets, pastries and desserts of all types, all white flour products including breads, crackers, biscuits, macaroni, spaghetti, pizza, most all soups, canned meats and vegetables and fruits and cereals. I jokingly tell my patients they can eat the box or cans, bottles or cellophane packages, but don't eat the processed foods in them. Truly, these cationic foods are very detrimental to your health and ideally should be avoided. The best safeguard to avoid these bad foods is to read all labels of any foods purchased and totally stay away from those items when food labels list the chemicals and additives that are put in the foods. Remember, fresh foods are the best to purchase, frozen or home canned are second best and bottled or packaged foods are the worst.

"And don't forget that most artificial sweeteners are also cationic and are not the best for you. The best sweeteners would be unprocessed honey (with some honeycomb in the bottle) and blackstrap molasses. White sugar or any ingredients ending in "ose" (glucose, fructose, maltose, etc.) as well as all white flour products tend to create an acid medium in the colon which is destructive to the good germs found in the colon. The good germs play a vital part in preventing yeast overgrowth, parasites and other harmful germs that try to grow in the colon.

"Also, remember refined foods and sugars are usually depleted in fiber and this simply slows the progress of the foods passing through the intestine which makes one more susceptible to constipation, hemorrhoids, varicose veins, colon and rectal cancers. Also, with a slower transit time through the colon, more time is allowed for putrefaction (rotting) of the refined foods to occur in the colon which allows more toxic substances to be absorbed into your system.

"And finally, please remember that all commercial wheat flour is prepared so that it can be stored for long periods of time without spoiling. To do this, 'the life' is removed from the wheat in the processing. Fresh whole wheat flour spoils rapidly. Unfortunately, except for those fortunate enough to possess a household flour mill, truly fresh flour is unavailable and this also applies to whole wheat breads found in most supermarkets. Probably your best choice under these circumstances is to purchase whole wheat bread from your local health food store and make sure that the bread purchased from your grocery store has written on the package 100% Whole Wheat or 100% Whole Grain. Eat no food products prepared from commercially processed wheat flour.

"All raw foods (except meats) are much more nourishing than cooked foods. The cooking process destroys or changes many vitamins, minerals and especially enzymes (cell produced catalysts involved in vital cell functions) which can severely compromise your digestion and the availability of these important nutrients. Raw fruits and vegetables are more cleansing and detoxifying than cooked foods, and their roughage or fiber value helps keep your food moving through the intestine efficiently. This plays a strong part in preventing hemorrhoids, varicose veins, diverticulosis and other colon diseases, as well as colon cancer. Also, the natural vitamins, minerals, amino and fatty acids in the raw foods are readily available for absorption and therefore play a major part in preventing deficiencies of these substances. The super abundance of natural enzymes in raw foods will ensure good digestion and absorption of essential nutrients.

"Many people go for weeks with no more raw food in their diet than perhaps a small amount of lettuce or an occasional glass of fruit or vegetable juice. Ideally, at least 75 % of our fruits and vegetables should be eaten raw and uncooked. This principle of nutrition is one that is most often overlooked and neglected in our American society.

"You should understand that raw fruits and vegetables are 'live' foods, and cooking them makes them 'dead' foods. Life diminishes in all fruits and vegetables in direct proportion to the time elapsed since picking. Life involves receiving live nutrients like vitamins, minerals, enzymes, amino acids and fatty acids and cooking makes many of these elements dead. We originally ate living food — that is right after picking or harvesting and even as recent as 30-40 years ago most people obtained much of their food from their own gardens and livestock. Dead foods are devitalized of most nutrients. Even though they will fill your stomach, they do not nourish your body and give good health. Therefore, dead foods like cooked fruits and vegetables produces death, and live foods like raw fruits and vegetables produce life.

"Our Creator with His omniscient wisdom made our foods whole and placed within each type of whole food the proper and adequate nutrients that are necessary for our body to digest, absorb and use these particular foods. This is why different foods contain different essential nutrients. Then humankind comes along trying to make a profit, refines the food, and removes many of the nutrients and adds chemicals to enhance taste and appearance and to preserve shelf life. This refining then destroys the God-intended value of the food. It's common sense to ask yourself, 'How can any given food be assimilated and used by our body when the refining process robs that food of its vital nutrients.'

"Let me explain why the above is so critically important. In researching and studying why the chronic degenerative diseases were increasing and what treatment methods could be applied to halt this onslaught on the health of America, I came to several conclusions. Of these conclusions, there were three that were certain primary sources that greatly contribute to the epidemic of cardiovascular-renal disease we are seeing today. My conclusions were influenced greatly by T.C. McDaniel, D. O. of Cincinnati, Ohio, and published work completed by the late physical chemist, Thomas M. Reddick of New York.

"These three vital contributing factors causing the cardiovascular-renal disease epidemic are:

1. Excessive mineral salts (strongly cationic) intake that is happening to most all Americans today.

2. The reversal of the God-provided natural sodium-to-potassium ratio that is directly caused by food processing today.

3. The ingesting of these excessive mineral salts are overworking, overwhelming and critically harming our kidneys which results in colloid particle imbalances in the blood, and then intravascular coagulation begins. Degenerative diseases result.

"As Dr. T.C. McDaniel concluded, I agree that a major factor contributing to the excessive mineral salts in our food supply lies in the basic misconception and lack of knowledge on the part of the [employees of the] FDA concerning the physical chemistry of food processing. Although the FDA

limits certain chemical additives to food to 1% of the amount demonstrated to be without harm to experimental animals, they permit virtually unlimited use of hundreds of chemicals that they classify as GRAS (Generally Recognized as Safe). I sincerely do not believe the FDA researchers fully understand the colloidal behavior of the excess salt, for example, found in our processed foods.

"In measuring the specific electrical conductance (mineral salts) in 8 fresh vegetables (asparagus, beets, carrots, corn, lima beans, peas, string beans and tomatoes), it was found that measurement of these foods in a fresh state resulted in an average of 7500 micromhos. These same foods measured from canned and processed sources gave an average reading of 17,500 micromhos. These readings show over 2-1/2 times the mineral salts found in these canned vegetables as compared to fresh forms.

"Another example was taken from the *Handbook of the U.S. Department of Agriculture* (No. 8) which shows the amounts of sodium and potassium and their ratios of these minerals in the natural God-given, fresh state, and also after being processed. Eighteen fresh natural foods were listed (including those mentioned in the specific conductance test). In the fresh, raw state, these foods averaged (after measuring total sodium and potassium content) 14% sodium and 86% potassium, giving a ratio of 1:6, or one part sodium to six parts of potassium. These same foods were listed after processing, and they showed 75% sodium and 25% potassium with a ratio of 3:1, three times as much sodium (added) to one part of potassium (most removed). These figures prove that the potassium was intended to be the major mineral with sodium the minor one. After processing, these ratios are totally reversed, which should give you the very best conclusions as to why you should eat as many of your fresh fruits and vegetables as you can, in the raw, uncooked, unprocessed form.

"3. Meat, Meat Products and Proteins in Your Diet

"Proteins are one of the seven food and nutrient groups that I've mentioned. Human muscle cells are composed primarily of protein and these proteins are made from chains of amino acids. Amino acids are molecules of chemicals that contain nitrogen bonds. Sources of these amino acids, of which there are twenty three known to be required in human nutrition, include meats from animals, fish, and poultry; dairy products; and non-animal sources — chiefly legumes (beans and lentils, etc.) nuts, seeds and sprouts. Proteins are also derived from the germ portion of whole grains. Our human body makes fifteen of these twenty three amino acids, and the additional eight are termed essential amino acids because they are not made by the body and must be included in adequate amounts in our diet. These eight essential amino acids are tryptophan, phenylalanine, leucine, isoleucine, valine, methionine, lysine, threonine, and, in children, histadine. Proteins are generally considered the building blocks in our body to make and repair new tissues, to make and repair certain cells and cellular parts, to make hormones, antibodies, enzymes and other necessary chemical compounds in the body. They also supply a certain amount of necessary anions in the body, although they are generally classed as amphoteric which means that they can act as an acid or an alkali, and may exhibit anionic or cationic properties.

"The largest concern regarding proteins surrounds the controversy of animal versus vegetable sources. One of the chief problems with animal protein intake is the excess fat content. Fats supply nine calories per gram compared to protein at 4.5 calories per gram; therefore, since each variety of meat varies in fat content, some proteins have more calories than others. For example, two ounces of baked chicken without the skin yields 284 calories and two ounces of broiled sirloin steak will yield 392 calories. It becomes very important in our diet that we try to choose meats that have the least amount of fat content in them. The highest fat content consists of pork and fatty red meats while the lowest calorie content includes chicken, fowl, and most types of fish and seafood products, as well as eggs and dairy products. "It should also be mentioned that dairy products like milk, cheese, yogurt, eggs and animal meats supply all eight essential amino acids. (Of course pasteurizing them destroys much food value.) Most vegetable sources do not supply all eight amino acids and thus must be combined to provide all essential amino acids together at the same meal. It has been shown in one study that excess proteins may contribute to calcium loss through the use of calcium as a binding agent or the excretion of nitrogenous waste products. Prolonged consumption of protein poor diets can retard brain development, modify the chemical composition of the brain, and produce long term learning and behavioral deficits.

"In the United States and Canada, it has been shown that about 40 percent of free living people over the age of 60, show evidence of protein malnutrition, or deficiencies of selective nutrients such as zinc and iron that are found in meats. This has a very detrimental effect on our immune system which makes us much more susceptible to infections of all types. Another study showed that 80 percent of women taking birth control pills have demonstrated abnormal tryptophan metabolism.

"To my patients, I recommend that pork (bacon, sausage, ham) be avoided at all costs. Pork not only contains extremely high amounts of saturated or bad fat but in Germany it has been shown that pork contains excessive amounts of certain bad germs that are often not destroyed in the cooking process. Pigs and hogs are scavengers and God even warned the Israelites not to eat pork. I have my patients avoid fatty red meats and use only the lean cuts of beef. I advise patients to limit lean beef to once a week and instead try to get their proteins from lean chicken, fowl, fish, low fat cheese, and low fat (unpasteurized) milk or yogurt and eggs.

"Excessive intake of proteins provides no more protein for the bodily needs than what is 'enough,' as the excess protein is used either as carbohydrate or fat. The more important factor to be considered is the digestion of a normal quantity of protein, so that a reasonable amount is supplied each day, and so I recommend to my patients that, if they are depending on meats for protein, they should limit their protein intake to one meal a day and preferably have an average serving of meat at the evening meal.

"Contrary to some opinions, the grinding of meat into small particles (like hamburger) does not increase its digestibility. Nor does the thorough chewing of meat. No protein digestion occurs in the mouth. Meat needs only to be chewed to the extent that it may be easily swallowed. On the other hand, grinding of meat can have deleterious effects. Ground meat spoils rapidly at room temperature and whole meat does not; in fact, a sort of 'predigestion' can occur. Nucleic acids are released in the grinding process and apparently this changes preservability. Similar action may occur when ground meat is introduced into the intestinal tract. Here the temperature situation for spoilage is ideal. If there is insufficient hydrochloric acid in the stomach or a lack of proteolytic (protein digesting) enzymes, the possibility of putrefaction (rotting) of proteins is greatly enhanced with ground meat as compared with whole meat. Preserved meats such as wieners, sausages, bologna, potted meat, luncheon meats, salami, and Vienna sausages do not have as much of a putrefaction tendency; however, they are absolutely loaded with chemicals and preservatives which play a very detrimental part in causing poor health. They simply should be totally avoided.

"4 . FOOD COMBINATIONS

"Poor food combining or food combinations can be a cause of toxicity in the body. The reason for this is that certain food groups do not digest well together. Some foods digest primarily in the stomach, others in the small intestine. Some foods digest in minutes while others take many hours. Some foods require an acid medium to digest in and others an alkaline medium. Therefore certain foods eaten together do not digest properly and thus tend to become toxic. For example, starches digest primarily in

the small intestine while protein digestion mostly occurs in the stomach. Eating the two together holds the starch in the stomach too long which leads to putrefaction. This is one example of how even the best food can become toxic to you. Fruits digest in a few minutes while starches require at least an hour or two to digest. When the two are combined, the fruit putrefies as it is unable to pass through the intestine quickly enough. Fruit with protein usually causes the same problem. The fruit needs to pass right through the stomach and the protein food needs to digest in the stomach for a much longer period of time, and when eaten together, this blocks the fruits' passage.

"Also sugar inhibits or retards the action of protein digesting enzymes. Therefore, sweet foods such as sugar and dessert foods should not be eaten at the same time as animal foods like meats. As an example, beans (pinto or navy beans) are an excellent vegetable source of proteins. In Mexico, the pinto bean is a major constituent of the diet and is eaten unsweetened. In this country, 'baked beans' are served which combine proteins and sugar. Baked beans are noted for the digestive flatulence (gas) that they cause. Most Americans are accustomed to finishing off a good protein meal (steak or other meat) with sweet desserts (like apple pie). Desserts should be eaten several hours after mealtime on an empty stomach for best nutrition. There are many sugar-protein combinations which may be avoided easily. The fact that most foods contain some protein must be taken into consideration of course. Also, a small amount of sugar does little harm if it is not eaten regularly. Even natural sugars such as honey and blackstrap molasses (which I usually recommend) are less harmful than any processed sugars, but they are best eaten at different times than with high protein meals. For example, orange juice that is high in natural sugars would not be an ideal combination with eggs (high proteins). A better choice would be tomato juice.

"We usually do not go into depth in the education of my patients concerning combinations of foods because I have found that the person who is in average good health can usually tolerate poor-food combinations without any serious or critical ill effects. However, in some patients who have a severely compromised immune system, I do encourage that they observe the following recommendations which have been shown through the ages to be the very best information concerning food combinations.

"1. Proteins generally do not combine with starches. This is probably the worst of the diseaseproducing habits. Of course, this really hits home 'with meat and potato' eaters, as well as those who excessively use sandwiches in their diet. In the digestive process, they tend to neutralize themselves and good digestion is impossible. The increased putrefaction and rotting takes place under these circumstances. Exceptions to this rule are avocados, which combine fairly well with grains.

"2. Fruits do not combine with starches. Fruits digest immediately in the mouth and small intestine, while starches require more of their digestive time in these areas. The fruit sugars are quickly absorbed into the intestine, while the starch requires digestion in the mouth, stomach, and small intestine. Ideally, one should eat a fruit meal by itself. Most people prefer to make breakfast their main fruit meal and this is a good idea.

"3. Fruits do not combine with proteins. Here again, the fruits go directly into the intestine, while protein requires much more time digesting in the stomach. If sugars are held back in the stomach while trying to digest protein, you can count on the fruit putrefying.

"4. Fruits do not combine with vegetables. A good way to remember this is that fruits are cleaners and vegetables are builders. It's very difficult to clean and build a house at the same time. One exception to this is tomatoes, a fruit. You can have tomatoes with most salad vegetables.

"5. Acid fruits do not combine with sweet fruits. These two food groups repel each other. Acid fruits include the citrus fruits like lemons, limes, oranges, pineapple, tangerines, and grapefruit, along with most available berries and tomatoes. The sweet fruits include bananas, dates, dried fruits, including apples, apricots, figs, peaches, pears, prunes, and raisins.

"5. FASTING

"Food combining is usually recommended for patients in very critical health and especially those with a very compromised immune system. If you've spent years as a 'junk food junkie,' ideally, you need more than withdrawal from these foods and changing to a natural foods diet. With the accumulation of chemicals, preservatives, and additives in these junk foods and other harmful substances in your body, a detoxification program should be implemented. Even natural foods, especially fruits, certain vegetables, and their juices, possess a considerable detoxifying effect. Certain vitamins are very important in the detoxification process and especially vitamin C. Fasting is the fastest way of bringing about elimination of toxins in the body and the quickest way of getting toxic materials out of the body.

Fasting on just water or perhaps juice greatly enhances body detoxification. During such a fast, the body can 'live off itself' and burns up dead cells, waste materials and excess fat to supply energy. Since many toxins end up stored in the fatty tissues, the benefits of fasting for detoxification is simply logical. I'm convinced that regular fasting one day per week produces great benefit in maintaining a clean system. Some authorities recommend longer fasts of three days or more, to be taken 3 or 4 times each year, which induces more thorough body detoxification, and this can be compared to a quarterly 'spring cleaning.'

"It is common knowledge that fasting has thousands of years of reputation as the ultimate form of detoxification. Let me briefly explain what fasting does and how it can help your health. When I speak of fasting, I am talking about the total abstinence from food but not water, for a certain period of time. When one fasts, no food is being converted into energy and the body must live off of itself, a process called autolysis. There's nothing harmful about this since the body must go for several weeks without food as it burns up dead cells and fatty tissues where most toxic chemicals are stored in the body. Fasting is really sort of an internal operation without using surgery. When the digestive and elimination systems shut down in fasting, more energy is available for detoxification and repair. Therefore, when one fasts, one usually sees a greater increase in one's energy on the third day of a fast, than what it would be when eating normally.

"I believe personally that short term fasts, such as one day per week, can be an excellent benefit to your health. I have also learned from research done in Germany that one should never fast more than ten days, however, as this could be very detrimental to your health. By abstaining from two or three meals one day each week, this gives you a sort of weekly 'house cleaning' inside your body. If you decide to fast, please remember that it can be very beneficial to your health, but you should certainly exercise some care by following the guidelines listed below.

How To Fast Properly

"1. When you begin to fast, the detoxification will often cause headaches, tiredness, fatigue, and even nausea. This is normal and it simply means that you are eliminating harmful toxins and substances from your body. When these side effects are seen, it merely shows that your body needs the fasting experience and these symptoms usually disappear after the second or third day.

"2. If you decide to fast, you should begin your fasting experience gradually. You should start with a one day a week fast and probably skip only two meals. Later on, you can skip three meals on your weekly fast, and after several months of this kind of fasting, you can then handle a two or three day fast if you desire. Never begin a long fast unless your body is accustomed to fasting.

"3. Once you begin your fasting program on a-one-day per week basis, you will soon notice that there is very little to no discomfort because of the successful elimination of most of your accumulated toxins.

"4. You should keep in mind that you should not fast if you are pregnant, have an advanced chronic degenerative disease or even diabetes.

"God Recommends Fasts

We must not forget that fasting is recommended by God in the Bible in many places and fasting is one of God's greatest gifts for man's health. It is probably the very best method to eliminate the toxins that have accumulated in your fatty tissues over a period of years.

"6. FERMENTED FOODS

"Fermentation was one of the first methods of preservation discovered for foods. Because of the fermentation process, foods such as sauerkraut, pickles, yogurt, cheeses, buttermilk, and cottage cheese came into existence. All of these foods in their natural form have a long history of use and are highly acceptable in dietary items. I've learned from researchers in Germany that there are two kinds of lactic acid produced by the body. When all body processes are functioning properly, the body produces a

form of lactic acid called L-lactic acid, and when the body is overly stressed and not functioning properly, a bad form of lactic acid called D-lactic acid is produced. Even today, with many of my patients with chronic degenerative diseases, I have found that by supplementing extra L-lactic acid for these patients, their improvement is greatly enhanced. As the fermentation process acts to produce primarily L-lactic acid, this natural acid is common to the previously named foods. This L-lactic acid seems to have a "preservative" effect on the intestinal tract as well. Such foods as yogurt and buttermilk thus have an enviable reputation for being favorable to intestinal environment. The fermentation process also seems to act somewhat as a 'predigesting factor.' Tough fibers are made softer; nutrients may be released from their biological hold, such as lactose (milk sugar), which is richer in buttermilk than in sweet milk. It has also been found that lactose favorably influences and enhances the absorption of calcium.

"Two Good Fermented Foods

"There are two foods that are outstanding in the fermented food class: buttermilk and sauerkraut. They are easily available and both are very rich sources of L-lactic acid. Buttermilk is preferred, of course, because of its high protein and calcium content.

Keep in mind that once pasteurized, the buttermilk's calcium is not available.] But those who do not care for buttermilk should consider sauerkraut as a source of L-lactic acid. It would be a good health practice to try to include some fermented foods in your diet each day, like buttermilk, yogurt, sauerkraut, or cottage cheese.

"7. Exercise and Physical Activity

"Did you know that some years ago a Gallop Poll reported that only 24 percent of the citizens of the U.S. exercise regularly? Because of the mechanization of our society over the past 100 years with machines and household appliances, and since only a very small number of people now earn their living in jobs requiring persistent physical activity; physical inactivity for the majority of Americans has become the rule and not the exception. I've asked many patients 'What is the most strenuous exercise that you have engaged in the past two weeks?' And the great majority states that actually their exercise has been no greater than walking up a flight of stairs, walking from their car across a parking lot to their place of business, or maybe even just pushing a grocery cart. What we should understand is that 'running around all day,' whether it be at home or at our place of work is definitely not exercise and should not be considered as such.

"There have been many new studies completed the last thirty years which have fairly well proven that lack of exercise or habitual inactivity very often contributes to high blood pressure, chronic fatigue, premature aging, poor muscle tone and lack of flexibility, which in turn aggravates low back pain, mental stress, coronary artery disease and especially obesity. Prolonged inactivity also slows bowel function, decreases male hormone production in men, as well as decreases sperm counts. Without proper physical activity, there is very inefficient transfer of oxygen in the lungs, and it also has been shown to aggravate and make us more susceptible to developing softening of the bones or osteoporosis. We have seen that lack of exercise causes rapid deterioration of muscle tissue, as well as connective tissue in our ligaments and tendons. If you want to age faster, then do not exercise because, when you

don't use your muscles; it is true that 'if you don't use it, you lose it.' Exercise also increases the good cholesterol in the body and lowers the bad cholesterol and total cholesterol levels.

"A person doesn't have to be a marathon runner or chop wood three hours a day in order to become more active. There are many forms of exercise that a person can perform and these range from walking to jogging, bicycling, swimming, rebounding, or getting involved in some sport activity such as tennis, volleyball, or possibly even playing golf or dancing. The most important decision for you, however, is to make a definite decision that you are going to exercise at least five days each week and begin *some* program. I'm going to briefly discuss two types of exercise programs that I will recommend for the great majority of my patients, and they involve brisk walking and rebounding.

"For those patients who are entering their 'golden years,' a simple routine involving a brisk, daily walking is quite sufficient for the initial part of the exercise regime and may be all that a lot of patients ever need. The usual response to my walking prescription is that walking makes a person hungry. This is not true. When the body is walking briskly, the body's fat deposits are tapped freely for energy in order to supply fuel for the muscles so the blood becomes loaded with these fuel materials. The net effect is that, not only does the muscle tissue have readily available fat to burn, but the hunger mechanism is short circuited, and there is actually less hunger than if there had been no activity. A prolonged walk at a steady pace with constant stress on the circulatory system and the heart is beneficial in many ways. The primary concern in exercise is to increase your pulse rate and get your heart beating faster. This increase should be from fifty to seventy percent higher than your normal resting pulse, but do not overdo it. You would be wise to get in the habit of exercising twenty minutes every day with your heart beating faster. Morning exercise is better for you because it will give you more energy all day long.

"In the beginning, the walk should be short and slow but gradually build up one's speed and distance. When asked how fast one should walk, I often use the following example: 'Imagine that you are wearing thin clothing and that the temperature outside is below freezing, the wind is blowing hard, and it is raining and you have to go to the bathroom very badly and you are a mile from home. How fast would you walk to get there?' Now, that's brisk walking!

"Of all the types of exercise available, in the past year I have concluded that the very best form of exercise is rebounding or using a small mini-trampoline, called a rebounder. This form of exercise is different from other physical activities because it puts gravity to work in your favor. It has many advantages over 'regular' exercise because it, in addition is a cellular exercise. By subjecting each of the sixty trillion cells in your body to greater gravitation pull, waste products are squeezed out and nutritional elements and oxygen are drawn into the cells. The cells function more efficiently, the metabolism increases to its maximum. With this form of exercise, the membranes around each cell become stronger as they demand more protein from the body. These thicker membranes are better able to fight off foreign invaders like germs, toxins, poisons, and other pollutants more effectively. Here, everything improves: the blood, the brain, the lungs, the muscles, all the internal organs, those of the senses, and even more.

"Rebounding exercise will increase the vital capacity (can handle more oxygen) in your lungs and more oxygen will be delivered to the body tissues and better absorption of oxygen will result. There appears to be a faster gaseous exchange within the lungs. The red blood cell count, as well as more blood, is pushed through these vessels. The heart muscles work more efficiently and collateral circulation improves. The result is that more oxygen is carried to the heart muscle. Elevated blood cholesterol and triglyceride levels tend to come down, and the good cholesterol levels increase. Rebounding also strengthens the adrenal glands so that more severe stresses may be handled by the body. Your metabolism is enhanced and there is better absorption or nutrients from food intake. Digestion, appetite and elimination all get better. This type of exercise also tends to decrease any tendency for blood clotting or coagulation in the blood vessels. Many scientists believe that a prime cause or contributing factor of

cancer is lack of oxygenation of the cells, and exercise is the main way to bring oxygen into the blood with which to bathe the cells.

"I feel the most important benefit of rebounding, however, is its effect on the lymph system. Most people are not familiar with what the lymph system really is. It is another circulatory system within the body and it is the system that drains and removes toxins, poisons, and waste products from between each individual cell and delivers these waste products to the lymph nodes and that part of the immune system that destroys and eliminates toxins, bacteria, poisons, and other products that get in your body. In one sense, the lymph system is the metabolic garbage can of the body. It gets rid of toxins, dead cells, cancer cells, waste products, trapped proteins, pathogenic bacteria, and viruses, heavy metals, and

assorted junk products that the cells need to get rid of.

"Your circulatory system (heart, blood vessels, and blood) delivers food and oxygen to your cells, and the products of cell metabolic breakdown must be drained away with its load of waste through the lymph vessels. Now, unlike the artery system, the lymphatics do not have their own pump. There are only three ways to activate the speed up of the flow of lymph away from the tissues it serves and back into the main circulation. Lymphatic flow requires (a) muscular contraction from exercise and movement (b) gravitational pressure and (c) internal messages to the one-way valves that are present in these lymph vessels.

"Arthur C. Guyton, M.D., Professor and Chairman of the Dept. of Physiology and Biophysics, University of Mississippi School of Medicine, is an internationally known expert on lymphology and the lymphatic system. He states, 'The lymphatic group becomes very active during exercise but sluggish under resting conditions. During exercise, the rate of lymph flow can increase to as high as three to fourteen times normal because of increased activity. An increase in tissue fluid protein increases the rate of lymph flow and this washes the proteins out of the tissue spaces, automatically returning the protein concentrate to its normal low level. If it were not for this continual removal of proteins, the dynamics of the capillaries would become so abnormal within only a few hours that life could no longer continue. There is certainly no other function of the lymphatics that can even approach this in importance.'

"As the lymphatic vessels have one-way valves in them, and the lymph flow only one way (towards the heart) when one jumps up on the rebounder, the lymph is thrown up also and cannot go back down the vessels because of the one way valves. This acts as a suction pump to pull out and suck out the lymph with accumulated toxins between the cells and return it back to the circulation where it is supposed to be.

"How to Rebound

"Jog on the rebounder for two minutes, then jump with both feet on the rebounder for two minutes and repeat this process over and over for twenty minutes in all. If you get dizzy at first, this is because the toxins are being pulled out of the spaces between your cells too rapidly. You should slow down or stop for a few minutes before continuing if this should happen. If you feel unsteady on the rebounder, you may want to hook a rope in the ceiling and let it hang down to hold onto or you could screw a little handholding hook in the wood door frame and simply hold on to this as you rebound.

"8. Drink Water, Water, Water — Live Longer, Longer, Longer

"The average person drinks nearly six times their body weight in water each year. In our bodies, water is absolutely vital for life. Our health becomes critical if we lose only 10% of our body water and death is certain if we lose 20%. Of our body weight, approximately 70% is water. Even our bones contain over 30% water. Our drinking water, beverages, and foods we eat are the sources of water for our bodies. Every cell in our body must have water or it dies. Water bathes the cells in our body and provides the medium or means of transportation for all metabolic elements which are food nutrients and body chemicals such as hormones, enzymes, vitamins, oxygen and minerals. In these cells, there are literally thousands of chemical reactions taking place at all times to use the food and water we take

into our bodies to produce our energy. These processes taking place in the cells are generally referred to as 'metabolism.' Water is actually produced during these processes. These metabolic elements in the body fluids (primarily water) are constantly flowing in and out of our body cells, and waste products flow out of the body cells into the lymphatic system where they are returned to the blood circulation system and then carried to the kidneys for disposal. The heart pumps about 2,000 gallons of this blood plasma through about 70,000 miles of blood vessels in our bodies each day, sometimes at the rate of 40 miles per hour. Actually about a quart of water flows through our kidneys every minute. The kidneys are continually filtering out the waste products from the blood, and these products are excreted in the urine.

"All body cells have a membrane or sac which completely surrounds the cells. The body water constantly bathing the cells is vital to maintain a delicate acid-alkali chemical and physical balance between the cells and all body organs. This delicate balance that must be maintained is referred to as homeostasis, and must be maintained or we will die. If we don't have enough water intake our body metabolism is depressed and when our metabolism slows down, our food has a tendency to turn into fat and we become much more fatigued.

"Water is essential to moisten the delicate membranes in our nose, throat, bronchial and breathing tubes, so that oxygen is brought to our blood and carbon dioxide (a waste product) excreted. Water must be available to lubricate our joints, as well as allowing absorption of our food nutrients in our digestive tract. Without adequate water, one will see constipation. Waste products and toxins are increased in the blood and are carried to the liver which puts additional stress on the liver. These accumulated waste products and toxins depress the function of most of our glands. Water is vital in regulating our body temperature. Water is needed for our muscles to function properly and to maintain the right tone in our muscles. Adequate water prevents wrinkling and sagging of our skin.

"It is extremely important that our body maintain a proper equilibrium between the intake and output of body water. This is called water balance. Our water intake comes from the fluids we drink (48%), from the solids we eat (40%), and from the metabolic processes taking place in the body (12%). The output water losses are from the kidneys (56%), skin (20%), lungs (20%), bowels or intestines (4%), and a small amount from tears. Proper water balance must be maintained by having the water intake equal the water output.

"The water in the body is distributed in two main compartments. Water outside the cells is called extracellular water, and the water inside the cells is called intracellular. Intracellular water (about 9 gallons) makes up 50% of our total body weight and extracellular water (about 4 gallons) makes up

20%. The extracellular water is further divided into the water around the cells (interstitial, 10-11 quarts) and the blood plasma (intravascular, 3-4 quarts).

"When we think about fluid retention, we are primarily concerned with the extracellular water, the water stored in the tissue spaces between the cells and water in the blood plasma. The chemical — sodium chloride (plain table salt) plays a very important part in determining whether fluid is retained or not. The concentration of sodium in the blood is carefully regulated by various hormones and chemical reactions in the body. When we take in too much salt, the kidneys begin to excrete more sodium in the urine in an effort to bring the delicately balanced sodium concentration back to normal. Sodium holds onto water and with excess sodium in our bodies, we become thirsty. When we then drink water, the sodium concentration is diluted and a delicate balance returns. When a person has swelling in the tissues, it generally means they have too much sodium in their body and in order to get rid of this sodium, we must make more water in our kidneys. To do this, we must make more urine; the best way to make more urine is to drink more water. This is the main way to get rid of any fluid retention without the use of drugs. This sounds paradoxical, but it is true: *You must drink more water to get rid of water*. If you

have fluid retention, drinking less water will not help, but may aggravate it. If you have fluid retention, drinking more water will not worsen it, but help cure it.

"You may be asking at this point, why not take a diuretic? Diuretics only cause water to leave the body in an abnormal and often dangerous manner. Besides, the water loss is only temporary. The body learns to depend on diuretics like many people are habituated to laxatives, when over a period of time they have had to increase the strength of the laxative for it to be effective. They must then depend on laxatives. I don't want this to happen to you.

"A Major Problem Today; Most Drinking Water is Polluted

From the above discussion, you can easily understand that water is the key to all bodily functions: digestion, assimilation, circulation, elimination, lubrication, and temperature control and other important factors. Because of this, I'm sure you can understand that the purity and quality of the water you drink is vital to your body's well being. Another very important point that few people stop to think about, is that the Earth does not make any new water. In fact, only one percent of the Earth's water is suitable for drinking. The other 99% is either ice or unusable salty water. This same one percent is recycled over and over with all the potential exposure to chemicals, toxins, and poisons. (Also think of homeopathic influences on water; i.e., magnetic imprints derived from negatives such as drugs, pesticides, herbicides, etc.)

"More and more, every day throughout our nation, magazines, television, and newspapers warn about the dangers of drinking polluted water, and many of the pollutants in the drinking water are tasteless, odorless, and colorless, but they are dissolved in the water. Unfortunately, for many generations, the oceans, rivers, and ground waters, have been a catch-all for waste products. The main sources of these waste products are AGRICULTURAL (fertilizers, insecticides, pesticides, herbicides, arsenic, nitrates), INDUSTRIAL (heavy metals, chemicals, solvents, mercury, organic waste, lead, rust, asbestos, dioxin, phenolics), and MAN-MADE (detergents, dissolved solids, sewage, algae, viruses, fungus, parasites, bacteria, hydrocarbons, chlorine). You should easily be able to see the seriousness of this problem when you stop to consider that over 66,000 chemicals are used in the United States and 45,000 pesticides are on the market. I saw in an issue of *Sierra Magazine*, an article which reported that of

1,200 different ingredients found in pesticides that are labeled 'inert,' only 300 are considered

'safe,' 100 are known to be dangerous and the risk for the remaining 800 are 'unknown.' The seriousness becomes even more apparent when one realizes that there are over 19,000 hazardous waste dumps, 95,000 landfills, tens of thousands of reservoirs, or pits that contain liquid waste, and millions of underground storage tanks and septic tanks. There are over three and a half billion gallons of liquid waste created each and every day, which potentially can pollute our water supply.

"It's quite obvious that Big Brother knows the danger of this polluted water in our society and wants to keep us ignorant of this fact. Would you believe that legislative action has made it *illegal* to claim that any municipally treated water is detrimental to your health? Can you believe this? *Ralph Nader's 1988*

Report states, 'Nationwide, 2,110 organic and inorganic contaminants have been identified in drinking water at various levels by Federal Land State Survey programs since the Safe Drinking Water Act was passed in 1974. Of these, the vast majority, nearly 2,090 of the over 2,100 contaminants are organic chemicals.' This Ralph Nader report presents a national portrait of the real drinking water contamination crisis that local, state, and federal officials have been unwilling or unable to manage. The Environmental Protection Agency only tests for 33 contaminants, and if the standards for these are met, the water is considered safe. What about all the contaminants not tested for? Another factor is that, some of the most hazardous contaminants like asbestos and lead usually enter the water after leaving the water treatment plants. Also, not realized by most people, is that the majority of water treatment facilities use aluminum sulfate to precipitate the cloudiness in our drinking water, and according to Colloidal Chemistry Laws, 3 parts per million of this aluminum will cause severe coagulation in our blood.

Therefore, since many contaminants are not even tested for and others enter the drinking water after treatment, we all are potentially at great risk from these very harmful substances.

The only way you can protect yourself is to drink distilled water (dead water), or reverse osmosis filtered water or, as I reported earlier, a combination of ceramic filter, activated carbon filter, reverse osmosis, ultra violet light and magnetic ring to rid homeopathic influences. I will refer to water treated by this multiple means as

'pure' water.

To attain the best of health, it is essential that we all use 'pure' water in our drinks of all types. I recommend that all my patients bring a sample of their water to the Clinic where I can check that the water is bad for your health if it is water that has been treated by a municipality. When

most patients see what comes out of their water, I don't have to say anything because it is obvious that there is pollution present. Now, what are your options that you can follow to ensure that you get 'pure' water for your family?

"No matter what type of water you use, whether it is reverse osmosis (RO) filtered water, distilled water, well water or municipally treated water, it is very important that you try to drink a least three quarts of water each day. I also recommend that you add the juice of a lemon (very high anions) to a

gallon of water that you drink. Another option here is that you may prefer some Zeta® crystals which

you can add to your water. This will also increase anions in your system very effectively. For those who want the absolute best, I recommend that you purchase Zeta crystals. Every cell in the body has an electrical potential. It is the electrical energy that differentiates life from death. As we age or become ill, our zeta potential drops and so does our energy. This is one reason why it is difficult to get out of bed, exercise or maintain self-motivation as we either become toxic, older or unhealthy. Without energy, without cellular electrical potential, we not only lose our health, youth and drive, we have a difficult time absorbing nutrients. By 'charging' distilled water with electrolytic minerals or Zeta Crystals, it not only reenergizes our cells, it lowers the surface tension of the water making it wetter and better absorbed and allows nutrients to be more bio-available.

"The sole purpose of Zeta crystals is to help balance electrolytes in the body fluids; this will allow a person's natural filtration system, the kidneys, to help get rid of unwanted cations in body fluids. These crystals have the added advantage of being very highly concentrated with good anions, as well as providing extra magnesium to your system. I am convinced that magnesium deficiency is probably the most common mineral deficiency in America today. Most physicians, when they measure magnesium blood levels, cannot get a true picture of magnesium levels since magnesium is an intracellular mineral, and just measuring blood levels can give a false picture of the true levels in the body. Zeta crystals added to drinking water simply help one reach homeostasis faster and more efficiently.

"Catalyst-activated water is an additional additive that seems to give more 'life' to the water you drink. It increases the surface tension of the water, and the water becomes 'wetter.' By coating the formed elements in the blood (red blood cells, white blood cells, and platelets) with this increased surface tension liquid, the cells become more slicky and simply flow through arteries and capillaries faster and easier, improving circulation.

"Clinic Visits

"I like all my patients to get a urine sample each visit and carry the urine sample to our laboratory to check the dissolved solids in their urine. This tells me if they are eating the right things and drinking the right water. It also tells a great deal about how body elimination is functioning. For all patients receiving intravenous injections, it is very important to have their effects checked in terms of dissolved solids in the urine. It would be helpful to devise a system where patients could check their own urine to motivate following diet and water intake properly.

"Better health with proper water intake decreases cations and increases beneficial anions. This plays a tremendous part in helping prevent and treat over 64 different diseases.

"'Pure' water for drinking and cooking cannot be emphasized enough. It's up to you to correct the problem.

"9. The Spiritual Life

Religion can have an important place in healing. You don't have to believe as I do, nor do you need to believe to make yourself healthy through proper diet. But I have learned that the best physical health flows from a dynamic relationship with God. Nothing counteracts emotional stress more effectively than spiritual insight and its resultant strength. Spiritual strength is one of the most powerful assets you can have to combat emotional stress and give you the best of health. God's word tells us, 'Let Him

(God) have all your worries and cares for He is always thinking about you and watching everything that concerns you' (Peter 5:7). Nearly three thousand years ago, the wisest man who ever lived, King Solomon, stated the relationship between spiritual and physical health in Proverbs 3:7-8, 'Trust and reverence the Lord and turn your back on evil; when you do that, then you will be given renewed health and vitality.' "Many people go through their entire lives never realizing the tremendous, powerful, ever-reaching light of God that can flood out all their black and gray places and allow them to step out of the darkness where many people dwell all their lives. God can cleanse you from top to bottom, inside to outside. God's ways are good, and they are not only good, but they are far above man's ways. In every area of your life, God can show you what is right and what is wrong, what will bring good and what will bring bad, what will bring sickness and disease, and what will bring good health. If we trust in Him, He will show us which things are really part of his intended ways for us and which are not. This can give us balance in our life. There are many things that must be put together in proper balance to achieve consistently good health. I have tried to bring out many of these important things in this chapter that I feel God has shown me. These are elements that work together to bring about and preserve health and

well-being.

"The Bible says, 'My people are destroyed by lack of knowledge.' This is so true. Sickness and premature death are commonplace all because we have no knowledge of the Lord's ways. We live so very far from the way that God intended us to live. That's one of the reasons there is so much pain and sickness, so many heart attacks, headaches, bad tempers, mental illness, and just plain lack of joy. We suffer a great deal just because of our own ignorance about God's ways. I think that most of us drift away from God's ways because of our wishes to satisfy our own desire. This is why you or I get into health trouble today. We want to gratify our flesh and desires more than we want to serve our God. I'm convinced that God has provided a remedy for every disease that might afflict us. It's possible that almost every disease is caused by some kind of violation of the natural laws of God. We don't obey them because we don't understand them.

"It appears that many of us are simply jaded and have become content to live a life of mediocrity. Some of us have never been taught God's ways; we certainly don't see them in the world around us.

"We have become so perverted now that we call evil good and good evil. We cannot blame it on others because we all do it. Now, maybe we aren't as bad as some people who are extremely perverse and evil, but we do it in little things and that's where it all starts. We live in a society that wants to push our children to be super human beings instead of teaching them God's ways and how to live in true freedom and simplicity, at peace with God and with our fellow men. Some of us *have* been taught the right way to do things, but we have chosen not to follow these instructions. We have this inner voice of knowledge that shows us the way, but we would rather ignore it and serve our own selfish desires. Many of us simply do not listen to this inner voice that really tells us what to do.

"I do not think it is wise to be preoccupied with your body's looks, but it is wise to value your body as the temple of the Holy Spirit which God has given you. The Holy Spirit of God dwells in and works through that wonderful body of yours. Now, how do you treat it? Do you feed it poorly, never allowing it to have any exercise, keeping it shut away from fresh air and sunshine, filling it with poisons of

unforgiveness and bitterness, never allowing it to rest and then being critical of it because it doesn't look good or can't do what you want it to do? You must, to gain the best of health, make up your own mind to have respect, appreciation, and love for the body that God gave you, no matter what shape it is in at this moment. You should remember God in your prayers, as David did when he said in Psalms

139:14, 'I praise you because I am fearfully and wonderfully made.' Paul tells us in Romans 12:1,

'Give your body to the Lord as a living sacrifice, holy and pleasing to God.'

"Our physical condition can influence our spiritual lives far more than most of us realize. If we are disciplined in the care of our physical bodies, we are far more likely to be disciplined in our spiritual lives too. Sickness detracts from our relationships and service far more than we imagine. God designed our body to be self repairing and self healing if we treat it properly. The great majority of Americans today do not have the advantage of learning good nutrition and the knowledge of God's ways. Some wonderful news is that your body can be rebuilt in a matter of months if you give the body the proper tools to work with. That is what I have been trying to do here. I'm giving you the knowledge that you can use if you want to apply it to achieve the maximum health possible. Just as there are physical laws such as the Law of Gravity or the Law of Cause and Effect, there are also Spiritual Laws. We usually have a good interpretation of these physical laws, and we have learned that when we go against them we will get hurt or must suffer the consequences. With the Law of Gravity (what goes up will come down), no right thinking person would jump off a building because they knew they could fall to their death. They would suffer the consequences of breaking the law. There are equally important spiritual laws concerning the preservation of good health, but few there are that follow them, and they will suffer the consequences because they are breaking spiritual laws. Read the Bible and pray to God to reveal these laws to you and He will.

"In our medical schools today, all doctors are taught to give out drugs and chemicals to treat symptoms of disease. It is true that many drugs have been developed that have saved millions of lives, but they are certainly used to great excess in our society all over the world. I believe that if God wanted us to use drugs and chemicals to treat symptoms, he would have provided them to us in some way other than the way they are provided today, 'to make a profit and get rich.' Over 99% of drugs and medications given today are cations and can be very harmful to our health if taken over a long period of time. In Revelations 18:23, where John is discussing the fall of Babylon, which represents evil, in the latter days, he makes the statement, 'And the light of a candle shall shine no more in thee; and the voice of the Bridegroom (Jesus) and of the Bride (true believers) shall be heard no more at all in thee; for thy merchants were the great men of the earth; for by thy sorceries were *all* nations deceived.'

"When one looks up the Greek meaning of the term sorceries, this word means pharmacies. Of course, we all know that pharmacies are responsible for giving us our drugs and chemicals to treat diseases. I personally do not believe that John is referring to narcotic type drugs, but drugs in general, and in these latter days, we are being deceived about good health because of drugs and chemicals. I believe this because I am seeing more and more people suffering from various illnesses that are tremendously aggravated by taking too many drugs. In fact, it's been estimated that 20% of the people admitted to hospitals are there because of iatrogenic medicine, and that means reactions and side effects of drugs and chemicals given to patients by their doctors. This is why I try to get patients off drugs as much as possible in my practice, and I sincerely believe this is what God wants us to do. This includes all types of drugs and chemicals.

"I know that all my efforts that have been dedicated to develop a deeper spiritual life and a closer relationship with God have paid off tremendously for me and given me strength that I could never find anywhere else.

"In the past 3 years, God keeps sending me more and more information, research studies and proven knowledge about the wonderful benefits of various herbs and how they can be used to restore health and fight disease. I ask God to guide me daily in treating all patients, and the Holy Spirit is telling my spirit that there is coming a revolution in the use of herbs and natural substances to treat and cure all types of diseases. As I remember you in my prayers, please remember me and ask God to send me the Truth so that God can use me as his instrument and vessel to heal all patients that he sends to me to treat, advise, and educate, and may Jesus Christ be glorified with every healing.

"10. Mental Attitude and Self Image

"With a good positive mental attitude, you will look better, feel better, and heal better. Our libraries are full of all types of books that will help you develop a better positive mental attitude. God tells us,

'As a man thinketh in his heart, so is he,' Proverbs 23:7. I have rephrased this proverb to make it a little easier to us to understand: 'We become what we think about.' Because of this, we need to try to force ourselves to think good positive, goal-oriented thoughts at all times. By doing this, because we truly become what we think about, we will soon find ourselves actually becoming whatever these thoughts are that we have been forcing ourselves to continually think about.

"The truth is that every circumstance of your life can be looked upon from a positive or negative viewpoint — it's entirely up to you. Dr. Robert Schuller gave an excellent example of this in the following story. He said:

"'One of my favorite stories is the classic story of the Chinese who had one horse and one son. One day his horse broke out of the corral and fled to the freedom of the hills. The neighbors came around that night and chattered. 'Your horse got out? What bad luck!'

" 'Why?' the old Chinese said. 'How do you know its bad luck?'

"'Sure enough, the next night the horse came back to his familiar corral for his usual feeding and watering, leading twelve wild stallions with him. The farmer's son saw the 13 horses in the corral, slipped out and locked the gate. Suddenly, he had 13 horses instead of none.

"'The neighbors heard the good news and came chattering to the farmer. 'Oh, you have 13 horses. What good luck!'

"'The old Chinese answered, 'How do you know that's good luck?'

"'Some days later, his strong young son was trying to break one of the wild stallions, only to be thrown off and his leg broken. The neighbors came back that night and passed another hasty judgment.

'Your son broke his leg? What bad luck?'

"'And the wise farmer answered again, 'How do you know it's bad luck?'

"'Sure enough, a few days later, a Chinese War lord came through town and conscripted every ablebodied young man, taking them off to war, never to return again. But the young man was saved because of his broken leg.

"Only God knows what's good for us and what's bad for us.

"Another important factor is for you to try to always feel good about yourself and have a positive self image. Do you have basically positive feelings or basically negative feelings about the person you see in the mirror? Do you love yourself or hate yourself? King Solomon put it this way: 'A joyful heart is good medicine, but a broken spirit dries up the bones' (Proverbs 17:22). Without a positive self image, you will not properly digest and assimilate your food or the nutrients in your food. If this happens, the foods can become toxic within your intestine and a negative self image, as well as other emotional and spiritual stresses interferes with our digestive system from functioning properly. Some researchers are convinced that the colon (large intestine) is a manifester of the emotions. So much so that a wise doctor in Philadelphia some years ago remarked that 'the colon is the mirror of the mind and when the mind gets tight, the colon gets tight.' On the other hand, positive feelings toward yourself relax the intestines, stimulating the proper functioning which will give you the best possible digestion and nutrition.

"It is also believed by most authorities that when you have relationships that are not good with other people, they usually result from a negative self image. If we don't get along with ourselves, we tend not to get along with others. Other people tend to react to the negative image that we project. Negative relationships affect our bodies just like a negative self image. For these reasons, we should all strive to develop a good positive mental attitude at all times and to keep a good self image concerning ourselves. I've seen so many people who live their lives according to what other people may think about them. Frankly, this is a rather stupid attitude, because when the real facts are known, most of the people you meet do not care that much about you or what you are or what you think unless it affects their own pocketbook. The important thing is to be genuine yourself, and we all know what we really are inside because we cannot fool ourselves. So don't live your life according to what you think people may think about you, but live your life in truth and be genuine to yourself. Then, you will always maintain a good positive self image about yourself.

"11. Stress and Stress Management

"Many human illnesses are directly related to stress, isolation, emotions, pressures from society and the negative effects of the social, political and industrial choices we are required to make each day. Stress therefore affects us physically, mentally, emotionally, and influences all our behaviors. Stress may be defined as a demand for adaptation. It has been shown, however, that we humans respond to demands not as they actually are, but as we perceive them to be. A stress may be real or imagined.

"There are many types of stress we constantly face. These stress factors may be physical (exposure to the extremes of temperature, injuries, or accidents), chemical (exposure to pollutants, allergens, poisons, toxins, and drugs), microbiological (germs, bacteria, viruses, fungus, and other microorganisms), psychological or extreme emotional states (fear, anger, sadness, or a sense of loss), mental functioning (suppression or repression), as well as inborn drives to hurry, to succeed, to compete, as well as sociocultural (work pressures, crime, IRS, regulations, financial crisis and peer and parental pressure). Stress affects practically every organ in the body and if not controlled can certainly aggravate and complicate most any known disease or illness. The intention of this paper is to summarize for you some suggestions on how you can better cope with stress and methods that have been proven to help relieve stress in your life. These methods help you reduce stress, relax better, and enjoy life more.

"Stress is the response of your mind, emotions and body to whatever demands are being made on you. So the important thing is that it's not so much *what* happens to you that determines the effect on stress upon your body, but the way that you respond to it. The ideal response is a relaxed, carefree and positive thinking reaction. This in itself will prevent many problems when you are faced with stressful situations. And don't forget, there are two kinds of stress, positive and negative. Positive stress is happy, desirable, controllable, easygoing good stress like being informed that you've just had an increase in salary. Negative stress, however, is maddening, sad, disturbing, uncontrollable and depressing like having an argument or being in an accident or losing a loved one. This is the worst type of stress you can have, and if you can learn to face it in a relaxed, carefree, positive thinking manner, it will not cause nearly the harm to your system as to the average person.

"a. **Develop a positive attitude about everything you do.** The Bible tells us, 'As a man thinketh in his heart, so is he.' We become what we think about. If we constantly think about negative, bad problems and thoughts, we are simply going to create more of these bad situations to face from now on. The Public Library is full of books that will show you how to think positively.

"b. Tell yourself to relax totally. By simply sitting down and taking some deep abdominal breaths and closing your eyes, try to relax all over. Sit in a comfortable chair and tell yourself that you are totally relaxing as you visualize in your mind — your feet relaxing, then your lower legs relaxing, then your upper legs, then your pelvis, then your stomach, then your chest and your hands, and your lower arms, your upper arms, your neck, and your head. Then, visualize yourself in your mind's eye as being totally relaxed. A few minutes of this will do wonders to relieve stress in your entire system.

"c. Practice breathing exercises to relax. You should use abdominal breathing to relax totally. Sit in a very relaxed position in a comfortable chair with your hands on the arms of the chair and your feet on the floor. Breathe in slowly through your nose as you expand your abdomen and imagine that you have a balloon inside your abdomen, and, as you inhale, you are slowly inflating the balloon which will cause your abdominal area to swell. Then, breathe out slowly through your nose. Pull your abdominal muscles in as you press all of the air out of your lungs. You should take several breaths in this manner, and it will help relax you. Another variation of this type of exercise is to use abdominal breathing as you inhale deeply through your nose. Then, exhale through your puckered mouth as if you were blowing out a candle. Repeat this several times.

"d. Cultivate a good sense of humor. Laughing always relieves stress. If you know yourself, you know what things make you laugh. If you would try to do these things more often, this will help you relieve stress. Remind yourself to have fun. This may mean going to a comedy movie or picking up a book of funny jokes to read to get you laughing. You may even consider keeping a laugh scrapbook where you can keep a record of all letters, funny jokes, poems, limericks, or anything you have collected that made you laugh. Read through these in times of severe stress.

"e. Listening to relaxing music will dissolve your tension. Listening to your favorite music is an excellent way to relieve stress. Instrumental music like that performed by the harp, piano, string ensembles, or the flute tend to be more soothing than vocal pieces which may distract you.[But for some folks relaxing music is fast tempo with a definite rhythm: Dixieland, rock, country and western, ragtime]. While enjoying the relaxing music, you will notice that you are breathing more slowly and deeply which means you are relaxing more.

"f. Call a relative or friend. When hit with any type of stressful situation, an excellent technique is to call a close friend or family member and discuss the situation with them which can help you get a clearer picture as to how you may solve any existing problem. Do not keep it pent up inside of you as it can build and grow within.

"g. Exercise or take a brisk walk to lift your spirits. Any type of exercise and especially brisk walking will result in very effective stress reduction. The faster you walk, or the harder you exercise, the more your stress will be relieved. This is because certain neurotransmitters are released during the exercise process for about 20 minutes. Try not to think about your problems while you are walking or exercising.

"h. Stretch or yawn for better relaxation. Yawning itself is a very effective way to relieve stress. If you yawn and try to stretch your muscles as far as you can, this will add effects to the stress relieving techniques. If you develop tension in your neck, shoulders and upper body, the simple shoulder shrug will help relax these muscles. Bring your shoulders up to your earlobes for three or four seconds, and then drop your shoulders down and think — shoulders up, shoulders down. Do this 3 or 4 times. Another simple exercise is 'reaching for the sky.' Try to push your arms upward and slightly backwards, and feel these muscles in your shoulders and upper back stretching. Hold this position for 10 to 15 seconds as you breathe normally. Stretching any muscles in your body will help you relax more.

"i. Take a nature break. If there is any way you can get out in the country, or out in the woods to get away from your present problems, even for a short time, this can do wonders for your stressful situation. It may be that going to the river and just sitting and watching the clouds go by and admiring the scenery will be of benefit to you. Even watching a video or going to a movie involving the great outdoors can be very relaxing.

"j. Take a vacation or a weekender. Getting away from your stressful environment is always relaxing. However, you should try not to feel guilty about not working when you 'get away from it all.'

When you do this, you should relax mentally, physically, and emotionally and learn to let everything go. Tell yourself that it's okay not to work at times. The best form is a vacation that lasts for at least a week to get maximum benefits however.

"**k. Get proper rest.** Sound sleep each night is a perfect antidote to stress. To do this, stick to a regular sleep schedule and try to begin relaxing about an hour before you go to bed. Don't eat a big meal before going to bed, and be sure that you sleep in a very comfortable environment. Also, taking a 15 minute nap in the afternoon if you can arrange it will be very stress relieving.

"**l. Prayer will break the anxiety cycle.** Praying can strengthen your religious beliefs and provide you with strength during times of loss or hardship which may include the death of a loved one, an injury or illness, or financial problems. Praying can teach forgiveness, patience and understanding and relieve some of the negative emotions like anger, bitterness, and hostility. This is an excellent stress reliever.

"Of course, there are other stress-relieving techniques such as getting a pet (excellent for many), but the important thing is to do something to try to relieve the existing situation.

"**12. Miscellaneous Nutritional Gems and Pearls**

" **a. Tea and Coffee.** Caffeine is one of a number of biochemically active compounds found in tea and coffee. Caffeine is also found in chocolate, cola based drinks, and a number of medications. An average cup of strong tea contains 50 mg of caffeine and coffee, 100 mg, although these can vary from brand to brand. Because of the biological activities of caffeine and related compounds, excess tea and coffee consumption may have a number of adverse effects on your health. Caffeine can cause anxiety and nervousness, depression, insomnia, and aggravate any pre-existing psychiatric states. Caffeine can affect your physical body by causing you to pass an excessive amount of urine, diarrhea, bloating, indigestion, shakiness and tremors, migraine headaches, rapid and irregular heartbeats, high blood pressure, restless legs at night and even high blood cholesterol. Excess caffeine can also affect women who have fibrocystic breast disease, as well as PMS. If you drink it at meal time, the caffeine can decrease the amount of iron absorbed from the vegetables eaten. Caffeine also interferes with zinc absorption. One of the worst things about caffeine is that it stimulates your body to produce excess insulin, and this can aggravate a person's condition who may have hypoglycemia or a carbohydrate intolerance. All of us would be wise to decrease the amount of caffeine in our system.

"**b. Soda Pop and Colas.** Soda pops and colas, including diet colas, are one of the worst things that have ever happened to health in America. The great majority of these drinks are loaded with sugar. They act as total cations because they are sticky, and most of these drinks are loaded with caffeine. In addition, all colas, soda pops, and diet drinks, are loaded with other chemicals that are totally cationic in nature and detrimental to your health. A person would be wise to leave out all these drinks in their lifestyle.

"**c. Alcohol.** Alcohol is probably the most acceptable 'social poison' after tea and coffee. Most beers average about 4% alcohol; wine contains about 6%, whereas, brandies and whiskies contain about 40%. We should not forget that alcohol is a food and provides calories in the form of carbohydrates. For an overweight person this can be detrimental. Alcohol has adverse effects on almost every vitamin and on many minerals. In particular, vitamin B1, B2, B3, B6, folic acid, calcium, magnesium, and zinc is depleted in the body in those who consume excessive quantities of alcohol. Deficiencies of these nutrients affect one's general health and one's mental health in particular. Alcohol interferes with fatty acid metabolism. The effects of long term consumption of alcohol on the body can be devastating. Liver damage, nervous system, and brain damage, as well damage to the heart can occur and be equally serious. We are learning now that the risk of certain types of cancer is increased as a result of alcohol consumption, especially cancer of the liver, esophagus, larynx, and mouth. Any woman who drinks alcohol while pregnant is an absolute fool. It's quite common for children who are born of mothers who consume substantial amounts of alcohol during pregnancy to suffer from facial deformities and be mentally retarded. If you are not pregnant, some studies have shown, however, that one drink a day can be beneficial to your circulation. This should be no more than one beer a day, an average glass of wine, or one ounce of spirits.

"d. Smoking. Cigarette smoking has a powerful anti-vitamin C effect, and most smokers have a lower than normal level of vitamin C in their blood. Smoking affects the workings of the pancreas, which is important in the digestion of our food, and in some people, can cause poor digestion.

"e. Drugs and Drug Abuse. The problem with drug addiction and drug abuse seems to be increasing all over our nation. Hundreds of thousands of people take medications to relax them or to sleep every day and, in particular, drugs such as Valium®, Librium®, Atvium®, Xanax®, Halcion®. It is

widely accepted that many people become physically and psychologically addicted to such drugs. They are unable to live without them, and their withdrawal from them when they try to get off them produces both physical and psychological symptoms. The medical profession has been slow to recognize and respond to this problem. It is therefore advisable that any person try to abstain from taking any of these drugs if at all possible.

"A Vital Message to My Patients

"I sincerely desire that all my patients and their families enjoy the best health possible. During the past five years, there has been an explosion of research and knowledge that can vitally affect the health of each of us. This chapter was written in an effort to educate you and convince you to change some of your eating habits so that you and your family will enjoy a healthier life and have fewer health problems. Some authorities may question some of my conclusions, but when I daily observe the health of my patients improve from following these suggestions, I must speak out and share this information with you.

"Today's number one health hazard is arteriosclerosis or hardening of the arteries. This causes heart attacks, strokes, and peripheral vascular disease which leads to more misery and suffering than any other disease known today. This does not count the expenditure of billions of dollars and the loss of millions of days of productive work from our work force.

"Before 1900, this disease was hardly known and was extremely rare. In fact, the first 'heart attack' was described in the medical literature in 1912. Dr. Paul Dudley White, President Eisenhower's heart specialist, saw a heart attack for the first time in 1929. The disease began with the advent of hydrogenated oils, margarine, and the processing of our grain foods such as wheat, corn, rye, barley, and oats. All the vital fatty acids are removed from these grains. The food companies must remove these fatty acids so that the grain foods do not turn rancid and spoil, otherwise the foods would not last long on the shelves of our supermarkets. Our great-great grandparents and their parents had very little arteriosclerosis even though their diets included foods known to be high in cholesterol such as eggs, butter, lard, and sow-bellies. However, they did not eat any hydrogenated oils and their grain foods were homeground and not processed. Processed foods are the primary villain, causing degenerative changes.

"I've known for 20 years that dietary cholesterol cannot be the cause of arteriosclerosis for several reasons. First, the dietary (20%) cholesterol in the stomach is broken down into its tiny component parts, and although some is absorbed through the intestinal wall, 80% of the cholesterol in our system is manufactured by our own body. The problem of arteriosclerosis develops because our bodies do not use properly the cholesterol that it makes. The Eskimos, whose diet by the way, is ten times higher in cholesterol than ours, have very little arteriolosclerosis. If dietary cholesterol intake caused arteriosclerosis, their death rate would be much higher than ours. But they do not suffer from heart attacks, strokes, and poor circulation in their extremities unless they move to more 'civilized' areas of the world and begin eating as we do. In two ways, the Eskimos' diet differs from ours: (1) they do not eat hydrogenated oils and (2) they eat a great deal of non-farmed cold water ocean fish which is high in essential fatty acids.

"In the early 1940s when the Germans overran Norway, the incidence of arteriosclerosis, cancer, and schizophrenia was quite high in that country. The Germans took away all the margarine from Norwegians, and the incidence of these diseases dropped significantly. After the Germans left and the Norwegians began to again eat their margarine, the incidence of these diseases increased to its former level.

"In America, we are developing arteriosclerosis at earlier ages than ever before, even though there is a greater effort on the part of most of us to decrease our cholesterol intake in our diets. Autopsies performed on soldiers killed in the Korean War showed approximately 30% of these young men suffered from advanced atherosclerosis. About 20 years later in the Viet Nam War, autopsies performed on soldiers killed, showed approximately 60% suffered from advanced arteriosclerosis. We must do something about this trend and that's the purpose for this paper.

"Recent research has proven that all hydrogenated oils block the chemical pathways that are necessary for our bodies to use the cholesterol that our own bodies manufacture. Our bodies must have certain essential fatty acids, now being removed from our foods, to assimilate and use our cholesterol, as well as to manufacture certain hormone-like chemicals called prostaglandins, which are vital to nearly all processes of cellular function in the body. Without these prostaglandins our cells cannot function properly and will be subject to disease. I believe that this is one of the main reasons that we are seeing an explosion of many chronic degenerative diseases such as arteriosclerosis, arthritis, diabetes, and lupus. Other conditions such as skin disorders and allergies, premenstrual syndrome, and systemic yeast infections can also benefit from these dietary changes.

"What You Can Do

"1. Totally avoid *all* hydrogenated oils like margarine and all deep fried foods such as doughnuts, French fries, potato chips. *Read food labels.* Our foods are being poisoned today with hydrogenated oils in our boxed foods, mayonnaise, and salad dressings. Use cooking oils with 'Cold Pressed,' 'Expeller Pressed,' or 'Non-Hydrogenated' written on the label. If these terms are missing, the oil is hydrogenated. The best is Virgin Olive oil which is naturally cold pressed. Even non-hydrogenated oils become hydrogenated at 350 degrees F, except for Virgin Olive oil which requires 400degrees F of heat. Use low temperatures and cook a little longer when frying foods. Extra Virgin Olive oil may be too strong in taste, and 'pure' olive oil is inferior, so use Virgin Olive oil, unless you enjoy the taste of the Extra Virgin. *Remember, avoid hydrogenated oils.* (See "Essential Fatty Acids Are Essential," http:// www.arthritistrust.org.)

"2. You must increase the proper fatty acids in your diet by eating non-farmed cold water ocean fish

3-4 times weekly. Cold water ocean fish include salmon, cod, mackerel, herring, tuna, orange ruffie, and sardines (pour off the hydrogenated oil). Fresh fish is the best, but canned fish is okay as they do still have the good oils in them. Warm water fish (snapper, flounder, catfish, bass, and perch) do not have much of the 'good' oils in them. Eat 3 teaspoons of Virgin, not pure, olive oil daily as on salads, but keep oil refrigerated after opening. Walnuts are high in fatty acids and make good snack foods. Eat only breads and cereals that have 100% whole wheat or whole grain written on the label. Most brown breads are not whole grain but have coloring added. Avoid processed or refined cereals or white flour products such as breads, crackers, macaroni, and spaghetti.

"3. With any illness at all, you should follow the above and add the following supplements and follow the directions below. (a) Purchase some salmon oil capsules (MaxEPA®) from a health foods store, and take 4-6 capsules daily. If you can't eat the fish mentioned above, you should take these capsules regularly. (b) Purchase some Borage oil and take 1 capsule daily or purchase Evening Primrose Oil capsules and take 4-6 capsules daily. Extreme care must be taken when buying these products as they are made only in England and many health food store products claiming these ingredients contain only soy oil. Efamol® is one acceptable brand. (c) Decrease your red meat intake since red meats contain arachidonic acid which can provide too much of a bad prostaglandin plus a substance called leukotrienes which will aggravate any disease condition. (d) Avoid all sugars, sweets, desserts, and all white flour foods. (e) Get a good hypo allergic non-yeast multivitamin and mineral tablet and take 3-4 tablets daily. Be sure you get at least 1,000 mg of vitamin C, 50 mg of B-3 and B-6, 50 mg zinc, 100 mcg selenium, and 400 mg of magnesium in your supplements. The above mentioned vitamins are necessary in the fatty acid chemical reactions.

"If you and your family will follow the above recommendations in your dietary habits, you will enjoy a longer, healthier life with much less chance of developing any chronic degenerative disease. Please read this paper carefully, several times and pass the information on to friends and relatives.

"SUMMARY FOR A SUPER NUTRITIOUS DIET PLAN WITH THE BEST LIFESTYLE CHANGES

"1. WATER.

Drink only pure water as I defined it earlier. Ideally, one should drink 3-4 quarts of this water, and to increase the anions in your blood, squeeze the juice of a lemon to a gallon of water. For even better results, get some Zeta® water (very high anions) and dissolve them *according to directions* in your 3-4 quarts of drinking water. Drinking this water will help your kidneys get rid of the excess cations you may take in without realizing it. All metabolic processes will function more efficiently by drinking this extra water.

"2. SUGAR AND REFINED OR PROCESSED CARBOHYDRATES.

This includes table sugar, sucrose, white, brown, or other sugars, glucose, honey, sorbitol, or any additive that ends in "ose" (maltose, lactose, and fructose). Many foods like cookies, pies, cakes, ice cream, soft drinks, chocolates, puddings, jams and jellies or any sweet-tasting foods contain *large* amounts of sucrose or other refined carbohydrates. Any white breads or white or refined flour products are used by your body like sugar, and they have a lower content of vitamins, minerals, and fiber than unrefined flour products and again should only be consumed in small quantities. [Blackstrap molasses and raw unfiltered honey are said to be exceptions;

they are not refined products and carry with them all the nutrients necessary for digestion.]

"3. ANIMAL AND VEGETABLE FATS SHOULD BE MODERATED.

Ideally, we should reduce our fat consumption to about 50 to 60% of present levels. The goal to strive for should be that fatty foods and oils should make up no more than 20% of our diet. Especially important is to avoid relatively poor quality foods with a high fat content like fried foods, pies, pastries, sausages, preserved and tinned meats, and especially all pork products. Most dairy products are also high in fat, and low fat forms. They should be preferred or eaten sparingly.

"4. ENSURE A DAILY INTAKE OF FRESH VEGETABLES, ESPECIALLY GREEN LEAFY VEGETABLES (HIGH ANIONS).

Such foods are rich in the nutrients that are most commonly found to be lacking in many ill and elderly people. Keep in mind that ensuring a good intake of raw or wokcooked vegetables and salads will help protect against some of the more common and more serious diseases in our society.

"5. EAT A WIDE VARIETY OF FOODS.

Eating the same foods over and over makes it very difficult to obtain adequate amounts of all the essential nutrients required for proper nutrition. Also, eating the same foods regularly makes one more susceptible to becoming allergic and addictive to these particular foods which can add stress to your already overstressed system. A wide variety of foods simply makes good common sense.

"6. ENSURE AN ADEQUATE INTAKE OF FIBER.

Ideally, our system needs 30-40 grams of fiber daily whereas the average person in our society only gets 8-10 grams of fiber each day in our fiberdeficient diet. High fiber foods include all beans, salads, fresh fruits, fresh vegetables, 100% whole grain cereals and breads such as wheat, oats, barley, rye, millet, corn and brown rice (never white rice). You should not rely too heavily on any one type of fiber such as wheat or bran. One of the best forms of good fiber is ground psyllium seed husks as found in *sugarless* Metamucil®. All persons having constipation should add this fiber to their diet each day.

"7. STRIVE TO EAT ONLY FRESH FOODS (HIGH ANIONS) AND TOTALLY AVOID ALL FOODS CONTAINING ADDITIVES SUCH AS PRESERVATIVES, COLORINGS, FLAVORINGS, OR CHEMICALS (ALL CATIONS).

All additives to foods such as all preservatives, coloring agents, emulsifiers, texturizers, flavorings, or any chemicals added, will have adverse effects on your health now and in the future. You will invariably find these additives in most all foods found in cans, bottles, boxes, or cellophane packages, and to avoid these very high cationic chemicals, you must read all labels on foods before purchasing. Fresh foods without additives or chemicals are greatly preferred.

"8. STRIVE TO EAT PROTEIN EACH DAY BUT NOT EXCESSIVELY

Ideally, you should eat your protein foods at the evening meal. These proteins are found in *lean* meats, eggs, low fat cheeses, poultry (without skin), nuts, seeds, peas, beans, lentils, sprouted beans, and 100% whole grains and especially 'cold water' non-farmed fish such as salmon., mackerel, cod, orange ruffee, trout, tuna, and sardines are all rich in proteins, vitamins, minerals, and good fatty acids. Unfortunately most salmon is now farmed, fed the same diet as land animals, and contains the same fate as land animals and contains no healthy fish oils.

"9. LIMIT YOUR INTAKE OF SALT IN COOKING OR IN FOOD.

Salt is sodium chloride (NaCl) and sodium is by far the primary cation found in our blood and all bodily fluids. Excessive intake of sodium or salt causes fluid retention, high blood pressure, heart strain and numerous other detrimental effects on our body physiology that only aggravates and compounds poor health. A wise individual will make every effort to limit and avoid any excess salt intake. [Genuine sea salt or Celtic sea salt, with their high and complete mineral contents, are said to regulate excessive sodium in the blood, raising or lowering it as needed. Unfortunately, most salt that is labeled as genuine sea salt or Celtic Sea salt has resulted from the refining of genuine sea salt, where all the minerals have been removed and sold to vitamin and mineral supplement suppliers. See The Grain & Salt Society, 4 Celtic Drive, Arden, NC 28704

"10. ALCOHOL CONSUMPTION SHOULD BE MODERATE AND LIMITED.

Recent studies conclude that a *maximum* of two drinks daily is a safe recommendation. One drink means one half a pint of beer or ale, one measure of spirits (bourbon, vodka, gin, scotch, whiskey), or one glass of wine. Women who are pregnant or who are trying to become pregnant and men or women with liver disease of any kind should not drink any alcohol at all.

"11. AVOID ALL HYDROGENATED OILS.

Avoid all margarines, processed cooking oils (unless cold pressed, expeller pressed, or non-hydrogenated) and avoid all processed foods that have hydrogenated oils listed on the container label. Ideally, one should use only Virgin [or Extra Virgin] olive oil for cooking purposes, and also avoid all deep fried foods which are all hydrogenated, no matter what oils are used to deep fry in. Coconut oil is also highly recommended.

"12. AVOID BECOMING OBESE BY NOT EATING EXCESSIVELY, ESPECIALLY FRIED OR FATTY FOODS, SWEETS, DESSERTS, WHITE FLOUR FOODS, OR REFINED CARBOHYDRATES.

This is especially important concerning high cationic water and foods as it appears that one's body is overloaded with cations; a primary defense is for one's body to store the excess cations in the fat or adipose cells which greatly encourages excessive fat to accumulate. Being significantly overweight reduces life expectancy and aggravates many conditions such as diabetes, hypertension, gout, arthritis, gall bladder problems, and other diseases. So lose weight if you are overweight, and try eating the high anionic foods (slicky) and avoid the processed cationic (sticky) chemically laden foods. Pure water should be used to decrease the cations and add lemon juice to increase your daily anion intake.

"ADDITIONAL RULES FOR HEALTHY LIVING

"1. AVOID TOBACCO PRODUCTS IN ALL FORMS.

Tobacco has many harmful effects whether in smoking, chewing, or using snuff.

"2. TAKE PRESCRIBED MEDICAL DRUGS AND OVER-THE-COUNTER DRUG-STORE MEDICATIONS ONLY IF ESSENTIAL.

All medications or drugs are 98% cationic in nature and should be taken only if prescribed by your physician. It is your job to remind your physician to try to decrease or stop any unnecessary medications. Remember, *drugs are drugs* and are not essential to health unless there is a defined medical problem. You will never find a person whose body is deficient in Tylenol or Valium.

"3. DO NOT TAKE ILLEGAL DRUGS.

Considerable harm and tragedy is caused by the illicit use of drugs. The dangers far outweigh any possible benefits that might result from their use.

"4. TAKE REGULAR PHYSICAL EXERCISE.

Regular physical exercise is absolutely necessary to maintain good physical health. I highly recommend the use of a rebounder or mini-trampoline for at least 20 minutes in the mornings — at least 5 days a week. Other forms of exercise such as brisk walking, swimming, cycling, or any sporting activity are acceptable, but above all, GET YOUR PHYSICAL EXERCISE. Do some form of exercise you enjoy doing.

"5. TAKE REGULAR MENTAL EXERCISE.

Our mind, like our muscles, needs exercise and with both, if you don't use it, you'll lose it. The mind affects the body in many known and unknown ways, and good mental health is necessary to enjoy good physical health. Various mental activities like reading, writing, and creative arts and hobbies can be very stimulating to your mind and should be engaged in. Stop watching too much television.

"6. MAINTAIN A WIDE VARIETY OF INTERESTS AND ACTIVITIES AND KEEP YOUR HOME AND WORK ENVIRONMENT TIDY.

A wide variety of interests and activities stimulates your mind and physical body. Working in a clean and tidy environment helps you to be more calm and relaxed. Both of these important areas are stress relieving and foster better health.

"7. FOLLOW DEFINITE GOALS AND PURPOSES IN YOUR LIFE AND BE SURE TO COMPLETE YOUR RESPONSIBILITIES YOU HAVE TAKEN OR PLANNED.

We are all involved in 6 areas of our lives all 24 hours of each day. These areas are your physical health, mental attitude, business, family, social, and your religious life. If you have set your goals in all these areas or if you have agreed to do something for anyone, make sure you act responsibly and complete these vital issues. This will relieve stress and cause an increase in your own self respect as well as enable you to enjoy a much fuller life. This will place you in a situation where you will be playing a vital part in creating your own future.

"8. TAKE NUTRITIONAL SUPPLEMENTS.

Concentrated vitamin and mineral supplements are generally necessary for a healthy individual living a stress-free lifestyle and consuming a natural wholesome diet. However, for the average American who eats on the run, fights deadlines, is subjected to pollution, radiation, heavy metal intoxicants from smoke and auto exhaust, food contaminants, and is generally on a treadmill, a conservative supplement program is probably a good preventive adjunct. To combat the destructive effects of free radicals (which can accelerate premature aging, produce liver defects and cancer) caused by food processing and environmental poisons, certain anti-oxidants (nutritional compounds which combat cellular oxidation and rancidity) should be included. Recent studies show that at least 90% of the American people are deficient in one or more nutrients. The only wise course of action is to take supplemental vitamins, minerals, anti-oxidants, trace minerals, and fatty acids. This will simply eliminate the possibility of nutritional deficiencies from these vital nutrients.

"9. TRY TO ELIMINATE STRESS FROM YOUR LIFE.

Stress aggravates all diseases and can only hamper any healing process. Study the section on stress relief and initiate some of the stress relieving techniques to help attain better health.

"10. STUDY AND LEARN GOOD NUTRITION AND APPLY THIS KNOWLEDGE TO YOUR LIFE.

Your future good health or poor health depends on you and you alone. I've told you what you must do to attain the best of health, but you alone must put this knowledge to use. I CANNOT DO THIS FOR YOU. YOU MUST PUT THE KNOWLEDGE INTO ACTION YOURSELF.

"11. GET A PET.

Having a pet to love and love you can do wonders to help relieve stress in every facet of your life. Recent studies show that pet owners live longer and their quality of life is better.

"12. PRAY TO GOD EVERY DAY.

This suggestion is probably the most important of all. I also recommend you invest a little time in your happiness and read the Book of John.

13. EAT RIGHT FOR YOUR TYPE.

We would also point to Peter D'Adamo's *Eat Right for Your Type*, a book that advises to follow a diet according to blood type. Peter J D'Adamo ND is a naturopathic physician noted for his popular books on the Blood Type Diet. His series of books suggest that appropriate diet and lifestyle depend in part on an individual's blood type

"DESIRABLE PRACTICES FOR HEALTHY FOOD SELECTION AND PREPARATION

"1. Eat only when hungry. Eat only portion sizes you feel you can safely digest. Reason: Over eating taxes your digestion which results in undigested food.

"2. Consume a wide variety of different foods. Reason: A wide variety will provide your body with more adequate types and amounts of vitamins, minerals, and other food supplements. This will help prevent food allergies.

"3. Avoid eating or drinking the same thing two days in a row. (Exception: pure water.) Try to rotate your foods. Reason: Variety in food increases potential vitamin and mineral intake and reduces the chance of developing food allergies.

"4. Eat slowly and eat only until satisfied. Eat small portions more often and large portions less often. Reason: Digestion and assimilation is your key to nutritional health. Your body can digest small amounts eaten frequently more efficiently.

"5. Chew food thoroughly. Ideally, chew each mouthful 20-30 times. Reason: Digestion begins in the mouth with enzymes in your saliva.

"6. Drink liquids between meals, not with meals and preferably 2 hours after and 15 minutes before. Reason: Liquids dilute digestive juices.

"7. Drink a glass of water upon arising (preferably warm). You may add fresh lemon juice or apple cider vinegar and 1 teaspoon of raw honey. Reason: This will stimulate regular and normal bowel movements each day.

"8. Foods, especially liquids, should not be taken very hot or very cold. Reason: very hot or cold foods create more stress.

"9. Drink plenty of pure water daily, preferably 60-80 ounces. This is especially so with exercise, when perspiring, eating dry foods, and in hot climates. Reason: Water keeps all tissues well hydrated and flushes out impurities that can cause toxic effects. Adequate water also improves elimination. Make sure it is pure water.

"10. Raw foods, except meats, should comprise 50% of total food intake and preferably 75%. Reason: Raw foods provide more fiber, more vitamins, minerals, and food supplements, and they also have more enzymes to give better digestion.

"11. At meals, it is best to consume a variety of raw vegetables when you eat cooked foods. Reason: There is a greater abundance of enzymes and fiber in vegetables which will assist digestion and assimilation of the cooked foods.

"12. Avoid overcooking. Reason: Vitamins, enzymes, proteins, and fatty acids are all heat sensitive and can be destroyed or chemically changed by overheating.

"13. Do not be overly concerned about calories, proteins, fats, carbohydrates, vitamins, minerals, while eating wholesome foods. Reason: A normal metabolism is programmed to adjust its selection and absorption of food stuffs in the presence of a wholesome lifestyle and dietary habits.

"14. In a vegetarian meal containing no animal products, some legumes (lentils, beans) should be added when consuming primary grains. Reason: Legumes provide certain proteins needed for balance.

"15. For those with compromised or delicate digestion, generally avoid concoctions containing combinations of animal protein (i.e. flesh) and carbohydrates (such as dried fruits, bread, bananas, potatoes, grains) or acid fruits and carbohydrates (such as citrus, tomato, vinegar) or milk and animal proteins all in the same *mouthful.* Instead, lean more to individual foods consumed separately.

"16. Avoid foods to which you are allergic. Reason: Allergenic foods create a broad spectrum of chronic health problems and upset digestion of other foods eaten at the same time.

"17. Eat sweets (including fruits), nuts and seeds alone and between meals only. Reason: For maximum digestion and assimilation — fruits, nuts, and seeds are best eaten in moderation and alone. When eaten with a meal or other snack food, they may upset digestion.

"18. When emotionally upset, eat less and chew well. Reason: Emotional upset changes digestive chemistry and interferes with complete digestion.

"19. Avoid distractions while eating such as television, radio, driving, or reading. Reason: When attention is fully with a meal and those with whom you share the meal, you can focus on thoroughly chewing and maintaining a relaxed enjoyable mental state which assists digestion and assimilation.

"20. Read labels and ingredients on boxed, canned, and packaged food. When dining out, question your server as to ingredients used in the foods you are ordering. Reason: Know what is in the food you eat and choose foods that serve your better health.

“21. Keep a brief food symptom-feeling journal of everything you eat or drink. Reason: You will learn more about foods and how they affect you by recording them over a period of time and reviewing the records.

“22. Be sure to avoid all hydrogenated or partially hydrogenated oils. Cold pressed oils are the best for cooking. Reason: Hydrogenated oils can block the normal chemical pathways of cholesterol metabolism.

“ Remember that an excellent diet will emphasize raw fruits, vegetables, grains, seeds, nuts, and sprouts as well as raw dairy or cultured dairy products. The best source of animal flesh protein is from non-farmed cold water ocean fish such as salmon, mackerel, cod, herring, and sardines.

“Ten Most Frequently Asked Questions Concerning Diet, Nutrition, and Illness

“1. Question: I’ve always been told that diet doesn’t really have much to do with treating or preventing disease. As I understand it, the only important thing is to eat a well balanced ‘American’ diet. Is this still true?

“Answer: It never was true. Nutrition is not a philosophy or a religion and what we don’t know CAN hurt us. A recent report published by a major US health agency claims that diet is a major factor in 60-80% of all cancer in the US. That means that for this one illness alone, 300,000 to 400,000 deaths, not to mention a lot of suffering, could be avoided by diet alone. Proper nutrition is very important.

“2. Question: These days I see so many television and magazine advertisements for packaged cereals, sugary sweet desserts, and margarine made with oil that many doctors think is dangerous and convenience foods loaded with additives and preservatives. If these products are supposed to be bad for our health, why aren’t they barred from advertising?

“Answer: Many concerned groups are bringing pressure to force truthful labeling and more limited advertising claims, but this sort of thing takes time. Think how many years it took before the U.S.

Surgeon General was able to remove cigarette advertising from television and force the tobacco companies to print a special warning message on each pack. Until this same idea takes hold with packaged foods, your best defense is to become an informed shopper.

"3. Question: I've been eating the same way for 30 years, and I've never been sick a day in my life. Why should I change my diet?

"Answer: Mostly because improper diet has a cumulative effect. Sometimes it takes a long time before bad habits catch up with us. Picture yourself sitting on one end of a see-saw. Weights are slowly added to the other end. At one point, the weight builds up until you are no longer sitting comfortably at your end. Instead, the see-saw is moving, and you are in a whole new position . . . one you didn't choose, and one you don't like.

"The same idea follows through with diet. Although our bodies are remarkably strong with an amazing capacity to fight off neglect and abuse, there comes a time when even the toughest system can take no more. This is especially true with your immune system. It doesn't suddenly veer out of balance one day. The change has been a long time building. Even though the immune system keeps fighting to maintain your body's health, the job keeps getting harder as your system gradually becomes weaker. One day your immune system can no longer conquer the destructive forces and to your surprise, you are sick. It's important to establish and maintain good health habits as a regular part of your everyday life. In the same way that poor health patterns can gradually destroy your immune system, good health

patterns can strengthen it.

"4. Question: Why does improper nutrition have different effects on people? Some get arthritis or allergies while others develop obesity or other diseases?

"Answer: Each one of us has an Achilles heel as far as our bodily health is concerned. Because of this, we react to the same destructive force in different ways. Our body's weakest link gives way, and it may be hereditary.

"**5. Question:** My grandfather lived to be 95, was never sick and yet he lived a really tough life under what we would consider very poor conditions. Why are we suffering so much misery at half his age?

"**Answer:** The many stress factors in life build up slowly. We are affected by many dangers that grandpa never knew about. The list includes: Polluted water, chemical fertilizers, indigestible food additives, refined sugars and starches, processed vegetable oils, smoke, smog, other airborne pollution, radiation, synthetic fabrics, home heating fumes, cigarettes, meats laced with hormones and antibiotics, vegetables dosed with pesticides, herbicides, and fungicides, plus artificial flavors, artificial colors, and artificial food that has nothing but chemicals in it. No wonder we get sick.

"**6. Question:** If I change my dietary pattern, will I get well and be cured?

"**Answer:** That's a big order because there are no magic bullets in chronic disease. You can't expect overnight results. After all, most physical illnesses are well established. Yes, you will get better, but it may take time. And yes, you can stay well, but we must work together to create and carry out your own health plan for optimum health.

"**7. Question:** But aren't my physical health problems a result of the natural aging process? Don't we all deteriorate as we grow older? Answer: Yes, of course. None of us are Peter Pan and aging is inevitable. However, with a proper health plan, you can hold back the years to an amazing degree. You can't expect to go mountain climbing when you are 95, but you can look forward to vital, active, and totally happy times in your twilight years.

"**8. Question:** I'm not really sure that I have the discipline to stick with a rigid pattern of specified food, exercise. Does that mean there is no hope for me?

"**Answer:** Come on! We all have to live in the real world. While you will get the best results from following your health plan to the letter, we all know that this sort of behavior is not only always possible. Just do the very best you can. You will get results proportionate to the work and effort you put in.

"**9. Question:** Why are we seeing each year an increase in chronic degenerative diseases?

"**Answer:** Recent studies prove that there are 5 determining factors causing this increase: (1) poor nutrition and diet (2) environmental pollution (3) lifestyle factors such as no exercise, stress, inadequate rest, negative thinking (4) genetics and (5) accidents.

"**10. Question:** What do you believe is critical to attain and maintain better health?

"**Answer:** (1) Proper water (2) uncontaminated, nutritious, properly prepared food and diet (3) adequate exercise (4) sufficient rest and relaxation (5) taking vitamins, proper minerals, and fatty acids (6) learning to cope with stress (7) correcting chemical imbalance in patients."

STRESS

The Importance of Stress

A person's overall nutritional intake is the most important single factor for preventing sickness and achieving wellness, and it is fundamental to every disease condition. Good dietary habits are a

Most necessary condition for reversing or controlling all disease states, but may not, in themselves, be a sufficient condition.

Absence of stress, like the presence of a good nutritional status, is also a necessary condition for preventing and achieving wellness, and, like good dietary habits, may also not be sufficient.

There is such a strong interplay between many basic factors that none can be overlooked when seeking wellness. For example, one of the causes of stress can be poor nutritional habits, while poor nutritional habits can also lead to physical and emotional stress. Both fasting and long-term or chronically stressful lifestyles can lead to hormonal unbalances which lead to many different disease states Aside from the interactive, underlying and pervasive nature of good nutrition, however, stress becomes the most important single factor in virtually every disease state. It's also a subject that physicians tend to ignore, and patients wish to avoid.

Just as physicians are generally not taught nutrition, so they are not taught the skills of stress management in medical school. Most of their education is heavily oriented toward drug treatments.

Even those who later specialize in mental, emotional and psychic disciplines are not provided with techniques that work effectively; and so, having at best a failed technology, psychiatrists resort to the use of damaging, mood-altering drugs.

The best that drugs can do for a distraught mental/emotional state is to temporarily occlude painful effects, and delay the individual's need to confront "real-world" stimuli. A continual drugging of sensitive mental/emotional problems continually delays solutions to the problems.

Some physicians who do recognize the importance of stress reduction in bringing about the disease-free-state have learned to use techniques that might reduce their patient's stress. Among techniques used are bio-feedback training, visualizations or guided imageries, aroma therapy, light and sound therapies, meditation, Yoga, qigong, Alcoholics Anonymous, religion, and so on. All of these can be important, if they satisfy the patient, and if they work.

C. Norman Shealy, M.D., Ph.D. writing in *Miracles Do Happen: A Physician's Experience with Alternative Medicine*, says, "Nothing is more important or powerful in stress management than physical exercise."

It is no deep, complex psychological mystery that our greatest source of stress is from personal relationships and from our work. These, after all, thrust at the very heart of survival.

The impact of stress on our bodies was neatly demonstrated by Hans Selye,[152] who described the bio-physical details of the "flight or fight" syndrome, and the exhaustion of adrenaline and its effect on our systems.

In simplified form, what happens is that a threat to survival triggers production of cortisol, a substance from the adrenal gland (cortex) very much like cortisone. Cortisol activates the body to produce quick energy which we need during our emergency state. We are programmed to convert certain T-cells — microorganism protecting cells found in the blood stream that are also part of our immunological system — into a form of quick energy. While this T-cell conversion is excellent for a real emergency, like running away from a saber-toothed tiger or an automobile that is bearing down on us, the tragic effect of a sustained emergency state soon becomes evident.

If we continue to unbalance our immunological system by converting some of its defense factors (specialized T-cells) into quick energy, we also permit organisms-of-opportunity to utilize their new opportunity, and infection — a cold or other pathogenically "derived disease" — hits us.

There are also other effects, such as those which stem from an unbalanced hormonal system, and perhaps even other effects not yet categorized.

A continuous emergency state — threat to survival, flight or fight syndrome — is a continuing stress, and a continuing stress is damaging mentally, emotionally and physically.

How the Body Adapts to Stress to Create Disease

Canadian physiologist Hans Selye[152] described a generally accepted physical model of the effects of prolonged stress at different stages on the human body, called the general adaptation syndrome (GAS). There are three stages (1) Alarm Stage; (2) Resistance Stage; and (3) Exhaustion Stage.

Alarm Stage of Stress

A young person filled with vitality and health will often overwork muscles and come home with "aches and pains" that soon disappear as the ability to bring nourishment to individual cells, to dispose of excess cellular wastes and to repair tissue proceeds rapidly. An older person, however, may take considerably longer and if the muscles are continually overworked or subjected to additional strain from other stress factors the body will began to adapt in other mechanical and biochemical ways. One example of such adaptation has been described by Canadian Carl Reich, M.D., who has shown through his research and clinical practices that biological stress from persistent lack of vitamin D3, calcium, and sunshine causes the body to adapt to any of dozens of different disease states including various forms of disease.[153] Rex E. Newnham, N.D., D.O., Ph.D.,[154] England, has shown a similar result when the body lacks boron.

Repetitive stress factors beyond the individual's ability to swiftly compensate leads to the second stage, or the resistance stage in the general adaptation syndrome (GAS).

Resistance Stage

The middle aged man or woman who works two jobs and who also leads a very stressful life at home because of the absolute need to take care of small children during periods when rest, peace and recovery are demanded of the mind, emotions and body may think that, though often fatigued, s/he coping rather well. Years may go by with such super-stress at home and work as the body slowly uses up resources and also functions with less efficiency due to aging. Circulation decreases minutely year by year, as does the secretion of hormones from aging glands. The heart, kidneys, liver and pancreas function with less efficiency — meanwhile the body like a very good soldier continues to attempt to repair itself from daily stress.

Additional stress may be acquired in the form of nutritional deficiencies; emotional trauma such as loved ones who've died; toxicity from traditional drug therapy that treats symptoms and not the causes, thus providing the illusion that with the drug one is coping; surgeries that interrupt the natural flow of energy — qi — along meridian lines, or incapacitate organs by destroying or deleting them; and other forms of stress — all take their toll.

Soon minor symptoms are acquired and small complaints begin: "I feel tired all the time." "My skin has broken out, and nothing I use clears it up." "When I get up in the morning my joints ache and I feel stiff all over, but I'm OK after I've moved around a bit." "I get headaches at work, and my back and wrist hurt all the time." — and so on!

When treated by means (pills) that simply hide symptoms — which are a way of saying "left untreated and hidden" — a persistently overworked muscle manifests pain, stiffness, and often inflametion, becoming less and less elastic and more fibrous. Additional stress is placed on tendon and ligament attachments to bones and muscles, which creates additional pain and structural mal-adaptations.

Left untreated with appropriate rest and nourishment, muscles and joint structures finally reach the exhaustion stage of the general adaptation syndrome.[155] Muscles and joint structures finally reach the exhaustion stage.

Exhaustion Stage

Joints are not just places where bones move in well-oiled sacs. Joints consist of interacting bones, muscles, skin, nerve tissue, fluids and so on. All components must be healthy and working well with one another.

When certain peripheral nerves leading to joints become biochemically unstable, they can fire impulses that signal both as a spinal reflex action back to the joint and also to the brain and back to the same joint as a pain signal. This can create a condition in the joint of insufficiency of nourishment which factor, in turn, leads to cartilage degeneration, free radical chemical damage, and finally inflammation, swelling, and permanent joint damage. (See *Intraneural Injection for Rheumatoid Arthritis and Osteoarthritis*, http:www.arthritistrust.org)

Muscular imbalances that derive from tendon and ligament imbalances lead to further structural stress. Although we're not aware of the fact — as we have no internal sensing mechanisms to tell us — our body's attempt to compensate creates calcium spurs and further joint damage.

Two adverse factors also become evident at this stage, viewed especially in rheumatoid arthritis, but also seen in some osteoarthritis: (1) various forms of microorganisms gain entrance to bodily tissues. The resulting tissue sensitivity to the toxins or protein products of the microorganisms sets up an internal "allergy" reaction, an antigen/antibody response. If the protein substances have a DNA structure — a genetic sequencing of basic protein molecules — similar to the tissues infected, the body's immunological system apparently attacks both the foreign agents and its own joint tissues; (2) "external" immuno-complexes, substances formed from other forms of antigen/antibody combinations, usually from food allergies, also lodge in joint tissues creating additional irritating foreign substances that lead to pain, inflammation, swelling and general cartilage (that is, joint) destruction. (See "Allergies and Biodetoxification for the Arthritic," http:www.arthritistrust.org)

By this time the lymph system (designed to sweep out impurities) is often overloaded and backed up, like a clogged house drain, and the concentrated toxicity problem simply cascades, looming ever larger. (See "Lymph Drainage Therapy" and, "Lymphatic Detoxification," http:www.arthritistrust.org)

Pain, swelling, and joint destruction, of course, lead to more stress. Thus is established a well-known positive feed-back loop, where stress has initiated a physiological/emotional/ mental sequence which creates more stress.

The Many Faces of Stress: Stress Has an Infinite Number of Faces

No one knows how many life forms have inhabited our planet, Earth. There must be trillions, if not an order of magnitude or so more. Life has adapted to deserts and oceans; to extreme cold and excessive humidities; to the depths of long-buried oil pools and sulphur-bearing rocks; it is found amidst scalding heat and caustic chemicals spewed up by hydrothermal vents; life is found far beneath the earth in solid rock; it is present in oxygen deficient environments, algae live out their complete existence in the swiftly vanishing, fleecy white clouds above us — life is everywhere on earth, and, for all we know, may be a fundamental characteristic of the universe itself.

The powerful engine that drives life into every niche and cranny is stress: biochemical, mechanical, nutritional, mental and emotional, environmental, electromagnetic, radioactive, and so on. A supreme beingness has devised a small DNA molecule that through various mechanisms can adapt or change successive progeny so that survivors can live comfortably, indeed, demand, the particular factors that previously represented serious stress factors for their parents.

This powerful engine — stress — is a wonderful force for species' development and evolution, but an extremely costly one for individuals within the species. Billions of individual bacterium must die before one microbial form is produced that can survive the onslaught of a new antibiotic. This individual then propagates a whole new genus from which springs certain individuals that can only live in the presence of the formerly deadly antibiotic.

As each species' adapts in response to radically changing environments, eventually a totally new species is born, one that cannot cross-breed with the original, and so life spreads, filling every possible niche and cranny.

From the preceding perspective it's easy to visualize that now, today, all of us are undergoing tremendous stress factors that may be producing a human species that can live in an oxygen deficient environment surrounded by deadly automobile fumes, pesticides, fluorides and herbicides, nourished by foods without enzyme content, vitamins or minerals or essential fatty acids: eggless eggs, fatless fats, cream less ice cream, and so on being the norm of the diet for those who survive all the deadly present-day stress factors.

But, oh, at what a cost to each of us as individuals. . . !

Advice for the Sick

Stress factors are common to all diseases. There are some important mental and emotional problems that should be understood and ways to confront these problems that are appropriate for the arthritic. The only difference between stress-relieving principles that apply to the osteoarthritic as compared to those that apply to the rheumatoid arthritic may be a much higher incidence of infectious microorganism in the rheumatoid victim.

Seven physicians (Jack M. Blount, M.D., Ronald Davis, M.D., Paul Jaconello, M.D., Warren Levin, M.D., Rex E. Newnham, D.O., N.D., Ph.D., Gus J. Prosch, Jr., M.D. , John Parks Trowbridge, M.D.) were asked to review the subject of stress, and reduce advice for the arthritic to its most elemental form. Here is their consensus:

Physician-Approved Advice for Reducing Stress

Not only can controlling the stress in your life help prevent contracting arthritis or other diseases but if you get the disease, controlling stress can help lessen the pain and its impact on the body. Be conscious of stress in your life and use the following guidelines to reduce stress:

• Develop a positive attitude about everything you do; associate with "positive attitude" people,

• Learn to relax,

• Learn proper breathing exercises,

• Cultivate a good sense of humor,

• Listen to relaxing music,

• Visit with friends and do things that you enjoy,

• Exercise, get outside in the sunlight, take <u>really</u> brisk walks,

• Permit yourself to yawn when required, and to stretch from time to time,

• Take enjoyable vacations, at least get away from humdrum routine,

• Always get proper rest,

• Learn about your inner spirit, pray according to your conscience and beliefs. Stay in control, don't just become a drug user, as happens to many patients.

Drugs — any kind of drugs — contain a hidden danger that lay unknown until recently, with the work of biochemist Hermona Soreq of Hebrew University, and Alan Friedman,[158] physician at Soroka Hospital in Beersheva, Israel:

Fatty tissues surround the blood vessels that nourish the brain. These specialized layers prevent infectious agents and large chemical molecules from passing through what is called the "blood-

Brain barrier," adversely affecting brain cells, our health, and behavior. Medical scientists have assumed that most drugs taken by mouth do not pass through this protective barrier. Indeed, few, if any, drugs are tested with patients under stressful conditions. Now, it's clear from the work of Soreq and Friedman that under stress the fatty sheath around brain vessels is affected, and various drugs can pass through blood vessels, affecting brain cells, health, and behavior. It follows, therefore, that all of the carefully reported listing of possible adverse affects described in required FDA "counter-indications," is incomplete and may, in fact, be vastly understating the dangers of both common and uncommon drugs, especially whenever stress — a common life factor — is experienced simultaneously with drug usage.

Biofeedback Training

Biofeedback training is a means of learning how to control nerve impulses and muscles that we would normally not be conscious of controlling. Usually, safe electronic mechanisms are used that

Help bring to our conscious awareness what our thought and muscle patterns are doing under a given stimulus.

Although biofeedback training might be useful in eliminating headaches, controlling asthmatic attacks, reconditioning injured muscles, and relieving pain, it can be particularly useful for relieving stress and emotions behind the stress.

Before the 1960s it was a commonly accepted Western belief that autonomic functions, such as the heart rate and pulse, digestion, blood pressure, brain waves, and muscle behavior were beyond our awareness control."They just happened." Now it is well known that many of these functions can be placed under conscious control, or modified if desired, to the benefit of the body's health. Of course, a few seekers after spiritual mysteries, some Yoga practitioners (an ancient healing discipline using breathing exercises, physical postures, and meditation), some who follow the spiritual path of Qigong teachings, and others have been able to control their autonomic nervous system in centuries past, but it was only the few who placed themselves under intense, long, usually life-time study, who obtained the ability. Modern instrumentation makes this chore relatively easy, often pleasant, and swift.

For example, once the physical attribute — heart rate, pulse, skin electrical conductivity, etc. — is chosen, a training signal is wired into the desired attribute — such as a bell, moving needle, light, or other feedback stimuli — and these signals will change according to changes in the chosen physical attribute. The individual will observe the training signal, and through practice, an individual soon learns to "think" or otherwise change internal signals so that the formerly autonomic function can now be consciously controlled.

One way that biofeedback might help is in reducing the sensation of pain by reducing one's emotional response to the pain.

Biofeedback can also be used with visual imagery to reduce stress and also to reduce levels of destructive chemicals in the blood stream.

Exercise for the Relief of Stress

Exercise is absolutely essential for optimum bodily functioning. Physical exercise places demands on all of the body's systems, pumping blood faster, bringing nutrients to the cells, disposing of cellular wastes, breaking down and repairing tissues, and so on. When the metabolism operates efficiently throughout, suppressed emotions and other stress factors dissipate.

Sick folks are often pain-filled, and what is "moderate" exercise to such a person may be "excessive" exercise to another. Although the goal may be to exercise for the purpose of stimulating the overall metabolism, the over-production of undisposed cellular waste products and the tearing down of more tissue than is rebuilt can place the sick person in a position where the disease and its accompanying pain is increased, rather than decreased.

An additional factor must be considered in the event that sickness is actually a by-product of sensitivity to microorganisms (as is surely the case with many of those suffering from many diseases).

First Roger Wyburn-Mason, M.D., Ph.D. then Gus J. Prosch, Jr., M.D. would caution that exercising without first eliminating these potential organisms may serve to spread the disease faster, as increased blood flow enhances the rate of microorganism distribution.

Aside from the possibility of an infectious organism, however, exercise is a must for all individuals, even if it is no more than twisting and bending fingers and hands.

Although many health professionals will advise the employment of "moderate" exercise, the definition of what constitutes "moderate," may be between you and your health professional in consideration of your present health circumstances.

The best goal is to slowly, safely increase physical exercise without also creating further damage, and more lasting pain. Although pain may be present before completely healed, there should be continued improvement for every kind of exercise employed. Start with a pad and pencil and record your ability to exercise by, say, counting the number of finger bends, or wrist twists, or even the number of attempts to stretch and touch your toes. From this information:

1. Set yourself a first safe goal.
2. Tomorrow, equal or exceed the goal, but not by so much that you create more suffering.
3. The third day, equal or exceed the goal of the second day. If you can't, don't be disappointed, as everyone's body has ebbs and flows in efficiency. Simply go back to day one, equaling or exceeding your accomplishment, if possible.
4. Continue as above, always recording your accomplishment or even graphing it against the number of days of trial. Your graph will wiggle up and down, which is natural, but overall it will rise, giving the appearance of a jagged outcropping reaching toward the clouds.
5. When you're satisfied with what you've done with one set of exercises, choose another, but don't forget the first. Now record both of them.
6. Continue expanding your abilities as above, adding number of movements, or attempts, and new exercises as your body permits.

If you're one of the fortunate ones, you'll want to take up a more active form of exercise: trampolining (which moves lymph faster); walking fast, or even running, dancing, swimming, etc.

Taking individual differences into account, then, John Hibbs, N.D. of Bastyr College, Seattle, Washington, recommends what he calls tissue aerobic exercise: relaxing exercise that allows blood flow to continue to the tissues. "The heart rate should increase and you should wind up sweating, but many doctors are switching over to a lower heart rate now. You don't need to go up to 140."

Don't pick an exercise that you despise, or even dislike, pick an exercise you enjoy, but try never to overdo, never over-achieve. Pamper your body, pet it, be nice to it — and it'll one day return the favor with improved health, lessened suppressed emotion, and certainly lowered stress.

Guided Imagery for Stress Relief

After a stressful day at work, filled with withering emotions, it is sometimes difficult to fall immediately to sleep, no matter the urgency of sleep. Many have learned that they can invent a scenario inside their mind somewhat more complex than counting sheep, but rather including something quite pleasant they'd like to do. Placing all of one's attention on the play-acting inside the mind quickly dissipates the wrought-up energies, and often one will fall asleep before finishing the scenario.

so on, focusing entirely on an image which they chose, and which they described in however much detail they could.

The result of this little exercise was that the subject lost any possible residual restimulation from associated memories containing similarities to those painful memories confronted and alleviated, and the session was ended.

While nowhere nearly as beneficial as that obtained when releasing huge stores of undesirable, pent-up pain and emotion, the use of guided imagery by itself has been sufficiently positive to attract many health professionals.

Guided imagery relies on a natural function discovered to be common to all people from childhood upward: the ability to focus thoughts, and to either recall or imagine a specific time in numerous perceptics when the body and emotions were at ease.

Meditation for the Relief of Stress

The art of meditation is perhaps as old as modern man, for it is the tribal shamans (healers) and primitive tribesmen who learned its value for many purposes, including that of healing.

According to Joan Borysenko, Ph.D., pioneer in the field of mind/body medicine, meditation is defined as any activity which keeps the person's attention anchored in present time without being influenced by past memories, nor preoccupied with future considerations.

Another way of describing such meditation is that we learn to "key out," all currently functioning stimulus-response mechanisms of the body, whether these are triggered by past, recorded memories, or were conditioned under painful and emotional experiences.

There are many systems for achieving appropriate meditation which are beyond the scope of this book. Some will advise sitting quietly while concentrating on the breath, image, or a sound, while others advise becoming aware of our sensory impressions, such as feelings, images, sounds, thoughts, odors,

Many stimulus-response mechanisms — or as some have phrased it, "automatic circuits" — operate daily to cause us to move our hands, head, and other body parts in almost random, meaningless behavior patterns (such as the desire — sometimes overriding desire — to scratch a particular place on the face, or behind the neck). To some extent we've all identified our personality, our beingness, our awarenessof-being-aware unit with these patterns, and if asked why we scratched, we'd answer that "I itched there," which is more of a justification after the fact than a statement of cause.

One of the easily observed phenomena when attempting meditation is the number of these overwhelming distractions that must be ignored in order to be in present time without computing conclusions about past events, or analytically predicting future actions or probabilities.

At the point where all these distractions disappear — and they will — one has usually achieved a meditative state.

There are physiological, psychological, and spiritual benefits from the daily practice of meditation. Meditation lowers the body's core temperature, which is one of two factors that have been shown to

extend life, the other being restriction of calorie intake.

Stress is more easily confronted, or handled, when we permit ourselves to simply "be," the distinguishing outcome of meditation. Of course, with stress under control, all disease states are better handled, including pain and the emotional components of pain. Jom Kabat-Zinn, director of the Stress Reduction Clinic at the University of Massachusetts Medical Center, has taught meditation and Yoga to thousands of patients, mostly referred to him by other physicians. "In one study overseen by Dr. Kabat-Zinn, 72 percent of the patients with chronic pain conditions achieved at least a 33 percent reduction after participating in an eight-week period of mindful meditation, while 61 percent of the pain patients achieved at least a 50 percentreduction." Additionally these patients improved their self-esteem and held more positive views about their bodies.

Meditative practices are quite easy to learn, and once the discipline takes hold, with frequency and time, the more benefits are received.

Meditation is not a substitute for medical or stress-related physical disorders. Although people can easily practice meditation by themself, physical problems should be attended to by those best trained in the art of healing.

Stress in Personal Relationships: The Suppressive Personality

According to the research of L. Ron Hubbard,[151] often there is one or more persons in the close work or home environment who are suppressive to the one who is sick, such suppression expressing itself in a way that constantly invalidates the sick person's actions, thoughts or emotions. It is a negative stimulus that depresses our beingness, our will to want to engage in friendly exchange of ideas or activities. Hubbard called these people "antisocial personalities." He estimated that about 15-20% of all humans have characteristics that can be called antisocial. An individual's intelligence, educational level or manner of earning a wage has no relationship to whether or not he or she is antisocial. Judges, administrators, physicians, ditch-diggers, taxi-drivers, editors, homemakers, teachers, any nationality, any race, any creed, any or all walks of life may fall into the 15-20% category.

A person who is so affected by another will often suppress his or her emotions and behavior in ways that express outwardly in the form of hormonal changes and accompanying clinical sicknesses.

The medical terminology is "psychosomatic," indicating that the person's state of mind governs his emotions and bodily condition. This is true to the extent that a person permits suppressive conditions and "suppressive" people to influence his or her mind and body.

As few physicians have training in recognizing the causative patterns, and would probably be resisted by their patients if they mentioned them, interpersonal stress sources are often ignored in treatment, although they may be the largest component of all diseases, acute or chronic.

Yoga for Stress

Yoga, one of the oldest known systems for health, is the practice of physical postures, breathing exercises, and meditation. Its practice in modern times has demonstrated the lowering of stress and blood pressure, regulation of heart rate, and even retardation of the aging process.

Yoga teaches an integration of the mind and body. The mind and body are one and the same, and should be written with a new symbol, as mind/body. The modern view of psychosomatic medicine may have stemmed from this ancient art where whatever affects the body also affects the mind and viceversa. Spelling out such a cause effect relationship is, in itself, inaccurate, as the true Yoga practitioner would view physical disease of the body, or aberrated behavior patterns, as being symptomatic of our forgetting the unity known as mind/body.

The thyroid gland and its hormonal production is basic to the stoking up of our cellular metabolic engines, which in turn is basic to the efficient utilization of enzymes which is fundamental to good health for all disease states. Indeed, many symptoms do stem from insufficiency of thyroid hormone or in its conversion to a form that slows down the metabolic heat engine. The practice of Yoga has been shown to normalize the production of thyroid hormone.

As the thyroid is the master regulator of all the other glands (with the pituitary being the master gland over all, including the thyroid), and as the glands are intimately tied in with stress and emotion, the ability to increase or decrease thyroid activity without taking drugs can be an important self-help process. There have been more than a thousand well-designed studies (since the 1970s) of meditation and Yoga. These studies have demonstrated that Yoga can bring about stress and anxiety alleviation, blood and heart rate reduction, improved memory and intelligence, pain alleviation, improved motor skills, relief from addiction, heightened visual and auditory perceptions, enhanced metabolic and respiratory functions, and many other benefits.[161]

Yoga can be ideally suited to the personal health maintenance program of all. To learn more, you can obtain numerous books at any book store.

Magnetism Truths: Selling the Magic Bullet

Billions of dollars spent each year intend to convince the public (and doctors) that a magic bullet "breakthrough" is in the offing. Just a few more billions, another decade or two for "proper" research, compose just the brightest research crew . . . "you could be saved any day now, hallelujah!"

We'll call this Magic Bullet, Type I.

"Just ask your doctor if blahblah is right for you!" Aside from a long list of whispered, damaging side-effects, it's really an alleged form of a magic bullet, too!

We'll call this Magic Bullet, Type II.

So we have two kinds of magic bullets huckstered daily, year in and year out.

Type I will cure most any kind of degenerative disease such as cancer, arthritis, diabetes, and so on. Just spend enough money for "research" and we'll get there together.

Type II will "cure" what ails you now! "Dr. So-and-so is really a bright man, and he said to take blahblah."

"I feel so much better now, and relieved that I no longer have to worry over. . . .!"

Whether the words are spoken or not, we are to understand that Magic Bullet Type I only requires money, time, and brains. Whereas Magic Bullet Type II will work immediately, never mind that it is not a true Magic Bullet, but only a symptom reliever, and that while the underlying biological disturbance is hidden and continuing, the treatment also adds on more biological problems for which additional Magic Bullet Type II's may be required.

Magic Bullet Type I is usually a con job, donated research funds normally going to support the very limited research laid out by domineering and all pervasive pharmaceutical companies who are not really interested in cures.

Magic Bullet Type II is a lie, passing itself off as a Type I finally completed.

Do Magic Bullets Exist?

Semmelweis developed a magic bullet. He washed his hands before delivering babies after having dissected cadavers. Childbed fever dropped "magically."

Vitamin C is a magic bullet against scurvy and numerous other problems!

Indeed, most of the vitamins are magic bullets against specific "lack-of" diseases. They are also magic bullets against many other potential health problems. For example, Vitamin A when taken by the pregnant mother can help prevent Spina Bifida in the newly born. Vitamin C, when taken in sufficient quantity, can strengthen the immune system so that many microorganism-based diseases are defeated.

Properly grown, stored and prepared foods are also magic bullets for a wide variety of ailments, especially when enzymes, vitamins and minerals are present and absorbed by the patient.

Specific antibiotics, such as penicillin, can be a magic bullet against bacteria that have not yet learned to adapt to its deadly influence.

A wonderful, woefully underused magic bullet is injectable dilute hydrochloric acid. It will stimulate macrophages and leucocytes to defeat virtually any bacterial invasion, whether they have adapted to antibiotics or not. Antigen specific colostrum is a fabulous magic bullet when properly used and administered. Complement prepared from any number of antigens surrounds and kills organisms immediately without passing thru the long, tedious, often defective process of vaccination, incubation and finally protection.

Heparin used externally and internally on recent burns, even severe ones, result in less pain, faster healing, and zero scar tissue.[162]

So, the answer is, YES! Magic Bullets do exist!!

But they are seldom Type I's and never, never Type IIs.

Primary Methods of Wonderful Cures from Alternative/Complementary Practitioners

Practitioners of alternative/complementary medicine utilize a wide variety of techniques to assist their patients toward wellness. To name just a few: kinesiology, electro-dermal screening, diet control along with determination of needed vitamins and minerals (orthomolecular medicine), Oriental medicine (herbs & diagnosis), acupuncture, electromagnetic frequencies, wave forms and polarities, biological dentistry, anti-Candida treatments, anti-allergy treatments, and so on.

All of these processes, and more, directly or indirectly have as an end result the literal formation of the same magic bullet which guarantees restoration of good health.

The Acidic/Alkalinity State

Let's consider diet control along with determination of needed vitamins and minerals and proper nutrition (orthomolecular medicine), to illustrate the problems faced by the practitioner and the patient.

Basic to everything is the physician's goal of having the patient achieve an alkaline systemic state. The problem of patient system acidity is a worrisome one for any doctor. Other than required stomach acid, system acidity promotes ill-health and prevents cellular repair. Tissue alkalinity promotes good health and assists cellular repair.

Litmus is a paper which has been impregnated with a chemical which changes color as the acidity, or hydrogen ion concentration of the fluid being tested increases or decreases. Using this test paper a blue of 7.5 to 7.0 test indicates a mild alkaline to neutral normal test. A green 6.5 to yellow 4.5 test indicates increasing acidic and abnormal tests.

Take a small piece of litmus paper and place some saliva on it at a time when the saliva is not dominated by either drink or food. Match the resulting color against the colors shown on the litmus paper spool. A dark purple color means one has sufficient alkalinity.

The closer the color matches the other end, yellow, the more acidity one has.

After you've tested yourself you probably won't be very surprised or excited. However, here's another simple test you can try:

Test the clean saliva of a baby, then a 2 or 3 year old, a 6 year old, a 12 year old, a 20 year old and so on, up to your age. Unless the testee is unhealthy, generally you'll find that your litmus paper begins as dark purple and by a continuous spectrum grades itself thru green and yellow as you pass from the baby to you. Contrary to your first possible surmise, other than dark purple is not really healthy!

Most alternative/complementary health professionals know the importance of changing from an acidic to an alkaline condition. Regardless of what specialties the health professional prefers, the major method used to achieve the alkaline condition is through allergy-free, good diet and necessary enzymes, vitamins, minerals and essential fatty acids.

There certainly is no reason or valid argument to change this approach, but it does have stressful pitfalls.

1. The patient cannot stay on the diet.

2. Tension, worry and emotional upset, physical injury or over-stressed muscle, fascia, tendon or other tissues such as internal organs can switch the patient from alkaline to acid rapidly.

3. The length of time for reversal from acid to alkalinity works against the willingness of the patient to comply.

Considering all of the above factors, this magic bullet usually works at a pace that could never be fired from a gun!

Can Acid to Alkaline Change be Faster, Safer and Effective?

William H. Philpott, M.D.[163] believes that during his forty years of medical practice and many years of experimentation with static magnets, he's isolated the rules for more rapidly and safely bringing about an alkaline condition. Many of his conclusions are surprising, but all are easily testable.

Dr. Philpott was a founding member of the Academy of Orthomolecular Psychiatry (remember Linus Pauling, Ph.D.), fellow of the Orthomolecular Psychiatric Society and the Society of Environmental Medicine and Toxicology and life member of the American Psychiatric Association, author of *Brain Allergies*, *Victory Over Diabetes* and numerous articles and booklets on food allergies and magnetics. He received the Linus Pauling Award in 1998 from the Orthomolecular Health Society.

His experimental work using magnetics on humans was preceded by Robert R. Becker, M.D. and

Becker's work by Harold Burr, M.D. Let's look at Dr. Philpott's conclusions:

1. During sleep our bodies are supposed to return to an alkaline condition; during waking hours we build up an acidic condition. A healthy body should balance the two conditions.

2. Sleep is our primary healing period.

3. Magnets have two poles, called South (S) and North (N) poles. To avoid confusion, Dr. Philpott sometimes calls the magnetic compass South pole the "South-seeking pole," and the magnetic compass North pole the "North-seeking pole." More accurately, he says, "A magnetometer is used to identify positive (+) and negative (-) magnetic poles. A magnetometer is a scientific instrument, which identifies magnetic polarity in terms of electromagnetic polarity, which is positive (+) and negative (-) rather than the geographic compass needle identification of north and south."

Dr. Philpott explains, "There is a need to understand the navigational error in identifying the magnetic poles as well as the parallel identification in identifying DC electrical current poles and DC static field permanent magnet poles made from the DC current. To those who have examined for and identified the distinctly opposite biological responses to opposite magnetic fields, the separate identification of the magnetic poles is an important must. To those not experienced in the knowledge of separate biological responses to opposite magnetic poles, the magnetic poles and the gauss levels needed for these responses is what is making biophysics become a predictable science parallel to the predictable industrial application of magnetics."

4. Other than those studying atomic forces, students are not taught the biological difference or any other difference between the effects of one pole or another; and, indeed, there appears to be no difference when a piece of iron is exposed to either pole. Both attract the iron.

5. However, there is a very important difference of these two poles on cellular biology as well as direction of rotation of electrons and ions. The South-seeking pole sets up conditions to alkalinize the body, whereas the North-seeking pole sets up conditions to acidify the body. Alkalinization leads to healing of many illnesses, while acidification leads to setting the stage, the terrain, for establishment of many illnesses.

He says, "This is paralleled and demonstrated to be true in an electrolysis unit. The positive electric pole is surrounded by a positive magnetic field. The pH of the fluid at that area becomes a pH of 2 which is markedly acidic and the pH around the negative electrode with its negative magnetic field surrounding it becomes a pH of 8. Therefore, we do have evidence that this is correct. That the negative electromagnetic pole, with its negative magnetic field or negative ions is alkalinizing and that a positive electromagnetic field with its positive magnetic field and positive ions is acidifying. . . . It was of interest that the doctor of whom I treated his heart and resolved the atheromatous plaques in his arteries had a blood pH of 8. A blood pH of 7.5 is the usual, normal pH. It doesn't hurt if the pH is up to 8."[7]

6. Grave errors are made by those who sell or use magnets when they

(a) mix positive and negative static magnets, or

(b) use the positive pole on their bodies.

7. The positive magnetic field rotates ions clockwise, a dextrotatory motion. The negative magnetic field rotates ions counter-clockwise, a levorotatary motion. Human cells and their physiology much prefer levorotary chemicals. In fact, in most instances, the human body will reject the dextrorotary chemicals.[3] (Consider vitamins and supplements labeled as "d-" or "l-" and the damaging consequence of using the dform as opposed to the lform. For human use, amino acids and fats are required to be the levorotary forms.)

8. Except for a very short period of time, and for only specialized purposes — to stimulate neuronal and catabolic glandular functions — the positive magnetic pole should never, ever be used on cellular biology.

9. Both the positive pole and the negative pole seem to eliminate pain, but they do so in two fundamentally different biological ways.

a. Pain is reduced or eliminated by the positive pole by increasing endorphins, the body's natural pain opiate. Even wise medical doctors have been found hooked on their own endorphins (addicted) when relying daily on the positive magnetic pole for pain relief.

b. The negative pole reduces or eliminates pain by changing systemic acidification to that of an alkaline state.

10. Both the positive and negative magnetic field are "dose dependent," that is, the stronger the magnetic field, the faster their action — positive to destroy, negative to heal.

11. The biological response to a positive magnetic field is acid-hypoxia — acidification + reduction in oxygen availability.

12. The biological response to a negative magnetic field is alkaline-hyperoxia — alkalinization + increase in oxygen availability.

13. Acid-hypoxia leads to many forms of degenerative disease. Thus, the almost superhuman effort of alternative/ complementary health professionals to flip their patient's acid-hypoxia to alkalinehyperoxia.

14. The human body does not need a frequency, polarity, wave form, et. al. from a Rife-type source, as the human brain establishes its own frequency from static magnetic sources — its own fields and the Earth's magnetic field. About 30% of human energy derives from the Earth's magnetic field; for sharks, it's about 90%.

15. Continuous (or long-time) exposure to negative polarity of reasonably high strength produces long-time alkalinity-hyperoxia, which has been shown to cure cancer and many other degenerative diseases.

16. Continuous (or long-time) exposure to negative polarity of reasonably high strength has been shown to kill every form of invasive microorganism (except the "good-guys" in the intestinal tract), whether or not embedded in the nerve structure, and to do so safely, without damaging Herxheimer effect.

17. A positive magnetic field is a signal of injury sent to the brain. But no healing-repair can occur due to the positive magnetic production of acid-hypoxia when a positive polarity is persistently used. When the brain receives the positive polarity signal it returns a signal of negative polarity, which is required for healing to begin, as it imposes an alkaline-hyperoxia for oxidative phosphorylation production of ATP (adenosine triphosphate).

Dr. Philpott's conclusions are consistent with and confirm the work of physicist Albert Roy Davis and medical doctor Robert O. Becker.

Extracts from Case Histories

Melanoma (Cancer of Skin): From "Magnetics and Melanoma: Katherine's Frightening Dilemma"

Dr. Philpott's wife, Katherine, developed a rapidly growing melanoma on the forehead which gave every evidence of being malignant.

Lessons learned: Treated only at night, first used neodymium disc negative magnet pole was under strength and too small an area. Apparently killed the melanoma where it covered but not at edges which were uncovered, and which continued to expand.

Using a 1-1/2" negative magnetic pole across the whole melanoma and 3/8" thick of 3,950 gauss, she was treated 24 hours daily, requiring one month. Ten weeks after daily treatment, the tumor had dried up and skin had grown under the tumor.

Candidiasis: Patient's stool sample contained multiple injurious disease-producing microorganisms including the fungus *Candida albicans*. Patient slept on 70 bed magnet for three months and then took another stool sample. Gastrointestinal symptoms had faded and her culture contained no injurious microorganisms but did contain the "good-guys" microflora.

Heart Attack: Doctor had heart attack and bypass surgery. One artery not bypassed was 50% closed. He wore continuously day and night a 4" X 6" X 1/2" negative magnetic pole. Nine months later artery left 50% closed was now 100% open.

Dr. Philpott's experimental work, including both rotation diets and magnetics and has covered many aspects of healing, including, but not limited to, addiction, Alzheimer's, allergies, cancer, detoxification, diabetes, emotional disorders, fibromyalgia, gastrointestinal problems, inflammation, liver disorders, major mental disorders, multiple sclerosis, osteoporosis, pelvic disorders, sleep, stress, universal sensitivity reactors, and viral encephalitis.

How can one treatment be so fundamental?

An acidic-hypoxia state deposits amyloidal tissue in the brain, plaques in the arteries, deposits in joints, gall bladder, kidneys and so forth.

An alkaline-hyperoxia state dissolves all of the above deposits!!!

Investigate New Drug Program

The story of Dr. Philpott's conversion from a strait-laced drug-oriented psychiatrist to one who actually solves problems via rotation diets and magnetics is extremely fascinating and reflects the inherent self-honesty of a physician who is most interested in patient wellness. This story can be found at http://www.arthritistrust.org, "Research" then "Research and Letters" tab, William H. Philpott, M.D.

But how did this doctor achieve such a broad range of research subjects?

Prior to approving a new treatment for a patient the FDA requires (1) assurance of safety and (2) review and acceptance by an institutional review board. Upon receiving these two factors, the FDA assigns an IND number to the patient test.

Once the MRI (Magnetic Resonance Imaging) was approved by the FDA as being essentially pronounced safe for human use, then Dr. Philpott knew that his magnetics program would also fall within the same approved category. He asked the FDA for an IND for use of magnetics on human problems. The FDA told him that he could precede without an IND and that the FDA had classified the application of magnets to humans as harmless, calling it "not essentially harmful." Since he was dealing with a non-injurious, non-prescription item, he did not need to report to them until sufficient data was successfully published in peer review literature. Then he could provide the FDA with reports and they would act on them to make a statement which would also satisfy insurance companies regarding safety and effectiveness.

Dr. Philpott did establish an Institutional Review Board consisting of experts who would be familiar with magnetics and medicine.

Dr. Philpott also disagrees with the FDA that open use of magnetics is essentially harmless, as he's satisfied himself through experimentation that the positive polarity can be quite damaging when applied in strength for lengthy periods. The positive polarity can be both addictive as well as acidifying, thus leading to the broad spectrum of health problems related to acidification.

Apparently the FDA has itself in a catch 22 on this one. Until a peer-reviewed medical magazine publishes Dr. Philpott's data, they will not be able to advise or protect folks from magnetic polarity misuse. They obviously consider positive polarity applications on human biology as "essentially safe," even though Dr. Philpott's data demonstrates that North-seeking polarity is not safe.

By means of experimentation with magnets Dr. Philpott has been able to cover a very wide range of health problems, and has learned a great deal about the need for a negative magnetic field by the human body. His motto is quite interesting:

"I do not claim that magnets cured you; you claim that magnets cured you."[5]

Polar Powered Magnets Catalog

Although it's possible to purchase magnets of the right size and gauss strength from numerous industrial magnet suppliers, Dr. Philpott, through his son-in-law, has over time conveniently worked out different magnetic flux delivery methods, magnet sizes and strengths for many different health protocols. The catalog, together with many articles and protocols can all be found at our website, http://www.arthritistrust.org, "Research" then "Research and Letters" tab, William H. Philpott, M.D.

So — Can Acid to Alkaline Change be Faster, Safer and Effective?

Apparently the answer is "yes!" acidic to alkaline systemic changes are a genuine Type I Magic Bullet available now, not in the future, and can be faster, safer and effective when assisting the patient to change from an acid-hypoxia to an alkaline-hyperoxia systemic state!

Apparently the only defect in this particular Magic Bullet Type I is that it doesn't require billions of dollars for research, nor a huge bureaucratic government board nor an intertwined medical establishment!

Dr. Philpott's following table clearly summarizes most of his major discoveries.

COMPARISON BETWEEN SUSTAINED BIOLOGICAL APPLICATIONS OF THE POSITIVE POLE AND NEGATIVE POLE

Negative Magnetic Fields

Attracts ferro-magnetic materials

Dose dependent; stronger gauss field produces stronger action

Brain's response is decreasing pulse frequency

A pulsing of:

12 cycles/second or less results in negative magnetic field

6-12 cycles/second results in relaxation

4 cycles/second results in disassociation

3 cycles/second results in lapse states

2 cycles/second results in sleep

Brain's pulsing frequency decreases as Gauss strength increases

Rotates ions and electrons counter-clockwise

Decreases pain by creating alkalinity (alkaline/hyperoxia) Is non-addicting with frequent use

No free radicals generated because of counter-clockwise spin No inflammation or stress because there are no free-radicals Anti-stressful

Governs cellular normalization and healing

Governs sleep by evoking melatonin in pineal gland

Strengthen thymus gland defenses Increase human growth hormone Non-compatible with cancer

Non-compatible with invasive microorganisms

Helps heal edematous and bleeding areas from acute injuries

when worn continuously for a week or two will heal local tissue, and will not harm the tissue, and will kill microorganisms

Activates alkaline-dependent oxidoreductase enzyme catalysis of oxidation-reduction production of ATP (adenosine triphosphate) necessary for human cell metabolism cancer cell metabolism

Detoxifies biological inflammatory free radicals (peroxides acids, alcohols and aldehydes) to non-inflammatory water and molecular oxygen

Destroys invasive microorganisms except "good-guys" microflora

Normal human cells have a negative charge, consistent with negative polarity magnetization

Reverses neuropathy, toxic neuritis, diabetic neuropathy, etc.

Positive Magnetic Fields

Attracts ferro-magnetic materials

Dose dependent; stronger gauss field produces stronger action

Brain's response is increasing pulse frequency

A pulsing of:

More than 12 cycles/second results in positive magnetic field Brain's pulsing frequency increases as

Gauss strength increases Rotates ions and electrons clockwise

Decreases pain by increasing brain opiates (endorphins) (acid/hypoxia) is addicting with frequent use

Free radicals generated because of clockwise spin Inflammation or stress because of free-radicals

Stressful

Governs cellular break-down and is destructive

Inhibits sleep by blocking melatonin in pineal gland

Weakens thymus gland defenses Decrease human growth hormone Compatible with cancer

Compatible with invasive microorganisms

Creates vasodilatation and unsuited for edematous bleeding areas from acute injuries

When worn continuously will produce an inflammatory red, raised, edematous area due to the acidevoked vasodilatation inflammatory reaction

When worn continuously for a week or two will create an acid evoked inflammatory vasculities (acid-burn), which is red, raised, edematous and itching with bacterial growth pustules

Activates acid-dependent transferase enzyme catalysis of fermentation production of ATP (adenosine triphosphate) necessary for microorganisms (viruses, bacteria, fungi, parasites) and cancer cell metabolism which also replaces the alkaline-hyperoxia necessary for oxidation-reduction enzyme catalysis production of ATP (adenosine triphosphate) Creates free radicals and inflammation

Provides excellent environment for invasive microorganisms, except for “good-guys” microflora

Abnormal cells such as cancer and invasive microorganisms have a positive charge, consistent with positive polarity magnetization

Produces peripheral neuritis of tingling, numbness, pain, loss of sense of pressure, etc.

Note: Whether positive or negative brains can also be driven by external pulsing field: using sight, sound, tactile, or brain stem using upper back of neck and low occipital

Diagnosis and Treatment of the Future

Would you believe that elements of future medical diagnosis and treatment began before 1122 B.C.?

Very few discoveries start from scratch and are thereafter full blown. Most major discoveries build upon predecessors. Let us tell you briefly about some of the predecessors...

The 1122 B.C. *Yi Jing* (*Book of Changes*) seems to be the earliest known reference to three natural powers embedded in every human being. Even prior to this significant publication, during the Shang dynasty from 1766-1154 B.C., archeological digs discovered 160,000 pieces of turtle shells and animal bones covered with written characters. This writing, called “Jia Gu Wen” (Oracle-Bone Scripture) was the earliest evidence of the Chinese use of the written word. While most of the writing was of a religious nature here was the earliest mention of acupuncture and other medical knowledge.[164]

And, as we mentioned above, 1122 B.C. was clearly a very early and significant historical monument toward building the medical diagnosis and treatment of the future.

Between 1756 B.C. and 1122 B.C. Buddhism entered China from India and several branches of Kung Fu flowered. Acupuncture became widespread but was in a rather chaotic mess until Dr. Wang Wei-Yi created what became a very famous brass human sculpture showing the 12 meridians that channel chi up and down the human body as well as pinpointing many acupuncture points. Dr. WeiYi pieced together the prior chaotic knowledge, its organizational value for medicine on par with

Dmitri Mendeleev's organization of the periodic table of the elements for chemistry.

"Chi" of course, was well accepted in China by then and generally defined as a kind of life force that traveled along the twelve defined meridians accessing all the parts of the human body and especially passing through all of the known acupuncture points which, in turn, accessed all tissues and organs in the body. Interestingly modern scientists with a knowledge of magnetic energy and electric current flow have been able to validate this ancient system. For one example, when measuring resistance from or near acupuncture points, electrical resistance clearly decreases at each acupuncture point and increases as the measuring tool moves away from the acupuncture point.

Numerous schools of medical treatment, religious interpretation and even martial arts absorbed this knowledge and there was created over the centuries different philosophies and methodologies based on the truth of meridians, acupuncture points and chi.

In 1833 Samuel Hunter invented an instrument to measure electrical resistance which was destined to play its part in the development of medicine of the future. Charles Wheatstone popularized it in 1843 and this device subsequently became known as the "Wheatstone Bridge," commonly studied in high school and college physics classes[165]

The next significant development, as the authors view it, came about in the late 1940s. A young man by the name of Lafayette Ron Hubbard began working with folks who had psychosomatic illnesses or some quirk in their thought processes called mental aberrations. Unlike psychologists and psychiatrists who tried to infer "correct" mental processes by observing outward behavior, and often dictating what they thought correct behavior should be Hubbard developed his knowledge via a set of axioms, or assumptions about the functioning of the mind. Those axioms were drawn from observations made from his research work with humans. We mention only one axiom as the 1950s published book, *Dianetics: The Modern Science of Mental Health,* and several hundred million words in other Hubbardian publications, details all of them

The exceedingly important axiom Hubbard formulated was this: "The mind knows how the mind works." By asking questions of a "yes" or "no" type a spontaneous answer was elicited from the patient. Whenever the axiom seemed to fail, Hubbard's directions sought to remove whatever was interfering with a clear answer.

Sometime during the 1950s Volney Matheson approached Hubbard with a modified Wheatstone bridge that he said would help Hubbard help people find moments of pain and travail in themselves. Hubbard experimented with this device which sent a small, unsensed DC battery current through the body. A dial moved backward or forward depending upon the amount of pain and anguish a remembered moment might have. Hubbard developed this device into what is now known as the "E meter," a device that makes it much easier for questions to be asked and answered from moments of anguish or pain similar to a lie detector.

That "the mind knows how the mind works" is not a trivial piece of philosophy because "the mind knows how the mind works" forms the next important step in the development of medicine of the future!

At this point in tracing the key developments of the medicine of the future there are two tracks both of them relying, more or less, on Hubbard's assumption that "the mind knows how the mind works" as well as on knowledge of meridians, acupuncture points and chi!

Independent of Hubbard — also in the 1940s — a German doctor, Reinhard Voll used an adaptation of the Wheatstone bridge and acupuncture points to develop an entirely painless system of diagnosis and therapy. According to Wikipedia, "Electroacupuncture following the Voll (EAV) method is an entirely painless system of diagnosis and therapy. Nowadays, this method is used to identify the precise focal point of the cause of disease and for selection of medication to be used in therapy.

"This form of diagnosis is particularly suitable in the case of chronic illness, because EAV is capable of isolating the toxins and environmental poisons which are the source of an illness. Various hidden inflammations and toxic deposits can be located by EAV, from dental materials such as amalgam, decaying food remains or environmental poisons. Subliminal diseases of the liver, gall bladder etc. can be detected and EAV can also identify psychological stresses.

"During the EAV test, the patient holds an electrode in his/her hand whilst readings at the most important of 1200 acupuncture points in the hands and feet are taken. Readings in the middle values (50-70 on the scale) are normal, higher or lower readings indicate abnormal pathological changes in the body. Fluctuations in the readings indicate the presence of hazards and focuses."

When this form of diagnosis was first developed it was used by medical doctors, chiropractors or simply lay people interested in helping others to wellness. A practitioner might cover the walls of her/ his office with every type of microorganism (in a bottle), or allergen or vitamins and minerals. When placing any of these items in the circuit the swinging needle would tell the practitioner whether or not a specific microorganism was affecting the patient, and where, or whether a particular brand of vitamins and minerals would be useful to achieve wellness, or if it would be helpful to create homeopathic remedies simply by imprinting proper electromagnetic imprints on liquids.

It seemed like the "yes" or "no" system applied with this device could answer almost any question about the patient's health — but it was terribly time consuming and tedious placing and removing different vials in the circuit.

The mind knows how the mind works, but the mind also controls the body — so it must know how the body works. An obvious extension of Hubbard's principle!

"There are more than 50 publications and dissertations from 912 universities in which the diagnostic possibilities presented by "Acupuncture according to Voll" method are confirmed."[165]

The next major milestone was the invention of the computer. Who invented the computer?

That's an ambiguous question because, like Topsy, it just grew, although credit is given to Konrad Zuse who, in 1936, created the first freely programmable computer, John Atanasoff and Clifford Berry who, in 1942, was first in the computing business, Howard Aiken & Grace Hopper who, in 1944 created the Harvard Mark I Computer, John Presper Eckert and John W. Mauchly who, in 1946, developed the ENIAC 1 Computer with 20,000 vacuum tubes, and so on with many more contributors until one reaches the present state of computers.

Had computers not come along when they did we'd still have Acupuncture According to Voll and the Hubbardian E-meter, but medical diagnosis and treatment would have forever remained slow and cumbersome, trying the patience of many patients and health professionals.

However, with the aid of computers another significant factor emerged. All objects, large or small, emit a resonance frequency when properly stimulated. For example Magnetic Resonance Imaging (MRI) creates detailed images of the human body using nuclear magnetic resonance. Protons located in hydrogen atoms (usually in water) forms small "magnets" under the strong magnetic field of the MRI. The MRI stimulates the body with radio waves to change the orientation of protons. From the scanning of electromagnetic changes the body's signals can be processed via computer to form the body's detailed image.

The MRI has become one of the mainstays of present-day medical practices, along with X-rays and CAT scans. However, the genius in putting together (1) The body/mind knows how the body/mind works, (2) acupuncture according to Vol, (3) that all objects have a unique resonance frequency, and (4) the phenomenal characteristics of modern day computers has brought about an invention often called "Computerized Electrodermal Screening" one of the diagnostic and treatment tool of the future available now through many practitioners.

James Hoyt Clark developed the software and hardware for Electroacupuncture According to Voll (EAV) and is known as the Orion System®. He owns the patent for this technology (US Patent 6,142,927) with over 90 claims that involve methods and apparatus for treatment with resonant signals. The FDA has approved his device for biofeedback and is classified as a Category 2 Class 2 device, the same category and class in which the ECG is placed (which measures electromagnetic fields to show heart problems by disturbances in the fields).

The Orion device is a tool used to make observations about the body (usually before disease manifests overtly) through measurements of the resistance of electron flow through acupuncture points on the skin. Other examples of electronic diagnostic or treatment systems include: ECG, MRI, TENS, and NMES. No devices being used in the US, whether Orion System or other non-patented systems derived from Jim Clark's devices, are approved by the FDA to diagnose or treat disease — but they very nicely and accurately can be instrumental in determining the body's needs at the moment!

What these devices do very well is measure electromagnetic signals generated outside the body as they pass through various channels of conduction through the body and its organs, likely using acupuncture meridian pathways. What Dr. Reinhold Voll, a German practicing preventive medicine for industry and child welfare, discovered in the late 1940's was that the resistance of the body to electron flow is not the same everywhere. Indeed, at the traditional Chinese acupuncture points, and several other points he himself found, the resistance is markedly less. He and an engineering friend created an instrument to measure that resistance, known originally as the galvanic skin resistance at the acupuncture points. Through clinical research with thousands of patients over the next decades, by Dr. Voll and others, it became clear that either too high, or too low of a resistance through the acupuncture meridians correlated closely with disease processes in the body, and usually these differences could be detected weeks, months or years before the clinical symptoms relating to those meridians and their associated organ systems became apparent. Normally, the skin has a resistance of about 1 to 2 million ohms, whereas at the acupuncture points, the resistance is only 100,000 ohms (a reading of "50" on Voll's calibrated scale). Therefore, too much energy flow through a meridian (which correlates with inflammation and more acute conditions) will read closer to 0 ohms (a reading of "100" on Voll's scale), and too little energy flow through a meridian (which corresponds to degeneration, cancerous-type, more chronic conditions) will read closer to 2 million ohms (or a reading of "0" on Voll's scale).

After establishing the baseline of the 12 meridians for a person, Voll, and other researchers were able to demonstrate that the introduction of a substance into the electromagnetic field of that person disturbed the energy flow through the meridians, and showed up as a change in the reading through the ohmmeter. In this way, they established that by "testing" the electromagnetic interference caused to a person's energy fields, through the proximity of an object with its own, unique energy field to that person, they could find which objects (whether viruses, bacteria, foods, heavy metals, toxins or any of various other substances) were causing the imbalance. Likewise, by testing vitamins, nutrients, pharmacological drugs, homeopathic remedies, or any number of other substances, they were able to balance the disturbed meridians (return it to the homeostasis of 100,000 ohms resistance at an acupuncture point). Clinicians since then, first in Europe, and subsequently in the United States, have used EAV (Electroacupuncture according to Voll) successfully in determining energy imbalances in patient's electromagnetic fields, then finding substances that balance those disturbances, with good results in clearing up disease symptoms, and, essentially, "curing" the disease.

That's the basic history behind Computerized Electrodermal Screening (CEDS). What Jim Clark did was to develop a way to reproduce the electromagnetic signature of the objects being tested (whether virus, vitamin or food) and store those signature frequencies in a digital coding in a computer. Now, by using a frequency generator, the electromagnetic field of thousands of objects can be quickly tested against a person's own unique electromagnetic field through the acupuncture meridians, just as though the object were physically there. Not only that, drugs, vitamins, herbs, or any substance being consumed or worn by a patient can be tested at the same time to indicate whether it is "good" or "bad" for the person, with respect to disrupting or balancing their energy fields.

Of course, the FDA has approved these devices as "biofeedback" devices, which they are, just as an ECG is a biofeedback device giving information about a specific electromagnetic field (that generated by the heart). Anyone being tested with a CEDS device should be aware that this information is suggestive of problems that may be "potential" only, in that they may not be clinically apparent for weeks to years in the future. Also, only a physician is licensed in this country to diagnose, and to prescribe remedies based on that diagnosis. Perhaps this will change in time, as the field of Vibrational, or Energy, Medicine becomes more familiar to the medical field at large, and to the policymakers trying to understand it.

A typical session with a CEDS device takes between an hour and two hours the first time (the baseline energy levels for the 12 meridians must be established first), and up to an hour thereafter, depending on the problems or severity of energy imbalances. Often, a session every two months or so to follow the course of the person trying different substances, on their own, is suggested until the imbalances are cleared. (From http://www.naturalhealthbridge.net/Clinic/CEDS2.html)

Just as lawyers have different knowledge and skills, or that doctors are not all equally knowledgeable, practitioners of this set of devices are unequal in their abilities. While the programmed computer may contain tens of thousands of unique frequencies, the practitioner operating the device must have a widespread knowledge of health factors. With such a knowledgeable practitioner one can reach the heart of their problem very rapidly — and it is never the body's need for a patented drug!

Computerized Electrodermal Acupuncture according to Voll is indeed a miraculous instrument and without questions the diagnostic and treatment facility of the future — available now!

Still there is a simpler method of utilizing the fact that "the mind/body knows how it works." No equipment is required and no medical degree.

George J. Goodheart, a chiropractor, invented "Applied Kinesiology" in 1964. Many other chiropractors were taught his findings until the knowledge spread widely throughout degreed medical professionals as well as through lay people.

Goodheart showed that the body's musculature system weakened or strengthened according to whether or not a substance was good for you or not good for you. Others refined his system to a high degree of diagnosis which, of course, leads to helpful treatments.

We're going to provide you with a simple method whereby you can test the truth of Goodheart's observations.

Choose a partner for this test. Have that person place a small amount of sugar in one hand and the other arm should be extended outward parallel to the chest. Ask your partner to resist your downward push of the extended arm. Push the extended arm downward. Now repeat the experiment with a small amount of salt placed in the hand that formerly held the sugar. What you will observe is that when you push downward on your partner's arm it will go much easier downward when the other hand contains sugar than when it contains the salt. This is another kind of "yes" or "no" test. Your partner's body/mind is telling you and her/him that the salt is OK for your body but that the sugar is not OK.

From this simple experiment others have devised more complicated tests that can determine many things immediately about the state of your health. But, like Computerized Electrodermal Testing according to Voll, the practitioner's skill can be important. They have to be sufficiently knowledgeable to know what questions to ask!

Applied kinesiology evaluates structural, chemical and mental aspects of health using manual muscled testing. Its premise is not shared by conventional "drug oriented" practitioners, which postulates that every organ dysfunction is accompanied by a weakness in a specific corresponding muscle, the viscerosomatic relationship.

In the hands of a good practitioner the subjective elements of this test fade away!

Finding a practitioner is easy -look among chiropractors, dentists, lay folks, medical doctors, osteopaths, wherever. . . .

Locating a superb practitioner of applied kinesiology may require more search.

The Naysayers

We can't leave you without mentioning that there is much criticism within the allopathic community of most of these techniques. After all, practitioners of allopathy have spent years learning what drugs to push and standard operating procedures for handling any health problem. They've also built up an "altitude" problem. They're the experts, you're not. Those who criticize the techniques described in this book generally have never studied them with an open mind and are greatly brainwashed by the billion dollar pharmaceutical industry.

You might want to check out through the internet the "Quackbusters" or "Quack Watch" sites. (We call them quack, quack busters). Read some of their comments about any of our recommended treatments. You'll soon realize that they speak primarily from the theories of allopathic medicine or that they quote so-called "scientific" studies that have been heavily compromised by the influence of patented drug companies. Indeed, some critics of quack, quack busters have gone so far as to state that these nay-sayers are financed by patented drug companies to reduce resistance against the sale of patented drugs! Unlike Fox News they are neither balanced nor fair. You'll note that they use the cherry picking method to make their points, that is, present only those things that support Big Pharma, and ignore those items that do not.

In an "Opinion by Consumer Advocate" Tim Bolen says "North Americans have known, or suspected, for some time, that there has been an organized assault by a group, against companies, and practitioners, offering alternatives to the drugs/surgery paradigm. That group calls itself the *"quackbusters,"* and they are a scam.

"I'm about to tell you WHY that assault was formally assembled, HOW THE SCAM works, and WHO the players are, and WHAT they're up to right now.

"If you know who they are, and how they operate, you can beat them."

Read the rest of the story at http://quackpotwatch.org There are literally hundreds of other excellent, surprisingly effective, low cost treatments for almost every disease, and complementary/alternative practitioners each have their favorites. We wish we could present all of them to you. Since we can't here's some references for you. Either search for them on the internet or go to http://www.arthritistrust.org and punch in the "Links" button:

Alternative Medical Connections

- About Arthritis Today
- Addictions
- Alkalize For Health
- Alternative Cancer Treatments
- Alternative Cancer Treatment (Flemish)
- Alternative Medicine Connection
- Alternative Medicine Directory
- Alternative Medicine Homepage (Univ. of Pittsburg)
- American Academy of Biological Dentists
- American College for Advancement in Medicine
- American Holistic Health Association
- Arthritic Association
- Association of Environmental Medicine
- Association of Naturopathic Physicians
- Bare, DC/Rife Technology
- Cancer (Ralph Moss)
- Cancer Decision (Ralph Moss)
- Cancer No More
- Charles Weber
- Cleansing and Cleanse (Colon Cleansing)
- Coconut — The Tree of Life
- Depression
- Disabilities
- Drugs

- Easy Immune System Health
- Edgar Cayce
- Environmental Pollution (Right-to-Know Network)
- Free Yurko
- Frety.NET
- Gary Null
- General Reference (English)
- Gilbert Ling, PhD.
- Health Association of Australia
- Health World Line
- Hyperbaric Oxygen Treatment
- Inflammatory Foods
- International Academy of Detoxification Specialists
- Karl Loren
- Life Extension Foundation
- Lyme Arthritis
- Lyme Arthritis Research Data Base
- Mike Adams
- Milk Healthy?
- Multiple Chemical Sensitivities; Myalgic Encephalomyelitis
- National Foundation for Alternative Medicine
- Natural Cures
- Natural Health Village
- Natural Health Bridge
- New York Rescue Workers Detox Project
- NutraSanus Natural Health, Herbal and Vitamin Supplements Guide
- Online Health Resources
- Optimum Magnetics Clinic
- Orthomolecular Medicine
- Price-Pottenger Nutrition Foundation
- Raw Milk
- Reuma in Beweging vzw (RiB vzw)
- Road Back Foundation
- Silver Lightning (Colloidal Silver)
- Society Links Directory
- Soma Health Association of Australia

- Supplement Guide (Vitamin & Mineral Guide)
- The Heimlich Maneuver
- The Insight Holistic and Integrated Medicine
- The National Foundation For Alternative Medicine
- Vaccination (Think Twice)
- Vaccination Debate
- Vaccination Links
- Vaccine Information
- Vitamn D
- Water Cure

Recmomended Health Publications

- Alternative Medicine
- Alternative Therapies
- Bolen Report (Health Newsletter)
- C. Norman Shealy, M.D., Ph.D.
- Defective Drugs
- Gallium for Arthritis (also see http://coldcure.com/)
- Health & Healing
- Health Freedom News
- Magnets
- Monterey Institute for the Study of Alternative Healing Arts
- Mycotoxins in Human Health
- Natural Healthline
- Nutrition & Healing
- News Target Insider
- Optimal Wellness Center
- Positive Health
- Second Opinion
- Townsend Letter for Doctors & Patients
- Truth in Labeling
- Whistle Blowers
- William Philpott, M.D.

Legal and Educational Foundations

- Advocates for Self Government
- Alliance for Natural Health (Europe)
- Australian Functional Medicine
- American Association for Health Freedom

- Bolen Report (Quack, Quack Organizations)
- California Health Freedom Coalition
- Campaign for Truth in Medicine (Australia)
- Citizens for Health & Campaign for Better Health
- Classified Directory of Society Web Links
- Coalition for Natural Health
- Complementary Alternative Medical Association
- Consumers for Dental Choice
- Dangerous Medicine
- Dietary Supplement Education Alliance
- Dietary Supplement Education Alliance Supplemental Info
- DirPedia: Dictionary, Encyclopedia, Web Directory
- Families Against Abuse
- Florida Health Freedom Action
- Fluoride Dangers
- Friends of Freedom (Canada)
- Foundation for Advancement of Innovative Medicine
- Georgia Complementary and Alternative Medicine Association
- Health Choice
- Health Freedom Advocates, Open Directory
- Health Freedom Massachusetts
- Health Lies Exposed
- Health Lobby
- Institute for Health Freedom
- Institute for Health Research
- International Advocates for Health Freedom
- Kevin Trudeau
- La Leva di Archimede (Europe)
- Law Loft Report
- Libertarian Party
- Medical News
- Minnesota Natural Health Coalition
- Monica Miller Health Lobby
- National Association for Alternative Medicine
- New Jersey Natural Health Coalition
- New York Natural Health Project

- News on New York
- National Health Freedom Coalition
- Oklahoma Health Freedom Network
- Oymaps A World Directory
- Protect Health Care Freedom
- Red Flags
- Skidmark Disease
- Society Links Directory
- Tennessee Integrative Medical Society
- Tim Bolen Reports
- Vitamin Lawyer News
- What's wrong with our health care system?
- Why Medical Insurance Does Not Pay for Workable Medicine (see page 4)
- Worst Pills.org

We sincerely wish you good luck in your search for wellness! References

1. *Racketeering in Medicine: The Suppression of Alternatives*, James P. Carter, M.D., Dr.P.H., Hampton Roads Publishing Co., 1993, ISBN 1-878901; *Elements of Danger*, Morton Walker, D.P.M., Hampton Roads Publishing Co., 2000, ISBN 1-57174-146-1; *Heart Disease, Stroke and High Blood Pressure: The Definitive Guide to Heart Disease*, Burton Goldberg, Future Medicine Publishing Corp.; A*lternative Medicine: The Definitive Guide*; Future Medicine Publishing Corp; *How to Spot and Handle Suppression in Medicine and Religion*; Anthony di Fabio; Kindle at Amazon.com; andmany other books.

2. *Alternative Medicine: Definitive Guide to Headaches*; Robert D. Milne, Blake More, and Burton Goldberg; Future Medicine Publishing Corp, 1997.

3. *Definitive Guide to Cancer*; W. John Diamond, W. Lee Cowden; 1997; Future Medicine Publishing Corp., 1997.

4. Personal conversation; http://brucehalstead.blogspot.com/2007/09/world-life-research-institutehistory.html

5. *Lipitor: Thief of Memory*; Duane Graveline, Kilmer S. McCully, Jay S. Cohen, 2006.

6. *How to Lie With Statistics*, Darell Huff, W.W. Norton & Co., 1993.

7. *Vitamin C, the Common Cold & the Flu*; Linus Pauling; Berkley Books; ISBN 0-425-04853-5; 1981.

8. See "Candidiasis: Scourge of Arthritics," http://www.arthritistrust.org.

9. Linus Pauling, Ph.D., *How to Live Longer and Feel Better*, Avon Publishers, W. H. Freeman and Co., 1986. (ISBN 0-380-70289-4); also see *Vitamin C and the Common Cold*, Op.Cit. (ISBN: 0-7167-0361-0); *Cancer and Vitamin C*, The Linus Pauling Institute for Science and Medicine, Menlo Park, 1979.

10. A. Kalokerinos, *Every Second Child*, Thomas Nelson, Australia; 1974 (ISBN: 0-879-83-250-9); Irwin Stone, *The Healing Factor*, Worldwide, New York, 1972 (ISBN:0-448-11693-6).

11. Robert F. Cathcart, "Vitamin C, Titrating to Bowel tolerance, Anascorbemia, and Acute Induced Scurvy, Medical Hypotheses 7:1359-13767, 1981.

12. Typically, stable molecules contain pairs of electrons. When a chemical reaction breaks the bonds that hold paired electrons together, free radicals are produced. Free radicals contain an odd number of electrons, which makes them unstable, short-lived, and highly reactive. As they combine with other atoms that contain unpaired electrons, new radicals are created, and a chain reaction begins.

13. *The Linus Pauling Institute of Science and Medicine Newsletter,* "How Vitamin C Can Prevent Heart Attack and Stroke," March 1992.

14. "Questionable Methods of Cancer Management: Hydrogen and Other 'Hperoxygenation' Therapies," CA: *A Cancer Journal for Clinicians*, 43 (1): 47-56, 1933.

15. International Bio-Oxidative Medicine Foundation, PO Box 13205, Oklahoma City, OK 73113-1205.

16. William Campbell Douglass, *The Cutting Edge*, PO Box 1568, Clayton, GA 30525. According to Douglass' paper, see: Docknell, *Inf./Immunity*, January 1983, pp. 456; Mallams, Finney & Balla, S.M.J., March 1962; Jay et. al., Tex *Rep. Biol.*

& Med., 22:106, 1964; Urschel, *Diseases of the Chest*, 51:180, 1967; Finney, et. al., *Angiology*, 17:223, 1966; *Hydrogen Peroxide — The Forgotten Miracle.*

17. Anthony di Fabio, *Chelation Therapy*, The Arthritis Trust of America/The Rheumatoid Disease Foundation, 7111 Sweetgum Road, Fairview, TN 37062-9384; http://www.arthritistrust.org.

18. Walter O. Grotz, ECHO, 300 South 4th Street, Delano, MN 55328. ECHO for a small fee can provide you with a listing of abstracts dating back to 1920; also see their *Progress Report*, 2nd Edition.

19. Dr. Paul K. Pybus, Anthony di Fabio, *The Herxheimer Effect*, The Arthritis Trust of America/ The Rheumatoid Disease Foundation, 7376 Walker Road, Fairview, TN 37062-8141; http:// www.arthritistrust.org.

20. Charles H. Farr, M.D., Ph.D., *The Therapeutic Use of Intravenous Hydrogen Peroxide* (Monograph). Genesis Medical Center, Oklahoma City, OK 73139, Jan. 1987.

21. T.L. Dormandy, "In Praise of Peroxidation," *Lancet*, II (Nov. 12):1126, 1988.

22. Charles H. Farr, M.D., Ph.D., "Physiological and Biochemical Responses to Intravenous Hydrogen Peroxide in Man," *JACAM*, 1:113-129, 1988.

23. "Why Hydrogen Peroxide?" *International Bio-Oxidative Medical Foundation Newsletter*, Vol. II, No. 1, Op.Cit., 1989.

24. Ed McCabe, *O2xygen Therapies*, Energy Publications, 99-RD1, Morrisville, NY 13408, 1988.

25. Leon Chaitow, "Bland Attacks `Fad' for Hydrogen Peroxide," *Townsend Letter for Doctors*," May 1988, p. 204; from *Journal of Alternative & Complementary Medicine* (UK).

26. Jonathan Collin, M.D., "The H2O2 Crusades," *Townsend Letter for Doctors*, Op.Cit., June 1989, p. 322.

27. Homeopathic Physician, 7315 E. Evans Road, Scottsdale, AZ 85260; (480) 998-9232; Out of state phone calls are not returned. Permission given for reproducing this booklet in full.

28. American College of Advancement in Medicine (ACAM), 23121 Verdugo Dr., Suite 204, Laguna Hills, CA 92653.

29. James J. Julian, M.D. ,*Chelation Extends Life*, Wellness Press, 1654 Cahuenga Boulevard, Hollywood, CA 90028, p. 31, 1982.

30. Halstead, Bruce, *The Scientific Basis of EDTA Chelation Therapy*, Golden Quill Publishers, Inc., 1979.

31. Farr, Charles H., M.D., PhD, White, Robert L. P.A.C., PhS., Schachter, Michael, M.D., *Chronological History of EDTA Chelation Therapy*, Revised October 1991.

32. John Parks Trowbridge, M.D., Morton Walker, D.P.M., *The Healing Powers of Chelation Therapy*, New Way of Life, Inc., 484 High Ridge Road, Stamford, CT 06905, 1991

33. Efrain Olszewer, M.D. and James P. Carter, M.D., Dr. PH, "EDTA Chelation Therapy: A Retrospective Study of 2,870 Patients," Elmer Cranton, Ed., *A Textbook on EDTA ChelationTherapy; Special Issue of Journal of Advancement in Medicine*, Volume 2, Numbers 1/2, Human Sciences Press, Inc, 233 Spring Street, New York, New York 10013-1578, p. 197, Spring/Summer 1989.

34. James P. Frackelton, M.D., "Letters to the Editors," *Townsend Letter for Doctors*, July 1992.

35. Personal Communication from Warren Levin, M.D. to Perry A. Chapdelaine, Sr.

36. Morton Walker, D.P.M., (Gary Gordon, M.D., Consultant) *The Chelation Answer*, M. Evans and Company, Inc., p. 18, 1982.

37. Arabinda Das, "Complementary medical Treatment for Coronary Heart Disease," *Townsend Letter for Doctors*, p. 419, May 1992.

38. American Heart Association, *Heart and Stroke Facts*, 1992.

39. Zigurts Strauts, M.D., *Townsend Letter for Doctors*, p. 382-383, May 1992.

40. E.L. Hannan, H. Kilburn, Jr., H. Bernard, J.F. O'Donnell, G. Lukacik, E.P. Shields, "Coronary Artery Bypass surgery: The Relationship Between Inhospital Mortality Rate

and Surgical Volume After Controlling for Clinical Risk Factors, *Med-Care*, Nov 1991, 29(11): 1094-107.

41. G.T. O'Connor, S.K. Plume, E.M. Olmstead, L.H. Coffin, J.R. Morton, C.T. Maloney, E.R. Nowicki, J.F. Tryzelaar, F. Hernandez, L. Adrian, et. al. "A Regional Prospective Study of In-Hospital Mortality Associated with Coronary Artery Bypass Grafting, "*JAMA*, Aug 14, 1991, 266(6): 803-9.

42. J. Zelen, T.V. Bilfinger, C.E. Anagnostopoulos, Coronary Artery Bypass Grafting. The relationship of Surgical Volume, Hospital Location, and Outcome, *NY State J Med*, Jul 1991 91(7): 290-2.

43. Baron, John, D.O. personal interview and unpublished documents.

44. H. Richard Casdorph, M.E., Ph.D. "EDTA Chelation Therapy: Efficacy in Arteriorslerotic Heart Disease," Elmer Cranton, Ed., *A Textbook on EDTA Chelation Therapy, Special Issue of Journal of Advancement in Medicine*, Volume 2, Numbers 1/2, Human Sciences Press, Inc, 233 Spring Street, New York, New York 10013-1578, p. 121, Spring/Summer 1989.

45. Efrain Olszewer, M.D. and James P. Carter, M.D., Dr. PH, "EDTA Chelation Therapy: A Retrospective Study of 2,870 Patients," Elmer Cranton, Ed., *A Textbook on EDTA Chelation Therapy, Special Issue of Journal of Advancement in Medicine*, Volume 2, Numbers 1/2, Human Sciences Press, Inc, 233 Spring Street, New York, New York 10013-1578, p. 197, Spring/Summer 1989.

46. Lau, Benjamin, M.D., Ph.D., *Garlic Research Update*, Odyssey Publishing, Inc. 2135 West 45th Avenue, Vancouver, B.C., Canada V6M 2J2, p.2-3, 1991.

47. Elmer Cranton, Ed., *A Textbook on EDTA Chelation Therapy, Special Issue of Journal of Advancement in Medicine*, Volume 2, Numbers 1/2, Human Sciences Press, Inc, 233 Spring Street, New York, New York 10013-1578, p. 18, Spring/Summer 1989.

48. Efrain Olszewer, M.D., Fuad Calil Sabbag, M.D., and James P. Carter, M.D., Dr. PH., "A Pilot Double-Blind Study

of Sodium-Magnesium EDTA in Peripheral Vascular Disease," *Journal of the National Medical Association*, Vol. 82, No.3, March 1990.

49. E.W. McDonagh, D.O., FACGP, C.J. Rudolph, D.O., Ph.D., and E. Cheraskin, M.D., D.M.D. "An Oculocerebrovasculometric Analysis of the Improvement in Arterial Stenosis Following EDTA Chelation Therapy," Elmer Cranton, Ed., *A Textbook on EDTA Chelation Therapy, Special Issue of Journal of Advancement in Medicine*, Volume 2, Numbers 1/2, Human Sciences Press, Inc, 233 Spring Street, New York, New York 10013-1578, p. 155, Spring/Summer 1989.

50. H. Richard Casdorph, M.D., Ph.D. and Charles H. Farr, M.D., Ph.D. "EDTA Chelation Therapy: Treatment of Peripheral Arterial Occlusion, an Alternative to Amputation," Elmer Cranton, Ed., *A Textbook on EDTA Chelation Therapy, Special Issue of Journal of Advancement in Medicine*, Volume 2, Numbers 1/2, Human Sciences Press, Inc, 233 Spring Street, New York, New York 10013-1578, p. 167, Spring/Summer 1989.

51. Personal communication from Warren Levin, M.D.

52. Walter Blumer, M.D., and H. Richard Casdorph, M.D., Ph.D. "Ninety Percent Reduction in Cancer Mortality After Chelation therapy With EDTA," Elmer Cranton, Ed., *A Textbook on EDTA Chelation Therapy, Special Issue of Journal of Advancement in Medicine*, Volume 2, Numbers 1/2, Human Sciences Press, Inc, 233 Spring Street, New York, New York 10013-1578, p. 183, Spring/ Summer 1989.

53. Personal knowledge.

54. Josephson, Emanuel M., M.D., "Glaucoma and Its Medical Treatment With Cortin," *JAQA*, Vol. 3, No. 1, p. 2-6, Oct. 1987.

55. Morton Walker, D.P.M., *Chelation Therapy,* Freelance Communications, 484 High Ridge Road, Stamford,Ct 06905, 1980.

56. "Radical Concerns Over Drinking Water," *Science News*, Vol. 141, No. 24, June 13, 1992, p. 398.

57. 16. Evers, Ray, M.D., "Chemo-Endarterectory Therapy and Preventive Medicine", *Townsend Letter for Doctors*, Feb/Mr. 1986. Issue #49.

58. Gordon E. Potter, M.D. "The Blood/Brain Connection,' *Townsend Letter for Doctors*, July 1992.

59. Butterfield, J.B, "Free Radical Pathology and its Involvement in Chronic Disease Processes", *Stroke* 9: 443-445.

60. Cranton, E.M., Frackleton, J.P., "Free Radical Pathology in Age-Associated Diseases", *Journal of Holistic Medicine* 6:1.

61. Collin, Jonathan, M.D., "Free Radical Pathology and Chelation Therapy", *Townsend Letter for Doctors*. 1984.

62. Carter, James P., Olszewer, Efrain, "EDTA Chelation Therapy in Chronic Degenerative Disease", *Medical Hypotheses* (1988) 27: 41-49. *of Holistic Medicine* 6:1.

64. Evers, Ray, M.D., "Chemo-Endarterectory Therapy and Preventive Medicine", *Townsend Letter for Doctors*, Feb/Mr. 1986. Issue #49.

65. Handbook of Chemistry and Physics, 26th edition, p. 1637 viscosity formula 1942.

66. *Protocol for the Safe and Effective Administration of Intravenous EDTA Chelation Therapy*, obtained from one of the semi-annual meetings of the American College of Advancement in Medicine (ACAM) 23121 Verdugo Dr., Suite 204, Laguna Hills, CA 92653.

67. Joseph Mercola, M.D. http://www.mercola.com, "Some Doctors Health Care Concerns," 3/5/2011.

68. Theron Randolph, M.D., Ralph Moss, Ph.D., *An Alternative Approach to Allergies,* Bantam Books, New York, ISBN: 0-553-29830-6.

69. Paul Reilly, N.D., "Natural Therapies for Autoimmune Diseases," *Townsend Letter for Doctors*, 911 Tyler St., Port Townsend, WA 98368-6541, Issue #42, 1986, p. 331.

70. Warren Levin, M.D., "Allergy/Addiction to Foods and Chemicals," *Let's Live Magazine*, 444 N. Larchmont Blvd., Los Angeles, CA 90004, June 1976. Used with permission of Warren Levin, M.D.

71. *Dr. Braly's Food Allergy & Nutrition Revolution*, James Braly, M.D., Laura Torbet, Amazon.Com.

72. For complete information on the foods to avoid, contact Arthritis Help Centers, phone (973) 361-1867; or see *Inflammation Nation* by Ed Wendlocher at Amazon.Com. What Harvard Medical School researchers seem to have concluded is as follows:

a. When chili peppers activate certain nerve receptors, this activation is also responsible for a burning sensation associated with inflammation, tissue damage and "arthritis."

b. When inflammation occurs, a "p 38" molecule switches on. This is an intracellular signaling molecule which causes a "cascade" of enzymes to increase the amount of heat that passes through a protein known as "TRPV 1," sometimes called the "ion-channel protein." It is also sometimes called the "chili pepper receptor."

c. The "chili pepper receptor" is very sensitive to capsaicin. Capsaicin causes chili peppers to feel "hot."

d. Regulation of the chili pepper receptor was not expected; according to Harvard anesthesia researcher professor Clifford Woolf as large increases in the amount of receptor from increasing inflammation does not change production of mRNA. However, "The gene itself is not being changed, the mRNA that is being translated is."

e. Dr. Woolf may perform further research in using p 38 inhibitors for treatment of inflammation and accompanying pain. Footnote from: "Hot research, burning pain: the protein TRPV1 is sensitive to capsaicin, found in chili peppers."

73. DIANETICS, SCIENTOLOGY, HUBBARD, CELEBRITY CENTRE, and PURIFICATION RUNDOWN are trademarks and service marks owned by Religious Technology Center. NARCONON is a trademark owned by ABLE (Association for Better Living and Education).

74. *The John W. Campbell Letters*, Vol. I, by Chapdelaine and Hay, (hc ISBN: 0-931150-15-9; pb ISBN 0-931150-16-7) and *The John W. Campbell Letters With Isaac Asimov and A.E. van Vogt*, Vol. II, AC Projects, Inc. 7111 Sweetgum Drive SW, Fairview, TN 37062-9384; (hc ISBN 0-931150-19-1)

75. L. Ron Hubbard, *Dianetics: The Modern Science of Mental Health*, Bridge Publications, Inc., 4751 Fountain Avenue, Los Angeles, CA 90029, published from 1950 thru present.

76. David W. Schnare, Max Ben and Megan G. Shields, "Body Burden Reductions of PCBs, PBBs and Chlorinated Pesticides in Human Subjects," *Ambio*, Vol. 13, No. 5-6, 984, p. 378. Also see Shields, Megan, M.D., "Hubbard Method of Detoxification Requires Niacin for Increased Effectiveness," Op. L., "PCB Reduction and Clinical Improvement by Detoxification: An Unexploited Approach," *Human and Experimental Toxicology*, 1990, p. 235-244; Norman Zucker, M.D., "Hubbard's Purification Rundown: A Workable Detox Program," Op. Cit., *Townsend Letter for Doctors*, January 1990, p. 54.

77. "Human Detoxification — New Hope for Firefighters," California Firefighter, Federated Fire Fighters of California, No. 4, 1984, p. 7.

78. Foundation for Advancements in Science and Education, Park Mile Plaza, 4801 Wilshire Blvd., Los Angeles, CA 90010.

79. Zane R. Gard, M.D., Erma J. Brown, B.S.N., P.H.N., Giovanna DeSanti-Medina, "Bio-Toxic Reduction Program Participants (Condensed) Case Histories," Op. Cit., *Townsend Letter for Doctors*, June 1987, p. 167.

80. C. Orian Truss, M.D., *The Missing Diagnosis*, PO Box 26508, Birmingham, AL 35226, 1983.

81. "Candida Albicans," *Capsulations*™, No. 15, Thorne Research, Inc., PO Box 3200, Sandpoint, ID 83864, October 1989.

82. Raymond Keith Brown, M.D., *Aids, Cancer and the Medical Establishment*, Trizoid Press, New York, 1993, ISBN0-9639293-0-5.

83. James P. Carter, M.D., Dr.P.H., *Racketeering in Medicine*, Hampton Roads Publishing, Inc., 891 Norfolk Square, Norfolk, VA 23502. p. 80, ISBN 1-878901-32-X.

84. Morton Walker, D.P.M., John Parks Trowbridge, M.D., *The Yeast Syndrome*, Bantam Books,1540 Broadway, New York, NY 10036-4094, 1986.

85. William B. Crook, M.D., *The Yeast Connection*, Professional Books, PO Box 3494, Jackson, TN 38301, Third Edition, 1986, ISBN 0-933478-11-9. Also see *Solving the Puzzle of Your Hard-ToRaise Child*, Op. Cit. 1987, ISBN 0-933478-12-7.

86. Dennis W. Remington, M.D., Barbara W. Higa, R.D., *Back to Health*, Vitality House International, Inc., 3707 North Canyon Road, #8-C, Provo, UT 84604, ISBN 0-912547-03-0, 1986.

87. Paul A. Goldberg, M.P.H., D.C., Personal Letter, May 18, 1994.

88. David R. Soll, Ph.D., The Rheumatoid Disease Foundation *Second Annual Medical Seminar*, Santa Monica, CA, 1986.

89. Personal visit with Phillip Hoekstra, Ph.D., 1985.

90. Lida H. Mattman, Ph.D., *Cell Wall Deficient Forms*, 2nd Edition, CRC Press, Inc., 2000

Corporate Blvd., N.W., Boca Raton, FL 33431, 1993, ISBN 0-8493-4405-0.

91. Gus J. Prosch, Jr., M.D., *Chronic Systemic Candidiasis*, Biomed Medical Center, Inc., 759 Valley Road, Birmingham, AL 35226, patient handout sheet.

92. Personal letter for Stephan Cooter, Ph.D., dated May 15, 1994.

93. S.M. Peck, H. Rosenfeld, "The Effects of Hydrogen Ion Concentration, Fatty Acids and Vitamin C on the Growth of Fungi," *J. Invest. Dermatol.* 1:237-265, 1938.

94. William (Bill) G. Neely, D.C., 512 E. Unaka Ave., Johnson City, TN 37601, personal communication, 1992.

95. Frederic Damrau, M.D., "The Value of Bentonite for Diarrhea," *Medical Annals of the District of Columbia*, Vol. 30, No. 6, June 1961, p. 328.

96. Benjamin Lau, M.D., Ph.D., *Garlic for Health*, Odyssey Publishing, Inc., 2135 West 45th Avenue, Vancouver, B.C., Canada V6M 2J2, 1991, ISBN 0-941524-32-9. Also see:

Tariq H. Abdullah, M.D., O. Kandil, Ph.D., A. Elkadi, M.D., and J. Carter, M.D., "Garlic Revisited: Therapeutic For the Major Diseases of Our Times?," *Journal of the National Medical Association*, Vol. 80, No. 4, 1988; Christopher L. Marsh, Robert R. Torrey, James L. Woolley, Gary R. Barker, Benjamin H.S. Lau, "Superiority of Intravesical Immunotherapy With Corynebacterium Parvum and Allium Sativum in Control of Murine Bladder Cancer," *The Journal of Urology*, Vol. 137, February 1987, p. 359; Benjamin H.S. Lau, M.D., Ph.D., Takeshi Yamasaki, D.V.M., M.S., Daila S. Gridley, Ph.D., "Garlic Compounds Modulate Macrophage and T-lymphocyte Functions," *Mol. Biother.,* Vol. 3, June 1991; Benjamin H.S. Lau, James L. Woolley, Christopher L. Marsh, Gary R. Barker, Dick H. Koobs, Robert R. Torrey, *The Journal of Urology*, Vol. 136, September 1986; Padma P. Tadi, M.S., Robert W. Teel, Ph.D., Benjamin H.S. Lau, M.D., Ph.D., "Anticandidal and Anticarcinogenic Potentials of Garlic," *Integrated Therapies*, School of Medicine, Loma Linda University, Loma Linda, CA 92350, 1990; address correspondence to Benjamin H.S. Lau, M.D., Ph.D.; Benjamin Lau, M.D., Ph.D., Garlic Research Update, Odyssey Publishing Inc. Op. Cit, 1991, ISBN 0-941524-32-9.

97. Dan Bensky, Andrew Gamble, *Chinese Herbal Medicine, Materia Medica*, Revised Edition, Eastland Press, Inc., PO Box 12689, Seattle, WA 98111, 1993, ISBN 0-939616-15-7.

98. Dr. Stephen Cooter, "Molybdenum: Recycling Fatigue Into Energy," *Townsend Letter for Doctors*, 911 Tyler St., Port Townsend, WA 98368-6541, April 1994, p. 332; an excerpt from *Beating Chronic Illness: Fatigue, Pain, Weakness, Insomnia, Foggy Thinking*, Pro Motion Publishing, 10387 Friars Rd., San Diego, CA 92120, 1-800-231-1776.

99. *Arthritis: Osteoarthritis and Rheumatoid Disease Including Rheumatoid Arthritis*, Anthony di Fabio, & Gus J. Prosch, Jr., M.D., *Rheumatoid Diseases Cured at Last* (1985); Anthony di Fabio, *The Art of Getting Well,* Anthony di Fabio (1988); *Intraneural Injections for Rheumatoid Arthritis and Osteoarthritis & The Control of Pain in Arthritis of the Knee,*

Dr. Paul K. Pybus, (1989), The Arthritis Trust of America/The Rheumatoid Disease Foundation, see Amazon.com at Kindle.

100. Jarisch, A. Wien. *med Wschr.* 45:721, 1895.

101. Herxheimer, K. Krause: "Uber eine bei Syphilitische vorkommende Quecksilerberreaktion. *Deutsch. Med. Wschr.* 28:50, 1902.

102. Herxheimer, K. and Martin, H.: So-called Herxheimer reactions. *Arch. Derm. Syph.* 13:115, 1926.

103. Heyman, A., Sheldon, W.H. and Evans, L.D.: Pathogenesis of the Jarisch-Herxheimer reaction. *rit. J. vener. Dis.* 28:50, 1952.

104. Millian, G.: Syphilis: Reaction d' Herxheimer. *Biotropisme. Paris nd.*: 37:91, 1920.

105. Robert W. Bradford, D.Sc., Henry Allen, "The HLB Blood Test as an Indicator of Oxidative Injry & Disseminated Intravascular Coagulation," *Townsend Letter for Doctors*, 911 Tyler Street, Port Townsend, WA 98368-6541, April 1995, p. 30. [From Morrison, D.C., et. al., The effects of bacterial endotoxins on host mediation systems, *American Journal of Pathology* 93 526 (1978).]

106. Jadassohn, J.: Beitrag zur Jarisch-Herxheimer Reaktion. *Z. Haut Geschlechtskr* 19:158, 1965.

107. Fleishman, K. and Kreibich, C.: Zum Wesen der Reaktion nach Jarish-Herxheimer. *Me. Klin.*
21:1157, 1925.

108. Mahoney, J.F., Arnold, R.C., and Harris, A.: Penicillin treatment of early syphilis. *Amer. J. Public Health* 33:1387, 1943.

109. Moore, J.E., Farmer, T.W. and Hoekenga, M.T.: Penicillin and the Jarisch-Herxheimer reaction in early, cardiovasculaar and nuerosyphilis. *Trans. Ass. Amer. Phycns.* 61:176, 1948.

110. Joulia, P., Pautrizell, R., Texier, L. and Sebra, De.: La chute des eosinophiles sanguines apre une premiere injeciton de penicilline au cours de la syphilis primo-secondaire: temoin du conflit antigene-anticorps. *ull. Soc. Franc. Derm. Syph.* 58:399, 1951.

111. Gudjonsson, Haraldur: The Jarisch-Herxheimer Reaction, Stockholm 1972 (A summary based on the following seven publications:

a. Skok, E. and Gudjonsson, H.: On the allergic origin of the jarisch-Herxheimer reaction. *Acta Dermatovfener* (Stockholm) 46:136, 1966.

b. Gudjonsson, H. and Skog, E.: The effect of prednisolone on the Jarisch-Herxheimer reaction. *Acta Dermatovener* (Stockholm) 48:15, 1968. *pallidum*. Jarisch-Herxheimer reaction? *Proc. 18. Meeting Scand. Dermatol. Ass.*, Turku 1968.

d. Gudjonsson, H. and Skog, E.: Fever after inoculation of rabbits with *Treponema pallidum. Brit. J. vener. Dis.* 46:318, 1970.

e. Gudjonsson, H., Newman, B. and Turner, T.B.: Demonstration of a virus-like agent contaminating material containing the Stockholm substrain of the Nichols pathogenic *Treponema pallidum. Brit. J. vener. Dis.* 46:435, 1970.

f. Gudjonsson, H. Newman, B. and Turner, T.B.: Screening out a virus-like agent from the testicular suspension of the Nichols pathogenic *Treponema pallidum. Brit. J. vener. Dis.* In press at time summary was written.

g. Gudjonsson, H.: Experiments to induce febrile Jarisch-Herxheimer reaction on syphilitic rabbits with penicillin and erythromycin. *Acta Dermatovener.* (Stockholm). In press at time summary was written.

112. Wyburn-Mason, Roger: *The Causation of Rheumatoid Disease and Many Human Cancers*, IJI Publishing Co., Ltd., Tokyo, Japan, 1978. [Summary available through The Arthritis Trust of America.]

113. Guy [study performed in South Africa by a Rheumatologist], reference source lost.

114. Prosch, Gus J., Jr, M.D..: Personal communication: Ed.

115. Jeon, Kwang: Research proposal and paper (based on arthritic knee effusion samples submitted by our referral physicians from their patients) submitted to The Arthritis Trust of America.

116. Pybus, Paul K. P, Davies, A.H.: Paper submitted to The Arthritis Trust of America (based on knee effusions submitted by our referral physicians.)

117. Wyburn-Mason, Roger: *The Reticulo-Endothelial System in Growth and Tumour Formation*, Henry Kimpton, London, England, 1958.

118. Personal letter from Russ McMillan, D.D.S., M.P.H., Dr. P.H. to The Arthritis Trust of America/ The Rheumatoid Disease Foundation, June 13, 1994.

119. *Three Years of Hydrochloric Acid Therapy*, http://www.arthritistrust.org, "Books and Pamphlets" tab.

120. Coley's Toxin formula is now found at our website at http://arthritistrust.org, "Research" and then "Research and Letters" tab, under Wayne Martin's name. Wayne Martin's thinking about medical treatment has been frequently reported in *Townsend Letter for Doctors & Patients* (911 Tyler St., Port Townsend, WA 98368-6541; http://www.towsendletter.com). It is there one should go for his articles.

121. Martin's recommendations for the safe easing of pain through the use of ginger can be found in our Arthritis Trust of America Summer 2001 Newsletter at http://www.arthritistrust.org, "Newsletters" tab.

122. "Three Years of HCl Therapy" as published in *The Medical World* is available from http://arthritistrust.org at the "Books and Pamphlets" button.

123. Wikipedia: http://en.wikipedia.org/wiki/Pasteurization.

124. Wikipedia: http://en.wikipedia.org/wiki/United_States_raw_milk_debate.

125. William Campbell Douglass, II, M.D., T*he Milk Book: The Milk of Human Kindness Is Not Pasteurized* by William Campbell Douglass II and MD, [See Amazon.com], Mar 9, 2004.

126. The U.S. District Court for the District of Columbia; Impro Products Co., Inc., vs. John R. Block Secretary of the United States (Civil No. 81-1284, July 9, 1982; July 28, 1982; Sept 2, 1982.)

127. Trevor Lyons, B.D.S. (U. Lond.), L.D.S., R.C.S. (Eng.), R.M. (C.C.M.), Eleanor Stanfield, B.A., Introduction to Protozoa and Fungi in Periodontal Infections, 45 Rosebery Avenue, Ottawa, Ontario, Canada K1S 1W1, 1989.

128. H. Hugh Fudenberg and Giancarlo Pizza, "Transfer Factor 1993: New Frontiers," Progress in Immunologic Significance of the Thymus in Adult Mouse." Nature 195, 1318 (1962).

129. Ibid; From H.S. Lawrence: "The Transfer in Humans of Delayed Skin Sensitivity to Streptococcal M Substance and to Tuberculin with Disrupted Leukocytes," J. Clin. Invest. 34, 219 (1955).

130. Ibid; Also from H.H. Fudenberg and H. L. Fudenberg: Past, Present, and Future in Annual Review of Pharmacology and Toxicology, p. 475-516, ed. E. Jucker, Birkauser Verlag; Basel, Switzerland (1989).

131. See "The Roger Wyburn-Mason, M.D., Ph.D. Treatment for Rheumatoid Disease," and "Thomas McPherson Brown, M.D. Treatment of Rheumatoid Disease," http://www.arthritistrust.org.

132. Morton Walker, D.P.M., "Bovine Colostrum Offers Broad-Spectrum Benefits for Wide-Ranging Ailments," Townsend Letter for Doctors & Patients, April 1999, p. 74.

133. Lida H. Mattman, Ph.D., Cell Wall Deficient Forms: Stealth Pathogens, 2nd & 3rd editions, CRC Press, Boca Raton, FL.

134. Personal correspondence from Lida H. Mattman, Ph.D.

135. Congressman Berkely Bedell, "Bedell Testifies Before U.S., Senate," Townsend Letter for Doctors, 911 Tyler St., Port Townsend, WA, 98368-6541, December 1993, p. 1229.

136. "Minnesota Milk-Cure Case Ends with Mistrial," Townsend Letter for Doctors, 911 Tyler St., Port Townsend, Washington, 98368-6541, August/September 1995, p. 81; from Minneapolis Star Tribune, 3/16/95.

137. T. Ebina, et. al., Med Microbiol Immunol, Springer-Verlag, 173:87-93, 1984.

138. H. Hugh Fudenberg and Giancarlo Pizza, "Transfer Factor 1993: New Frontiers," Progress in Drug Research, Vol. 42, Birkhauser Verlag Basel (Switzerland), 1994. From, F.F.A.P. Miller: "Immunologic Significance of the Thymus in Adult Mouse." Nature 195, 1318 (1962).

139. Ralph J. Stolle, Lee R. Beck, Ph.D., Stolle Immune Milk, Stolle Milk Biologics, Int., 6954 Cornell Road, Cincinnati, OH 45242, 1989.

140. Zoltan Rona, M.D., "Bovine Colostrum," Nature's Impact, August/September 1998, p. 57.

141. 37. Other Important Papers Used as Source Material:

142. Patents used as source materials:

142.a. U. S. Patent Office October 25, 1945; 628,987

142.b. Canadian Patent Office December 1, 1959; 587, 849

142.c. U. S. Patent Office April 2, 1968; 3,376,198

142.d. U.S. Patent Office April 18, 1981; 4,284,623

142.e. U. S. Patent Office September 6, 1983; 4,402,938

142.f. U. S. Patent Office March 28, 1989; 4,816,563

142.g. U. S. Patent Office June 27, 1989; 4,843,065

142.h. U.S. Patent Office April 2, 1991; 33,565

142.i. U. S. Patent Office April 7, 1992; 5,102,669

143. **We Provide These Additional References for Those Who Wish to Pursue "Immune Milk" Further**

(1.) Charles A. Janeway, Jr., M.D., "How the Immune System Recognizes Invaders," Scientific American, September 1993, p. 73.

(2.) Congressman Berkely Bedell, "Bedell Testifies Before U.S., Senate," Townsend Letter for Doctors, 911 Tyler St., Port Townsend, WA, 98368-6541, December 1993, p. 1229.

(3.) Personal letter from Berkley Bedell July 18, 1994; also personal interview.

(4.) "Picking Out the Lymes From the Lemons," Townsend Letter for Doctors, 911 Tyler St., Port Townsend, WA. 98368-6541, May 1993, p. 408; reprint from Science News. Tribune, 3/16/95.

(5.) Personal interview with, and correspondence from a scientist who chooses not to be identified.

(6.) See Gus J. Prosch, Jr., M.D., "Candidiasis: Scourge of Arthritics,"1994, see http:// www.arthritistrust.org.

(7.) Stephen Tobin, D.V.M., "Lyme Disease," Townsend Letter for Doctors, 911 Tyler St., Port Townsend, WA, 98368-6541, January 1993, p. 63.

(8.) See Fred S. Kantor, "Disarming Lyme Disease," Scientific American, 415 Madison Avenue, New York, NY 10017-1111, September 1994, p. 34.

(9.) Pearl Atkin, R.N., M.A., CS, "My Experience With Lyme Disease," Townsend Letter for Doctors, 911 Tyler St., Port Townsend, WA, 98368-6541, November 1992, p. 997.

(10.) Malcolm Ritter, "Whey Could Prevent HIV Infection," Wisconsin State Journal, January 31, 1996, quoting the February Nature Medicine.

(11.) Pearl Atkin, R.N., M.A., CS, "Treatment of Lyme Disease," Townsend Letter for Doctors, 911 Tyler St., Port Townsend, WA, 98368-6541., December 1993, p. 1220.

(12.) Burton Goldberg Group, Alternative Medicine: The Definitive Guide, Celestial Arts, PO Box 7123, Berkeley, CA 94707.

(13.) "Malaria Therapy: A Cure for Cancer and Aids?" Journal of Longevity Research, Vol.1/ No.2, December 1994, p. 8.

(14.) Anthony di Fabio, "Lyme Disease: Arthritis by Infection," The Art of Getting, 1994, , see http:// www.arthritistrust.org.

(15.) Textbook of Internal Medicine, J.B. Lippincott Company, East Washington Square, Philadelphia, PA 19105, 1989.

(16.) Personal communication with Herbert Saunders, Calvin Johnson, Atty. Bob Collins, Paul Weighner, MS patient, Herbert Struss, Ph.D., Diane Miller, Atty,

(17.) From references quoted in Patent 4,816,563, March 28, 1989.

(18.) T. Ebina, et. al., Med Microbiol Immunol, Springer-Verlag, 173:87-93, 1984.

(19.) Berry Campbell, William E. Petersen, "Immune Milk," Journal of Immune Milk, Volume 1, Number 1,

International Association on Immunity, 2651 University Avenue, St. Paul, Minnesota, p.3, June 1964.

(20.) E. Petersen, "Immunity From Milk," Ibid, p. 29.

(21.) B. Sekla, E. Holeckova, "Diathelic Immunization of Sheep Against a Rat Cancer," Journal of Immune Milk, Volume 1, Number 2, Op.Cit., December 1964; Reprinted from Nature, Vol. 185, February 27, 1960, p. 618-619.

(22.) Herbert E. Struss, "Immune Milk Treatment of Rheumatoid Arthritis — Review," Ibid, p. 23.

(23.) R.M. Porter, Ph.D., "The Protective Milk Concept," Certified Milk, Volume 35, No. 3, Certified Milk Magazine, 405 Lexington Ave., New York, NY, May-June 1960, p. 6.

(24.) H. Hugh Fudenberg and Giancarlo Pizza, "Transfer Factor 1993: New Frontiers," Progress in Drug Research, Vol. 42, Birkhauser Verlag Basel (Switzerland), 1994. From, F.F.A.P. Miller: "Immunologic Significance of the Thymus in Adult Mouse." Nature 195, 1318 (1962).

(25.) Ibid; From H.S. Lawrence: "The Transfer in Humans of Delayed Skin Sensitivity to Streptococcal M Substance and to Tuberculin with Disrupted Leukocytes," J. Clin. Invest. 34, 219 (1955).

(26.) Ibid; Also from H.H. Fudenberg and H. L. Fudenberg: Past, Present, and Future in Annual Review of Pharmacology and Toxicology, p. 475-516, ed. E. Jucker, Birkauser Verlag; Basel, Switzerland (1989).

(27.) Ibid; Also Peng, Li-yi, Yang Dao-li, QiFa-lian, Jia Bo-sen, Wang Bao-cheng Due GungDialyzable Placenta Extracts" in Recent Advances in Transfer Factor and Dialyzable Leucocyte Extracts, p. 354-5, ed. T. Fujisawa, S., Sasakawa, Y. Iikura, F. Komatsu, Y. Yamaguchi, Maruzen Co. Ltd.; Tokyo, Japan (1992).

(28.) Taken from instructions and capsule labels furnished by Herbert Struss, Ph.D. used in the original studies and also from article, Cyril M. Smith, M.D., "Immune Milk in the Treatment of the Rheumatoid Arthritis Syndrome," Journal of Immune Milk, Volume I, Number 1, International Association on Immunity, 2651 University Avenue, St. Paul, MN, June 1964.

(29.) Paul K. Pybus, Dr., "The Herxheimer Effect," see http://www.arthritistrust.org..

(30.) SymbioticHomepage (www.symbioticsllc.com.

(31.) Sarah Richardson, "Licking Infections," Discover, Vol. 17, Number 1, January 1996, p. 18. minophen," American Journal of Pain Management, Vol. 8, No. 3, July 1998.

(32.) The U.S. District Court for the District of Columbia; Impro Products Co., Inc., vs John R. Block Secretary of the United States (Civil No. 81-1284, July 9, 1982; July 28, 1982; Sept 2, 1982.)

(33.) Tom Tauke, "Iowa Woman Wins 20-year Battle With Bureaucracy," Des Moines Sunday Register, November 18, 1984.

(34.) Patents used as source materials:

(35a.) U. S. Patent Office October 25, 1945; 628,987

(35b.) Canadian Patent Office December 1, 1959; 587, 849

(35c.) U. S. Patent Office April 2, 1968; 3,376,198

(35d.) U.S. Patent Office April 18, 1984; 4,284,623

(35e.) U. S. Patent Office September 6, 1983; 4,402,938

(35f.) U. S. Patent Office March 28, 1989, 4,816,56

(35g.) U. S. Patent Office June 27, 1989; 4,843,065

(35h.) U.S. Patent Office April 2, 1991;
33,565

(35i.) U. S. Patent Office April 7, 1992; 5,102,669. Those who are interested in receiving copies of the above may order them from the U.S. Patent Office. 37 converted to 36 above.

(37.) Other Important Papers Used as Source Material:

(37a.) W.E. Petersen, "Immune Milk Treatment of Rheumatoid Arthritis — Review," Journal of Immune Milk, Vol. I, Number 1, W.E. Petersen Research Institute, International Association of Immunity, 2651 University Avenue, St. Paul, MN, June 1964 [Out of Print].

(37b.) W.E. Petersen, "A History of the Use of Immune Milk in the Treatment of Fall Pollenosis," Journal of Immune Milk, Vol. II, Number 1, W.E. Petersen Research Institute, International Association of Immunity, 2651 University Avenue, St. Paul, MN, June 1965 [Out of Print].

(37c.) Arthur E. Dracy [Brookings, South Dakota], "Immune Milk in the Treatment of Poison Ivy," Journal of Immune Milk, Vol. II , Number 1, W.E. Petersen Research Institute, International Association of Immunity, 2651 University Avenue, St. Paul, MN, June 1964 [Out of Print].

(38.) Ralph J. Stolle, Lee R. Beck, Ph.D., Stolle Immune Milk, Stolle Milk Biologics, Int., 6954

Cornell Road, Cincinnati, OH 45242, 1989.

(39.) Confidential Descriptive Memorandum, The Offering of Stolle Milk Biologics International, L.P., Dominick & Dominick.

(40.) Trevor Lyons, B.D.S. (U. Lond.), L.D.S., R.C.S. (Eng.), R.M. (C.C.M.), Eleanor Stanfield, B.A., Introduction to Protozoa and Fungi in Periodontal Infections, 45 Rosebery Avenue, Ottawa, Ontario, Canada K1S 1W1, 1989.

(41.) Anthony di Fabio, Gus J. Prosch, Jr., M.D., Arthritis: Osteoarthritis and Rheumatoid Disease, Including Rheumatoid Arthritis, 1997, p. 196, , see http://www.arthritistrust.org.

(42.) Lida H. Mattman, Ph.D., Cell Wall Deficient Forms: Stealth Pathogens, 2nd & 3rd editions, CRC Press, Boca Raton, FL.

(43.) Personal correspondence from Lida H. Mattman, Ph.D

(44.) Tables from early patent. **Also see Universal Oral Vaccine -With Patents, http://www.arthritistrust.org.**

(45.) Jesse A. Stoff, M.D., The Use of Dialyzable Bovine Colostrum Extract in Conjunction With a

Holistic Treatment Model for Natural Killer Cell Stimulation n Chronic Illness, 2122 North Craycroft, Suite 112, Tucson, AZ 85712, 1998.

(46.) Morton Walker, D.P.M., "Bovine Colostrum Offers Broad-Spectrum Benefits for Wide-Ranging Ailments," Townsend Letter for Doctors & Patients, April 1999, p. 74.

(47.) Zoltan Rona, M.D., "Bovine Colostrum," Nature's Impact, August/September 1998, p. 57.

150. Royden Brown, *How to Live the Millennium: The Bee Pollen Bible*, C.C. Pollen Company, 3627 E. Indian School

Rd., Suite 209, Phoenix, AZ 85018-5126. (Can be purchased at http://www.Amazon.Com)

151. Personal contact plus several dozen Hubbardian books and DVDs available through any Church of Scientology.

152. Scientist **Hans Selye** (1907-1982) introduced the **General Adaptation Syndrome** model in 1936 showing in three phases what the alleged effects of stress has on the body. In his work, Selye '*the father of stress research,*' developed the theory that **stress is a major cause of disease because chronic stress causes long-term chemical changes.** He observed that the body would respond to any external biological source of stress with a predictable biological pattern in an attempt to restore the body's internal homeostasis. This initial hormonal reaction is your fight or flight stress response and its purpose is for handling stress very quickly! The process of the body's struggle to maintain balance is what Selye termed, the *General Adaptation Syndrome.* Pressures, tensions, and other stressors can greatly influence your normal metabolism. Selye determined that **there is a limited supply of adaptive energy to deal with stress.** That amount declines with continuous exposure. (http:// www.essenceofstressrelief.com/general-adaptation-syndrome.html

153. See http://www.arthritistrust.org, "Research" tab, then "Research and Letters" tab. Find Reich in left hand alphabetical listing.

154. Rex E. Newnham, Ph.D., D.O., N.D., "Boron and Arthritis," http://www.arthritistrust.org.

155. See "Sclerotherapy, Proliferative Therapy, Reconstructive Therapy: Treatment of First Choice for Osteoarthritis and for Other Arthritic-like Pain" http:// www.arthritistrust.org.

156. See, Dr. Paul Pybus, *Intraneural Injection for Rheumatoid Arthritis and Osteoarthritis*, Amazon.com at Kindle.

157. See "Lymph Drainage Therapy" and, "Lymphatic Detoxification," http:www.arthritistrust.org.

158. *Stress — From Molecules to Behavior*, Hermona Soreq & Alan Friedman, Wiley-Blackwell.

159. L. Ron Hubbard, *Dianetics: The Modern Science of Mental Health,* Bridge Publications.

160. See Jon Kabat-Zinn http://www.mindfulnesstapes.com/author.html.

161. See "Thyroid Hormone therapy: Cutting the Gordian Knot," http:www.arthritistrust.org.

162. See "A Burning Issue," *Townsend Letter for Doctors & Patients*," October 2005, p. 66; also at http://www.arthritistrust.org, "Articles" tab.

163. For most of Dr. Philpott's publications on the effects of magnetism on human tissue go to http://www.arthritistrust.org. Thence click the "Research" button, and then the "Research and Letters" button. Find Philpott along the left side. Levorotary: turning toward the left or counterclockwise; *especially*: rotating the plane of polarization of light to the left — Dextrorotary: turning clockwise or toward the right; *especially*: rotating the plane of polarization of light toward the right.

www.ingramcontent.com/pod-product-compliance
Lightning Source LLC
Chambersburg PA
CBHW020725180526
45163CB00001B/106
* 9 7 8 1 5 1 4 1 4 5 9 8 2 *